How to Prevent
and Treat Diabetes
with Natural
Medicine

How to Prevent and Treat Diabetes with Natural Medicine

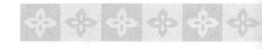

Michael T. Murray, N.D.
Michael R. Lyon, M.D.

RIVERHEAD BOOKS
a member of Penguin Group (USA) Inc.
New York 2003

Riverhead Books
a member of
Penguin Group (USA) Inc.
375 Hudson Street
New York, NY 10014

Copyright © 2003 by Michael Murray, N.D., and Michael Lyon, M.D.
All rights reserved. This book, or parts thereof, may not
be reproduced in any form without permission.
Published simultaneously in Canada

Food Guide Pyramid page 101 courtesy U.S. Department of Agriculture and
U.S. Department of Health and Human Services.

Library of Congress Cataloging-in-Publication Data

Murray, Michael T.
    How to prevent and treat diabetes with natural medicine / by Michael T. Murray,
    Michael R. Lyon.
        p. cm.
    Includes bibliographical references and index.
    ISBN 1-57322-259-3
        1. Diabetes—Alternative treatment.   2. Naturopathy.   I. Lyon, Michael R.   II. Title.
    RC661.A47M868   2004   2003058457
    616.4'6206—dc22

Printed in the United States of America
10 9 8 7 6 5 4 3 2 1

This book is printed on acid-free paper. ∞

Book design by Tanya Maiboroda

To Roland Gahler, for his steadfast devotion to evidence-based natural medicine and his tremendous commitment in supporting our message.

Acknowledgments

First, it is important for us to acknowledge all the researchers, physicians, and scientists who over the years have sought to better understand the role of diet and natural medicines in the prevention and treatment of diabetes. Without their work, this book would certainly not exist. Next, it is important to acknowledge the role that our agent, Bonnie Solow, played in linking us up with Amy Hertz and Riverhead Books. We are indebted to the team at Riverhead for having the perseverance to make our book as reader-friendly and practical as possible.

MICHAEL T. MURRAY, N.D.
Most of all, I would like to acknowledge my wife, Gina. Her love, support, and patience are the major blessings in my life, along with our two wonderful children, Alexa and Zachary.

MICHAEL R. LYON, M.D.
To Sandi. You are the love and light of my life.

Contents

Diabetes—
A Twenty-first-Century Epidemic

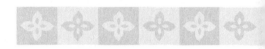

Diabetes is a preventable disease, even if it's in your family. If you have diabetes, it is treatable with natural medicine. In most cases, you can eliminate the need for drugs and, in some cases, dependence on insulin. You can also dramatically reduce the risk of serious complications of diabetes, such as heart disease, blindness, kidney failure, and amputations. Failure to use natural medicine in the treatment and prevention of diabetes is a mistake you can't afford to make.

Diabetes is not a new disease, but its relative rarity prior to the twentieth century coupled with its rather recent emergence as a major disease has led many experts to classify it as a disease of modern living. There are compelling reasons to justify this classification. Most important, diabetes is not just an inevitable result of "bad genes." In fact, diabetes arises from diverse causes—many that are indeed by-products of modern life. In this book we will provide practical and authoritative knowledge concerning these many factors leading to diabetes. In addition, we will carefully outline the steps you can take to prevent this devastating disease even if your family history indicates that you are at risk. Most important, to the 17 million Americans with diabetes and the 16 million with various stages of *prediabetes* (insulin resistance or glucose intolerance), we will present a cutting-edge system to manage the various manifestations of diabetes and to avoid its potential catastrophic complications. We have also outlined emerging evidence demonstrating that diabetes can almost always be significantly improved and in many cases it can be reversed altogether—a revolutionary concept indeed for the majority of diabetics who still believe that the diagnosis of diabetes is a life sentence.

Diabetes is one of our society's biggest drains of resources—both financial and human. The total economic toll of diabetes in the United States alone is staggering—more than $100 billion annually. To put this in perspective, the average annual health care costs for a diabetic are approximately $12,000, while health care costs for an adult without diabetes are about $3,000. Diabetes is responsible for more than 30 million doctor visits each year, along with more than 15 million days of hospitalization for diabetes-related issues.

Diabetes Is a Silent Killer

Approximately one-third of the 17 million people in the United States with diabetes are unaware that they have it. Many of these individuals first become conscious that they have diabetes when they develop one of its life-threatening complications, such as heart attack, stroke, or kidney disease. Overall, the risk for death among people with diabetes for these catastrophic complications is about four times that of people without diabetes. In addition to an earlier death, diabetes carries with it significant risks for serious complications such as blindness, the need for dialysis, and limb amputation.

Major Complications of Diabetes

- *Heart disease and stroke*—Adults with diabetes have death rates from cardiovascular disease that are about two to four times those for adults without diabetes.
- *High blood pressure*—About 75 percent of adults with diabetes have high blood pressure.
- *Blindness*—Diabetes is the leading cause of blindness among adults.
- *Kidney disease*—Diabetes is the leading reason why people need to go on dialysis, accounting for 43 percent of new cases.
- *Nervous system disease*—About 60 to 70 percent of people with diabetes have mild to severe forms of nervous system damage. Severe forms of diabetic nerve disease are a major contributing cause of lower-extremity amputations.
- *Amputations*—More than 60 percent of lower-limb amputations in the United States occur among people with diabetes.
- *Periodontal disease*—Almost one-third of people with diabetes have severe periodontal (gum) disease.
- *Pain*—Many diabetics have chronic pain due to conditions such as arthritis, neuropathy, circulatory insufficiency, or muscle pain (fibromyalgia).
- *Depression*—Depression is a common accompaniment to diabetes. Clinical depression can often begin to occur even years before diabetes is fully evident. As well, depression is difficult to treat in poorly controlled diabetics.
- *Autoimmune disorders*—Thyroid disease, inflammatory arthritis, and other diseases of the immune system commonly add to the suffering of diabetes.

The Need for Natural Medicine

Diabetes is a very serious disorder that needs to be treated effectively. Obviously, the best treatment for any disease is primary prevention. Can diabetes be prevented? Absolutely—and it is quite clear that the best way to achieve this goal is to follow the recommendations in Part I of this book. While current conventional medical treatment has undoubtedly helped many diabetics live healthier and longer, the most effective treatment of diabetes and other blood sugar problems requires the use of the lifestyle, dietary, and supplement strategies that we outline in this book. We want to stress that for chronic diseases like diabetes, relying on conventional drugs alone is a huge mistake. As you read *How to Prevent and Treat Diabetes with Natural Medicine* you will understand why we feel so strongly about the absolute need for incorporating natural medicine into your diabetes treatment plan.

Our goal in writing *How to Prevent and Treat Diabetes with Natural*

Medicine is to present a valuable resource that provides not only the latest information on dietary, lifestyle, and supplement strategies, but also the critical guidance you need in using this information. In this book, we have outlined a simple, practical, and yet comprehensive program of lifestyle and dietary measures while giving you authoritative guidance in the proper use of vitamins, minerals, herbs, and other natural measures based on your individual needs.

How to Prevent and Treat Diabetes with Natural Medicine will show you clearly how natural medicines can:

- Significantly reduce your risk for developing diabetes—even if many of your family members or ancestors are or were diabetic.
- Possibly reverse diabetes, even in many diabetics who are currently using insulin.
- Improve the sensitivity of cells to the action of insulin, thereby improving glucose tolerance and normalizing blood sugar.
- Promote weight loss and slow down or block the absorption of sugar from the intestinal tract.
- Effectively reduce the complications of diabetes, including heart disease and retinopathy.
- Improve the actions of drugs and insulin while reducing their side effects.

You will learn that the best diet in the management of diabetes and other blood sugar disorders is not the one promoted by the American Diabetes Association (ADA), but rather the diet outlined in our book. In addition, while diet is critical, diabetics have an increased need for many nutrients compared to nondiabetics. Therefore, proper dietary supplementation is the only practical solution. Supplying the diabetic with key natural products has been shown to improve blood sugar control as well as to help prevent or improve many of the major complications of diabetes.

We also incorporate important herbal medicines and "functional foods" in our program to help control blood sugar levels. Recent developments in these areas have led to natural remedies that are effective, are free of unwanted side effects, and have substantial documentation of efficacy.

Evidence-Based Natural Medicine— Our Clinical Experience

How to Prevent and Treat Diabetes with Natural Medicine presents what we call *evidence-based natural medicine*. This means that our recommendations are derived from scientific evidence, not folklore or marketing hype. Coupled with this reliance on published scientific research and clinical studies is our own clinical experience; proven recommendations will be given rather than some theoretical model. We have many years of experience managing diabetic patients by applying the principles outlined in this book. This experience has helped us learn firsthand what works and what does not.

In addition, we have interspersed many real-life case histories throughout the book as examples to inspire and educate you on the value of our program. While diabetes is often a challenging disease, the truth is that we actually get very excited when a new patient is a diabetic because we know that our recommendations will dramatically impact the quality of his or her life. You can imagine how wonderful that feels. This controlled euphoria is the motivation for many doctors to work so hard for their patients. We are no different.

Some Words of Caution

Although this book discusses numerous natural medicines and approaches, it is not intended as a substitute for appropriate medical care. Please keep the following in mind as you read:

- If you have diabetes, we want you to talk to your doctor about using the recommendations given in this book. Conventional medical doctors should embrace the recommendations given in the book because they will recognize that our recommendations are scientifically valid. To align your doctor with our program, we have provided extensive references from the medical literature.
- Do not self-diagnose. Proper medical care is critical to good health. If you have concerns about any subject discussed in this book, please consult a physician, preferably a naturopathic doctor

(N.D.), nutritionally oriented medical doctor (M.D.) or doctor of osteopathy (D.O.), or other natural health care specialist.

- Make your physician aware of all the nutritional supplements or herbal products you are currently taking to avoid any negative interactions with any drugs you are taking.
- If you are currently taking a prescription medication, you absolutely must work with your doctor before discontinuing any drug or altering any drug regimen.
- Diabetes is a multifactorial disease that requires a multifactorial solution: medical, nutritional, and lifestyle changes. Do not rely solely on a single area of focus. You can't just take pills and not change your diet, or do the diet and the pills but ignore the lifestyle issues. Any effective approach for diabetes must be integrated.

How to Use This Book

We have tried to make this book as reader-friendly as possible. As you will see, there is a massive amount of useful, practical information here. The book is organized into three major sections: prevention, treatment, and dealing with complications. We encourage you to read all three sections, but realize that many may simply read what they feel is the most pertinent to them. In particular, individuals with diabetes are likely to go straight to the sections on treatment and support. While we have tried to make each section separate to itself with little need to flip back and forth from one chapter to the next, key points are reiterated concisely and we always provide a page number for more information. We have also compiled a tremendous amount of useful information in the Appendices and the Resources section; physicians interested in our sources will find the References and Notes quite useful. We have also included an open letter for patients to take to their physicians (see Appendix D, page 306) to help align them with the program.

Our Hope

It is our sincere hope that you—or someone you care about—will use the information provided in the following pages to achieve greater health and happiness. We have witnessed firsthand the tremendous impact our program can have in our patients' lives and hope that you will experience the same.

Live in good health with passion and joy!

Michael T. Murray, N.D.
Michael R. Lyon, M.D.

P a r t   O n e

Prevention

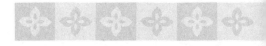

Chapter One

An Ounce of Prevention . . .

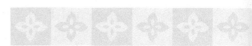

We've all heard it said many times: "An ounce of prevention is worth a pound of cure." When it comes to our health, that old saying carries a ton of truth. Unfortunately, there is not a great deal of emphasis on prevention in our current medical system. Can diabetes really be prevented? In most cases the answer is an emphatic YES! It is a very sad fact that the major killers in the United States are related primarily to diet and lifestyle. Diabetes is one of the diseases at the top of this list. As we'll explain in the first part of this book, by reducing or eliminating as many risk factors as possible, and by following key dietary, lifestyle, and nutritional supplementation strategies, you'll greatly reduce your chances of developing the disease.

At each moment, the human body tries to maintain the ideal internal conditions needed to carry out its many tasks. The technical term for this goal is *homeostasis,* which literally means "same standing." A lack as well as an excess of blood sugar (glucose) can be devastating, so extraordinary control mechanisms maintain blood sugar levels within a narrow range. If these control mechanisms are disrupted, hypoglycemia (low blood sugar) or diabetes (high blood sugar) may result.

Effective solutions for any disease reflect reestablishing the normal built-in controls that keep our body systems in fine tune. For blood sugar disorders, whether diabetes or hypoglycemia, the goal is to remove factors that stress the homeostatic control mechanism while at the same time working on enhancing the way in which these body "thermostats" work.

We believe in *functional medicine,* an approach pioneered by the nutritional biochemist Jeffrey Bland, Ph.D. Functional medicine does not focus on the isolated entity called disease, but rather on the specifics of the functional mechanisms that cause the disease to manifest.

Self-Assessment of Diabetes Risk

The key strategy in the primary prevention of diabetes (preventing the actual development of diabetes) is to identify the presence of risk factors and to use dietary guidelines, lifestyle practices, and nutritional supplements that are associated with a reduction in this risk. The term *risk factor* refers to anything that might increase your chance of developing the disease. The higher the number of risk factors, the greater the likelihood that diabetes will develop. On the other hand, reducing the number of risk factors increases the chances that primary prevention will succeed and the individual will never develop diabetes. Since the risk factors for type 1 and type 2 diabetes differ considerably, we will address them separately.

In assessing the likelihood that an individual will develop a certain disease, specialists in epidemiology (observational and statistical studies of people and diseases) use a concept known as *relative risk*. Relative risk (abbreviated RR) is a number that shows how much more likely it is that individuals who possess a certain trait will develop a condition, compared with individuals who do not share that trait. For example, someone whose RR is 1.5 is 1.5 times as likely, or 50 percent more likely, to develop a condition compared to someone whose RR is 1. An RR of 2 means you are twice as likely, or 100 percent more likely, and so on.

Self-Assessment of Risk for Type 1 Diabetes

We have constructed the following assessment of type 1 diabetes risk, based on many variables. Since type 1 diabetes affects primarily children, more than likely a parent or grandparent will be filling out this survey for his or her child or grandchild. By completing this survey, you'll generate a score that indicates the relative risk of type 1 diabetes. We will follow up this survey in Chapters 2 and 3 by taking a closer look at the processes that can ultimately destroy the insulin-producing cells and how we can prevent, slow down, and even potentially reverse the process.

A few words of caution: Relative risk is a statistic that's used to compare large numbers of people. So we cannot with any certainty predict the specific (absolute) risk as an individual. Our solution to this difficult task of determining risk was to insert as many variables as we possibly could into each questionnaire.

Self-Assessment of Risk for Type 2 Diabetes

We have constructed the following assessment of type 2 diabetes risk, based on many variables. By completing this survey, you'll generate a score that indicates the relative risk of type 2 diabetes. By reading the information in the "Rationale" column, you'll get a quick summary of the scientific data explaining why these variables are important. We will follow up this survey in Chapters 4 and 5 by taking a closer look at the processes that lead to type 2 diabetes and how we can prevent, slow down, and even potentially reverse the process.

Blood Sugar Regulation

Since diabetes is primarily a disorder of blood sugar regulation, we need to briefly discuss how the body controls blood sugar before we tell you how to prevent diabetes. We also need to point out that since diabetes

Instructions

For each of the following, please enter a 1 in the Score column if the risk factor does *not* apply. Otherwise, enter the risk number shown. (*Note:* Insert only one number for each factor.)

	FACTOR	RISK	SCORE
1	Twin with type 1 diabetes	12	
2	Father, mother, or nontwin sibling with type 1 diabetes	4	
3	Introduction of cow's milk within first year of life	2	
4	History of rotavirus or enterovirus gastrointestinal infection	2	
5	Two or more servings per week of foods preserved with nitrates (hot dogs, bacon, ham, smoked and cured meats)	2	
6	Live in northern latitudes or lack of sufficient exposure to sunlight	1.5	
7	History of celiac disease or laboratory-confirmed sensitivity to gluten	1.5	
8	Regular supplementation with probiotics (especially with Bifidobacteria)	−1	
9	Breast-fed for six months	−2	
10	Regular cod-liver oil supplementation during pregnancy or as a child (1 to 3 tsp daily)	−2	

Total Score: _____

Determining Type 1 Diabetes Risk

To determine the relative risk, add the scores in the Score column and write the total on the line indicated. (Remember that if a factor does not apply, you should enter a 1 in the Score column.) Divide the total by 10 and write the result here:

RR: _____

The result is an approximate guideline that indicates the relative risk (RR) of developing type 1 diabetes. Remember, a relative risk of 2 means the person is twice as likely to develop type 1 diabetes as someone with an RR of 1. If your RR is 0.75, you are 25 percent *less* likely to develop type 1 diabetes.

Instructions

For each of the following, please enter a 1 in the Score column if the risk factor does *not* apply. Otherwise, enter the risk number shown. (*Note:* Insert only one number for each factor.)

	FACTOR	RISK	SCORE
1	Family history of diabetes (parent or sibling with type 2 diabetes)	10	
2	More than 20 percent above ideal body weight	7.5	
3	A waist/hip ratio above 1.0 for men and above 0.8 for women	7.5	
4	Diet focuses on high-calorie, low-nutrient junk foods and sources of saturated fats (meat and animal products)	5	
5	Sedentary lifestyle and lack of regular exercise	5	
6	Hypertension (blood pressure > 140/90)	2	
7	Snore or have sleep apnea	2	
8	Over age 50	1.5	
9	Regular consumption of fish or fish oil supplements	−1.5	
10	Regular vitamin E supplementation (more than 100 IU daily)	−3	

Total Score: _____

Determining Type 2 Diabetes Risk

To determine the relative risk, add the scores in the Score column and write the total on the line indicated. (Remember that if a factor does not apply, you should enter a 1 in the Score column.) Divide the total by 10 and write the result here:

RR: _____

The result is an approximate guideline that indicates the relative risk (RR) of developing type 2 diabetes. Remember, a relative risk of 2 means the person is twice as likely to develop type 2 diabetes as someone with an RR of 1. If your RR is 0.75, you are 25 percent *less* likely to develop type 2 diabetes.

really refers to a *set* of diseases, there will be different risk factors and prevention strategies for each different form.

The majority of glucose in the body is derived from dietary carbohydrates. There are two groups of carbohydrates: simple and complex. Simple carbohydrates, or sugars, are naturally found in fruits and vegetables, but most of the simple sugars consumed in developed countries are in the form of refined sugar such as sucrose (white sugar). When high-sugar foods are eaten alone, blood sugar levels rise quickly, producing a strain on blood sugar control. The body responds to the rise in blood glucose levels after meals by secreting insulin, a hormone produced by the beta cells of the pancreas, a small gland that resides at the base of the stomach. Insulin lowers blood glucose by increasing the rate at which glucose is taken up by cells throughout the body. Declines in blood glucose, such as those that occur during food deprivation or exercise, cause the release of glucagon, a hormone produced by the alpha cells of the pancreas. Glucagon stimulates the release of glucose stored in body tissues as glycogen, especially the liver. If blood sugar levels fall sharply or if a person is angry or frightened, the adrenal glands may release epinephrine (adrenaline) and corticosteroids (cortisol). These hormones provide quicker breakdown of stored glucose for extra energy during a crisis or increased need.

Ideally, this is how the body controls blood sugar levels. Unfortunately, many Americans stress these control mechanisms through diet and lifestyle. As a result, diabetes and other disorders of blood sugar regulation are among the most common disease of modern society.

A Diabetes Primer

Although we think of diabetes as a blood sugar disorder, it actually affects much more than blood sugar. It is also characterized by abnormalities in fat and protein metabolism, inflammation, and immune system function.

The hormone insulin is at the center of diabetes. Diabetes can occur when the pancreas does not secrete enough insulin or if the cells of the body become resistant to insulin. Insulin promotes the uptake of blood sugar by cells throughout the body. When there is not enough insulin or when there is a lack of sensitivity to insulin by the cells, the blood sugar cannot get into the cells (see figure 1.1). This failure can lead to serious complications. Like most hormones, insulin also has a dark side. Too much insulin, through either injection or the body's own manufacture, also contributes greatly to the many long-term complications of diabetes.

Diabetes is divided into two major categories: type 1 and type 2 (see Table 1.1). Type 1, or insulin-dependent diabetes mellitus (IDDM), oc-

Figure 1.1. Insulin helps transport glucose into cells.

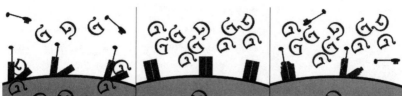

| Normal | Type 1 Diabetes | Type 2 Diabetes |

Key: Insulin receptor (open) —   Glucose — G   Insulin —
Insulin receptor (closed) —

curs most often in children and adolescents. For that reason it is often called *juvenile-onset diabetes.* Individuals with type 1 diabetes require lifelong insulin for the control of blood sugar levels. Type 1 diabetics must learn how to manage their blood sugar levels on a day-by-day basis, modifying insulin types and dosages as necessary, according to the results of regular blood sugar testing. About 5 to 10 percent of all diabetics are type 1. Type 1 diabetes results from destruction of the insulin-producing beta cells in the pancreas, coupled with some defect in tissue regeneration capacity. What ultimately destroys the beta cells are antibodies produced by white blood cells. Antibodies are designed to seek out and destroy infecting organisms such as viruses and bacteria. However, in *autoimmune diseases,* antibodies develop that are targeted for the body's own tissues. Antibodies for beta cells are present in 75 percent of all cases of type 1 diabetes, compared to 0.5 to 2.0 percent of people without the disease.

Type 2, or non-insulin-dependent diabetes mellitus (NIDDM), usually develops after age 40 and is often called *adult-onset diabetes.* It is generally thought that up to 90 percent of all diabetics are type 2; however, it is now thought that about 15 percent of adults diagnosed with type 2 diabetes actually have type 1. In type 2 diabetes, insulin levels are typically elevated, indicating a loss of sensitivity to insulin by the cells of the body. In type 2 diabetes there is usually plenty of insulin; it is just not doing a very good job of unlocking the cells to allow the glucose to enter. Later on, as type 2 diabetes progresses, insulin levels can drop and

Table 1.1. Differences between Type 1 and Type 2 Diabetes

FEATURES	TYPE 1	TYPE 2
Age at onset	Usually under 40	Usually over 40
Proportion of all diabetics	Less than 10 percent	Greater than 90 percent
Family history	Uncommon	Common
Appearance of symptoms	Rapid	Slow
Obesity at onset	Uncommon	Common
Insulin levels	Decreased	Normal to high initially, decreased after several years
Insulin resistance	Occasional	Often
Treatment with insulin	Always	Usually not required

insulin deficiency can magnify further the effects of insulin resistance. Obesity is a major contributing factor to this loss of insulin sensitivity. Approximately 90 percent of individuals with type 2 diabetes are obese. Achieving ideal body weight in these patients restores normal blood sugar levels in many cases, thus curing their diabetes. Even if type 2 diabetes has progressed to the point where insulin deficiency is present, weight loss virtually always results in significant improvements in blood sugar control and dramatic reductions in other health risks such as heart disease.

Other types of diabetes include *secondary diabetes,* a form of diabetes that is secondary to certain conditions and syndromes such as pancreatic disease, hormone disturbances, and side effects of certain drugs, and *gestational diabetes,* a form of diabetes that occurs during pregnancy. Gestational diabetes affects about 4 percent of all pregnant women—about 135,000 cases in the United States each year.

Prediabetes, Hypoglycemia, and Syndrome X

Prediabetes (also called *impaired glucose tolerance*) occurs when a person's blood glucose levels are higher than normal but not high enough for a diagnosis of type 2 diabetes. There are almost as many people in the

United States with impaired glucose tolerance (about 16 million) as there are diabetics. Although many of these people are reassured by their doctors or told that they just have "a touch of diabetes," research increasingly indicates that impaired glucose tolerance, even if diabetes never fully manifests, is accompanied by serious health risks and should be treated carefully. Many people with impaired glucose tolerance will go on to develop full-blown type 2 diabetes. Most important, it has become clear from research that impaired glucose tolerance is usually reversible and, in most cases, diabetes can be completely avoided. As well, impaired glucose tolerance is accompanied by many of the abnormalities of cholesterol, blood pressure, inflammation, and blood clotting that are typical of type 2 diabetes—perhaps on a lesser scale, but still associated with a serious increase in the risk of cardiovascular disease, stroke, and other health catastrophes. It is certainly not wise to ignore or minimize the seriousness of impaired glucose tolerance.

All told, roughly 40 million Americans have blood sugar disorders and many experts also consider *reactive hypoglycemia* a prediabetic condition. *Hypoglycemia* is low blood sugar. Reactive hypoglycemia, the most common form of hypoglycemia, is characterized by the development of symptoms of hypoglycemia 1 to 4 hours after a meal in individuals who are not on insulin or diabetic medications. Reactive hypoglycemia is thought to occur in those whose pancreas releases excessive amounts of insulin following the ingestion of carbohydrate-containing foods (especially sugary or low-fiber starchy foods). These people have cells that are somewhat resistant to the effects of insulin, and thus they need excessive amounts of insulin to keep blood sugar levels from going too high after meals. However, within 1 to 2 hours, this high amount of insulin has taken effect and blood sugar levels drop rapidly as cells rapidly "gobble up" all available blood sugar. To avoid dangerously low blood sugar levels, the body senses the rapidly dropping blood sugar and the adrenal glands release high amounts of epinephrine (adrenaline) and cortisol, stress hormones that stimulate the rapid release of stored sugar from the muscles and liver. The uncomfortable symptoms experienced by the "hypoglycemic" are not from low blood sugar, but rather from high amounts of stress hormones released to prevent seriously low blood sugar.

Drug-induced hypoglycemia is a potentially more serious or even deadly form of hypoglycemia that can occur in diabetics treated with insulin or certain diabetic medications. As in reactive hypoglycemia, the first symptoms of rapidly dropping blood sugar in hypoglycemia caused by medication are due to the release of the stress hormones epinephrine (adrenaline) and cortisol. Sweating, weakness, dizziness, shakiness, and rapid heart rate are examples of these symptoms. Since the brain is critically dependent upon blood sugar as its primary fuel, when hypoglycemia becomes more severe, the brain is seriously affected. In such cases, symptoms of hypoglycemia can range from mild to severe and include headache, depression, anxiety, irritability, blurred vision, excessive sweating, mental confusion, incoherent speech, bizarre behavior, lack of coordination, and later, if blood sugar goes below critical levels convulsions, coma and even death. Insulin- or medication-treated diabetics need to develop a keen awareness of hypoglycemia because serious hypoglycemic episodes can be dangerous and can cause permanent damage to the brain. Unfortunately, the bodies of many diabetics become less sensitive to the initial (adrenaline-related) signs of impending hypoglycemia over time (sweating, weakness, rapid heart rate, and so on). These individuals must develop an ability to monitor subtleties of their brain function instead in an effort to achieve good blood sugar control and avoid catastrophic hypoglycemic episodes.[1]

Syndrome X describes a cluster of abnormalities that owe their existence largely to a high intake of refined carbohydrates, especially in those who are genetically predisposed. The features of syndrome X usually include mildly to moderately impaired glucose tolerance, elevated insulin levels due to insulin resistance, high blood cholesterol and triglyceride levels, high blood pressure, and upper body obesity (around the waist more than around the thighs). The underlying metabolic factor in syndrome X is elevated insulin levels, which result from high intake of refined carbohydrates coupled with insulin resistance. Other terms used to describe this syndrome include *metabolic cardiovascular risk syndrome (MCVS), metabolic syndrome, Reaven's syndrome, insulin resistance syndrome,* and *atherothrombogenic syndrome.* While there is a push to abandon the term *syndrome X,* it has nonetheless persisted and has, increasingly, become the most accepted term.

Prediabetes, hypoglycemia, increased insulin secretion, syndrome X, and type 2 diabetes can be viewed as different facets of the same disease having the same underlying dietary, lifestyle, and genetic causes. The human body was simply not designed to handle the amount of refined

Hypoglycemia: A Historical Perspective

Both of us became interested in nutrition in the 1970s, when hypoglycemia was a popular self-diagnosis. A number of popular books (such as *Sugar Blues* by William Duffy, *Hope for Hypoglycemia* by Broda Barnes, and *Sweet and Dangerous* by John Yudkin) fueled this public interest. In these books, the dangers of too much sugar in the diet were clearly spelled out. Yet since those books were published, the per capita of sugar consumption has risen dramatically. The average American now consumes more than 100 pounds of sucrose and 40 pounds of corn syrup each year. This sugar addiction probably plays a major role in the high prevalence of poor health and chronic disease in the United States.

Research in the past two decades has provided an ever-increasing amount of new information on the role that both refined carbohydrates (sugar and low-fiber starchy foods) and faulty blood sugar control play in many disease processes. New terminology and descriptions (such as *syndrome X* and *impaired glucose tolerance*) are now used to describe the complex hormonal fluxes that largely result from ingesting too much refined carbohydrate. Reactive hypoglycemia is now considered just one manifestation of these other, more well-defined conditions of disordered blood sugar regulation (along with problems such as disordered blood lipids, elevated blood pressure, and inflammation).

sugar, salt, saturated fats, and other harmful food compounds that many people in the United States and other Western countries consume, especially in those who live a sedentary lifestyle. The result is that a metabolic syndrome emerges—elevated insulin levels, obesity, elevated blood cholesterol and triglycerides, and high blood pressure. Syndrome X is the label that modern medicine has chosen for a condition caused by poor dietary and lifestyle choices. It seems a bit silly for medical researchers to be spending millions of dollars in the development of drugs (or "magic bullets") to address these problems, when it would cost far less and be more effective to prevent them by teaching people how to choose a healthier diet and lifestyle. It is highly unlikely that there will ever be a drug that can properly replace the important dietary and lifestyle factors upon which the human body was designed to live and thrive.

Symptoms of Diabetes

The classic symptoms of diabetes are frequent urination and excessive thirst and appetite. In type 1 diabetes the symptoms are often quite apparent, but in type 2 diabetes, because the symptoms are generally milder, they may go unnoticed. For that reason and others, many people with type 2 diabetes do not even know they have the disease. The earlier diabetes is detected and addressed, the better the chance of avoiding the complications of diabetes. Because of this, it is vitally important to see a physician immediately if you are experiencing any of the symptoms associated with diabetes.

Symptoms of Diabetes
Frequent urination
Excessive thirst
Extreme hunger
Unusual weight loss
Increased fatigue
Irritability
Blurry vision

We also want to stress the importance of an annual physical exam and laboratory screening for diabetes, heart disease, cancer, and other major diseases.

Diagnosing Diabetes

The standard method for diagnosing diabetes involves the measurement of blood glucose levels. The initial measurement is generally a fasting blood glucose level taken after avoiding food for at least 10 hours but not more than 16. The normal reading is between 70 and 105 mg/dL (3.8 and 5.8 mmol/L in international or SI units). If a person has a fasting blood glucose measurement greater than 126 mg/dL (7 mmol/L) on two separate occasions, the diagnosis is diabetes. When a person has a fasting glucose between 110 and 126 mg/dL (6.1 and 7 mmol/L), he or she is said to be prediabetic (properly called impaired glucose tolerance).

An after-meal or postprandial measurement as well as a random glucose measurement is also quite helpful in diagnosing diabetes. A postprandial measurement is usually made 2 hours after a meal, while a random measurement is made anytime during the day without regard to the time of the last meal. Any reading greater than 200 mg/dL (11 mmol/L) is considered indicative of diabetes.

The "gold standard" in diagnosing diabetes, however, is the oral glucose tolerance test (GTT), a more functional test of blood sugar control that is performed in a doctor's office or a lab (see Table 1.2). The GTT is not the gold standard because it is the most accurate or convenient test, but rather because of its long-standing use. In fact, according to some studies the GTT is significantly less reliable than fasting blood glucose, especially if combined with a glycosylated hemoglobin level (or hemoglobin A_1C [$HgbA_1C$] as discussed shortly).[2, 3]

The GTT starts out just like a fasting blood glucose measurement in that after fasting for at least 10 hours but not more than 16, a baseline (fasting) blood glucose measurement is made. Then the subject drinks a very sweet liquid containing 75 grams of glucose (or 100 grams if pregnant). In the standard form of the test, blood sugar is rechecked once at 2 hours. In a more advanced method (which is especially helpful when also looking for evidence of hypoglycemia), blood sugar levels are rechecked at 30 minutes, at 1 hour, and then hourly for up to 6 hours, but usually only up to 3 or 4 hours. Basically, a blood sugar level increase to greater than 200 mg/dL (11 mmol/L) indicates diabetes. Levels that fall below 50 mg/dL (2.8 mmol/L) after 1 or 2 hours indicate reactive hypoglycemia.

The Glucose-Insulin Tolerance Test

Relying on blood sugar levels alone is often not enough in diagnosing blood sugar disorders, especially in atypical cases. Measuring insulin

Table 1.2. Glucose Tolerance Test Response Criteria

Normal—No elevation greater than 160 mg/dL (9 mmol/L); below 150 mg/dL (8.3 mmol/L) at the end of the first hour, below 120 mg/dL (6.6 mmol/L) at the end of the second hour
Flat—No variation more than +/– 20 mg/dL (1.1 mmol/L) from fasting value
Prediabetic—Blood sugar levels of 140 to 180 mg/dL (7.8 to 10 mmol/L) at the end of the second hour
Diabetic—Over 180 mg/dL (10 mmol/L) during the first hour; 200 mg/dL (11.1 mmol/L) or higher at the end of the first hour; 150 mg/dL (8.3 mmol/L) or higher at the end of the second hour

levels along with glucose during a glucose tolerance test often provides valuable information. In particular, many people at risk of diabetes will have normal blood sugar levels during fasting or with a glucose tolerance test, and yet have significantly elevated insulin levels in the fasting state and after ingesting the glucose drink. This usually indicates insulin resistance and is a key bit of evidence to support the diagnosis of syndrome X. Many diabetics will have elevated fasting and post-glucose-challenge blood glucose levels as well as elevated insulin levels. Case histories are presented later in the book to highlight the value of determining insulin levels.

We have found that simply determining the fasting glucose/insulin ratio is a useful screening technique for insulin sensitivity. Anything less than 7 indicates probable insulin insensitivity.[4] This test is particularly useful in determining the severity of prediabetes.

If a patient is going to endure a GTT we recommend also determining insulin levels. Doing so produces what is called a glucose-insulin tolerance test (G-ITT; see Table 1.3). Several studies have shown that the G-ITT leads to a greater sensitivity in the diagnosis of both hypoglycemia and diabetes than the standard GTT. In a study by Dr. Joseph Kraft reported in 1975, G-ITT tests were conducted on 3,650 patients suspected of having diabetes.[5] Surprisingly, when only the glucose data were considered, 1,713 of these patients were found to be normal. However, when both the glucose and insulin data were considered for these same subjects, 60 percent of them were found to have abnormal insulin secretion patterns consistent with what is now called insulin resistance. In cases that would now be considered prediabetic, borderline, or equivocal, the determination of insulin levels was also found to clearly indicate insulin resistance. Including insulin levels during a standard GTT makes a lot of sense, given the importance of insulin levels in contributing to syndrome X and diabetic complications. The downside to this test is that it takes time, involves multiple blood draws in a physician's office, and tends to be very costly. For example, G-ITT costs around $200 while a standard GTT is usually less than $30. Despite the inconvenience and expense, the G-ITT is often appropriate. Here are some specific examples and the reason why the test is important:

- For people with fasting blood sugar levels between 105 and 140 mg/dL (5.8 and 7.8 mmol/L), the goal is to determine what is occurring functionally and get an idea of how much insulin resistance there is.
- For thin or fit adults with poorly controlled type 2 diabetes, our experience is that these people often have significant reductions in pancreatic insulin production. A G-ITT can be used to determine whether insulin therapy (or medications that stimulate insulin production) is appropriate. (In actual practice a simpler test, a *C-peptide level* [see page 129 for a full explanation] is often used to differentiate type 1 from type 2 diabetics.) Adults who are true type 1 diabetics (that is, who produce little or no insulin) and who are not on insulin often develop extremely high blood sugar, severe dehydration, and highly acid blood (*ketoacidosis*). They are often identified as type 1 diabetics by becoming so sick that they end up in the hospital emergency department.
- For overweight children who have developed diabetes without the typical acute symptoms, the G-ITT can be used to clarify whether it is truly type 1 or type 2 diabetes. The importance of this determination is that type 2 diabetes can develop in children for the same reasons it develops in adults; if the child is already producing excess insulin, adding more fuel to the fire does not address the underlying issue of insulin resistance.
- For patients with longstanding type 2 diabetes there is often an eventual "burnout" of insulin production, requiring the patient to go on insulin. Again, a G-ITT can be used to determine whether insulin therapy is appropriate.

Table 1.3. Glucose-Insulin Tolerance Test Criteria

Pattern 1—Normal fasting insulin, 2–28 units. Peak insulin at ½ to 1 hour after a 50-gram glucose load. The combined insulin values for the second and third hours is less than 60 units. This pattern is considered normal, especially if glucose levels are also within the normal range.
Pattern 2—Normal fasting insulin. Peak at ½ to 1 hour with a delayed return to normal. Second- and third-hour levels between 60 and 100 units are usually associated with hypoglycemia and are considered borderline for diabetes; insulin values greater than 100 units coupled with normal to high glucose levels are considered definite insulin resistance and probable type 2 diabetes.
Pattern 3—Normal fasting insulin. Peak at second or third hour instead of ½ to 1 hour. Definite insulin resistance and probable type 2 diabetes.
Pattern 4—High fasting insulin. Type 2 diabetes or an insulin-producing pancreatic tumor.
Pattern 5—Low insulin response. All tested values for insulin less than 30 units. If this response is associated with elevated blood sugar levels, probable type 1 diabetes.

Glycosylated Hemoglobin

Another valuable laboratory test for evaluating blood sugar levels measures glycosylated hemoglobin (A_1C). Proteins that have glucose molecules attached to them (glycosylated peptides) are elevated severalfold in diabetics. Normally about 5 to 7 percent of hemoglobin is combined with glucose. Mild elevations in blood sugar result in an A_1C concentration of 8 to 10 percent, while severe elevations may result in concentrations up to 20 percent.

Since the average lifespan of a red blood cell is 120 days, the A_1C assay represents time-averaged values for blood glucose over the preceding two to four months. It is extremely valuable in providing a simple, useful method for assessing treatment effectiveness and patient compliance. A_1C determination along with a fasting blood glucose level can also be used in some cases to diagnose diabetes,[6] but we do not recommend it as the sole diagnostic criteria. About a third of diabetics diagnosed with the GTT have a normal A_1C.[7] We recommend that an A_1C be coupled with a fasting blood glucose level and a 2-hour after-meal (postprandial) glucose level for a more accurate diagnosis.

The A_1C assay is very helpful in determining the relative glucose load on the system and is also a way to monitor therapy. You will find that

What Urine Tests Measure

The presence of glucose in the urine is a source of concern, as glucose is not normally present in urine. But if blood sugar levels are too high (180 mg/dL [10 mmol/L] or higher), you may see glucose in the urine. Because urine glucose testing is only a very crude reflection of blood glucose and because it is of no value in determining hypoglycemia, it has generally fallen out of favor in the diagnosis or monitoring of diabetes. Even if it is used as a simple and inexpensive method to screen for diabetes, it is of little value as it will miss any diabetic whose blood sugar is less than 180 mg/dL (10 mmol/L) around the time of testing. Urine tests are a very useful way to measure *ketones,* substances that build up when blood glucose is very high in insulin-dependent diabetics.

the importance and value of determining glycosylated hemoglobin will be repeated throughout the book.

The Importance of a Regular Checkup

One of the most important aspects of diabetes prevention is getting a regular physical checkup as well as seeking appropriate medical care if any new symptom develops. Regular physical and laboratory exams are especially important if you have certain risk factors, such as a family history, for diabetes and other chronic diseases such as heart disease and cancer. The major benefit of regular screening examinations by a health care professional is that it can lead to early detection of diabetes, high blood pressure, heart disease, and cancer (Table 1.4).

Table 1.4. Recommendations for the Early Detection of Diabetes and Other Diseases

ITEM	RECOMMENDATION

Wellness checkup	A wellness checkup is recommended every year for children up to age 18; every 3 years for people age 19 to 40; and every year for people over age 40. This exam should include health counseling and, depending on a person's age and sex, a complete physical exam and screening for diabetes, cancer, and heart disease. Laboratory assessment should include at the bare minimum a complete blood count (CBC), fasting blood glucose, and cholesterol levels.
	
	    Beginning at age 50, men and women should follow one of these examination schedules:
	
	• A fecal occult blood test every year and a flexible sigmoidoscopy every 5 years
	• A colonoscopy every 10 years
	• A double-contrast barium enema every 5 to 10 years
	
	    A digital rectal exam (including prostate exam in men) should be done at the same time as the sigmoidoscopy, colonoscopy, or double-contrast barium enema. People who have a family history of colon cancer should talk with a doctor about a different testing schedule.

Special exams for women	All women age 18 and older should have an annual Pap test and pelvic examination. They should also have an annual clinical breast examination by a health care professional and should perform monthly breast self-examinations. Women with a family history of cancer of the uterus should have a sample of endometrial tissue examined when menopause begins. Women age 40 and older should have an annual mammogram. The clinical breast exam should be conducted close to the scheduled mammogram.
Special exams for men	To screen for prostate cancer, we recommend both the prostate-specific antigen (PSA) blood test and the digital rectal examination annually, beginning at age 40, especially for men in high-risk groups, such as those with a strong familial predisposition and African Americans.

Chapter   Two

A Closer Look at Risk Factors
for Type 1 Diabetes

Type 1 diabetes is a classic example of a "multifactorial" disease—many factors appear to contribute to its development. We know that ultimately the insulin-producing cells of the pancreas are destroyed in most cases by the body's own immune system, but what triggers this destruction can vary from one case to another. We also know that genetics plays a role in virtually all chronic diseases such as diabetes, cancer, and heart disease, but genetic factors generally play second fiddle to dietary, lifestyle, and environmental factors.

We find it interesting that most medical texts, diabetes organizations, and doctors tend to consider type 1 diabetes primarily a genetic disorder. We want to be very clear that while genetic factors may predispose the insulin-producing cells to damage through either impaired defense mechanisms, immune system sensitivity, or some defect in tissue regeneration capacity, genetic factors alone account for only a very small percentage of people who develop type 1 diabetes—perhaps as little as 5 to 10 percent of all cases. Dietary and other environmental factors are the chief factors that ultimately will determine whether the disease will develop.

Although genetic factors are obviously important, the entire set of genetic factors linked to type 1 diabetes have been termed "susceptibility genes," as they modify the risk of diabetes but are neither necessary nor sufficient for disease to develop.[1] Rather than acting as the primary cause, the genetic predisposition simply sets the stage for the environmental or dietary factor to initiate the destructive process.[2] The very term *predisposition* clearly indicates that something else needs to occur. Just as a parched forest may be predisposed to a forest fire, if there is a big rain, or no match or spark, then there is no fire. But if something ignites the fire it may burn out of control. Here is a statistic that is very important to focus on: Less than 10 percent of those with increased genetic susceptibility for type 1 diabetes actually develop the disease.[3]

Identifying the factors that predispose the insulin-producing cells to damage as well as those that trigger their destruction are some of our key goals in this chapter. After identifying these risk factors, we are going to provide an effective plan to prevent type 1 diabetes rather than leave you with the helpless feeling that a child developing type 1 diabetes is a cruel result of some sort of genetic Russian roulette.

As stated earlier, there is simply not enough focus on prevention in our current medical system. To illustrate this sad fact is to simply point out that while type 1 diabetes is a major disease of children, very few pediatricians, family practitioners, and other conventional doctors are aware of the risk factors for developing the disease. If you ask them what causes type 1 diabetes, they will almost uniformly answer "genetics." We find that appalling, based on the amount of good research examining risk factors for the disease. Remember, fewer than 10 percent of children with an increased genetic susceptibility for type 1 diabetes actually develop the disease. Instead of focusing on trying to identify the myriad of genotypes, we urge more researchers to focus on identifying and assessing risk factors more thoroughly so that we can improve the odds of not getting the disease.

Basic Facts of Type 1 Diabetes

- Results from damage to the beta cells of the pancreas that produce insulin
- Is characterized by dependence on daily insulin injections to maintain blood sugar control
- Accounts for somewhere between 5 to 10 percent of all cases of diabetes in the United States
- Has peak incidence during puberty, around age 10 to 12 in girls and age 12 to 14 in boys.
- Has a higher incidence in Caucasians than in other racial groups.

Twin Studies

The best evidence that environmental and dietary factors are the most important contributors to the development of type 1 diabetes comes from scientific studies performed on identical twins. There are two types of twins: *identical twins,* who have 100 percent of their genes in common, and nonidentical twins, who have 50 percent of their genes in common (on average). In diseases that are due primarily to genetic defects, both twins will develop the disease in most cases. This occurrence is referred to as *concordance.* If developing type 1 diabetes were governed only by genes, then every time one identical twin developed diabetes, the other should develop it, too. In detailed studies, the concordance rate for developing type 1 diabetes in identical twins was only 23 percent in one study[4] and 38 percent in another.[5] If one twin develops type 1 diabetes after age 24, then the concordance rate drops to 6 percent. These results indicate that environmental and dietary factors are much more important than a genetic predisposition in most cases. However, if that were the case, then theoretically we should see no difference in concordance among identical and nonidentical twins. But there is a difference, as the concordance rate in nonidentical twins is only about 5 to 11 percent—about the same percentage observed in the risk for other siblings.

The fact that the concordance rate in identical twins is significantly higher than in nonidentical twins makes it is easy to conclude that genetics are the dominant determinant of developing type 1 diabetes. However, if it were truly genetic, researchers would see a much higher concordance rate in identical twins—and why would only 10 percent of those who are genetically predisposed actually develop the disease? So, what is going on? Here are a couple of important considerations. First, since the environment and diet tend to be much more similar in identical twins raised together compared to nonidentical twins, a higher concordance rate in identical twins is now expected.[6] In fact, even in the absence of genetic factors, identical twins tend to have higher concordance rates for diseases linked to environmental and dietary factors.[7] Second, the fact that the concordance rate becomes weaker as the twins age also points to some sort of assault that initiated the diabetes in the one twin but not necessarily the other. Finally, more than twenty different genetic aspects (genotypes) have been implicated as the genetic factors that increase a person's susceptibility to developing type 1 diabetes.[8] It is most likely that genetics is the most important factor for some who develop type 1 diabetes, but remember that this number is probably in the neighborhood of only 5 to 15 percent of cases. Studies comparing genotypes suspected of playing a role in type 1 diabetes in concordant and discordant identical twins appear to bear this out.[9]

Additional Evidence

If you are still not convinced that dietary and environmental factors are the areas that we need to focus on for prevention, consider the following:

- There has been a three- to tenfold increase in the number of people with type 1 diabetes throughout the world over the last 40 years or so. Such a rise simply cannot be explained by an increased number of people genetically predisposed to type 1 diabetes. Changes to the human genetic code across large populations take more than one generation.[10]

A Peek into the (Very Near) Future—
Genetic Screening for Diabetes Risk

Although dietary, lifestyle, and environmental variables far outweigh genetics as the primary causative factors in both type 1 and type 2 diabetes, it is also clear that people can inherit various degrees of susceptibility to type 1 and, even more so, to type 2 diabetes. Now that the human genetic code has been completely broken, great strides are being made in the development of practical laboratory tests that will allow people to become aware of their risk for developing diabetes and a multitude of other diseases. The purpose of such testing is certainly not to increase people's paranoia, but rather, to give them increased awareness of the kinds of dietary, lifestyle, and environmental factors that they could modify in order to reduce their risk of developing diseases such as diabetes. In the future, a blood test taken at birth or in early childhood could be used to identify a child's risk of developing a wide range of conditions, from diabetes to coronary heart disease to Alzheimer's disease to various cancers. Accompanying this information would likely be a set of recommendations for dietary, lifestyle, and environmental factors that can greatly reduce the risk of these conditions. For example, if a child was found to have a high genetic risk for type 2 diabetes, special care could be taken to help that child become and remain athletic, to eat an optimal diet, and to maintain normal body composition.

Already certain labs are offering genetic risk profiling for some conditions through the measurement of simple risk factor genes known as single nucleotide polymorphisms (SNPs, pronounced "snips"). Labs such as Genovations (www.genovations.com) now offer medical or naturopathic physicians the opportunity to look for SNPs in their patients, allowing for sophisticated and individualized lifestyle and nutritional counseling in the interest of primary disease prevention. This kind of patient-centered medicine is really what functional medicine is all about—and it is why this innovative medical discipline is not some kind of alternative medicine. Functional medicine is really future medicine today!

Type 1 Diabetes Is Often Overlooked in Adults

It is generally thought that type 1 diabetes is a disease of children and young adults—thus, the term *juvenile-onset diabetes* has been used interchangeably with *type 1 diabetes*. While that may have been true years ago, recent studies now indicate that many patients initially diagnosed with type 2 diabetes, perhaps as many as 15 percent, may actually have type 1 diabetes.[11] These patients do not respond to oral hypoglycemic drug therapy and are unable to maintain adequate glucose control without the use of insulin. This new information reinforces the importance of measuring insulin levels in adults with diabetes to help differentiate between type 1 and type 2 diabetes. Measuring C-peptide levels, a by-product of pancreatic insulin production, is an even easier way to differentiate between type 1 and type 2 diabetes, especially in diabetics who are already taking insulin injections (see page 129 for further information).

- The rate of type 1 diabetes can increase dramatically when children in areas where type 1 diabetes is relatively rare move to developed countries.[12] For example, the rate of type 1 diabetes increased by nearly four-fold in one 10-year period in children of Asian origin moving to Great Britain, and the rate increased more than seven-fold in Polynesians migrating to New Zealand.[13, 14] Genetic factors simply cannot explain such a rapid change.

How Type 1 Diabetes Develops

Type 1 diabetes in most cases appears to be the result of some injury to the insulin-producing cells of the pancreas (the beta cells) coupled with some defect in the ability of these cells to regenerate properly. Types of substances that can damage the beta cells include *free radicals*—highly reactive molecules that bind to and destroy cellular components. Some of the key free radicals linked to type 1 diabetes are the nitrosamines—by-products of nitrates added to smoked or cured meats and found as a common contaminant in drinking water. Like tiny ornery BBs, these free radicals shoot through the cell's membranes, tearing gaping holes and putting the cell at risk. Once the cell has sustained considerable damage, it exposes proteins that the immune system then erroneously recognizes as foreign, thus causing white blood cells to do everything in their power to destroy what they think is an invading bacteria or virus. Individuals susceptible to type 1 diabetes may have a reduced capacity to deal with free radicals due to impaired antioxidant and repair mechanisms. In addition to free radicals, viruses can also damage the beta cells, either directly by invading beta cells, or indirectly by activating the immune system in a manner that allows for immune system damage to beta cells.

Regardless of the primary trigger, what destroys the beta cells is the immune system. A type of white blood cell known as a B cell attacks the beta cells or special white blood cells known as T cells that destroy beta cells without antibodies. The evidence to classify type 1 diabetes as an autoimmune disease is the fact that antibodies—proteins made by white blood cells—that bind to and destroy the beta cells are present in 75 percent of all cases of type 1 diabetes, compared to 0.5 to 2.0 percent of people without the disease. Although these antibodies to the beta cells develop in response to cell destruction due to other mechanisms (free radical damage, viral infection, food allergies, and so on), it appears that normal individuals either do not develop as severe an antibody reaction or are better able to repair the damage once it occurs.

Overview of Environmental and Dietary Risk Factors

We have already given you some clues to some of the nongenetic risk factors for type 1 diabetes, but there are others. Most of the recent information indicates that the function of the gut immune system is central in the development of type 1 diabetes, so we are going to focus on this aspect first. This involves looking at dietary factors that disrupt gut immune function as well as the role of certain viruses—specifically enteroviruses and rotaviruses—in the development of type 1 diabetes. The key dietary factors that have received the most attention are early exposure to cow's-milk proteins and intolerance to gluten (a protein in grains). We will also take a closer look at the role of nitrates in food and water as well as other compounds that can cause damage to beta cells.

The Gut Immune System and Type 1 Diabetes

Accumulating data indicate that abnormalities of the gut immune system may play a fundamental role in the development of the immune attack on beta cells and the subsequent development of type 1 diabetes.[15] The gut immune system serves a vital role in processing the many food and microbial antigens (particles that elicit the formation of antibodies by white blood cells) to protect the body from infection or allergy. In some cases of type 1 diabetes, the gut immune system develops antibodies that ultimately attack the beta cells. It is interesting to consider that one of the contributing factors to type 1 diabetes may be poor protein digestion.

In animal models, diet can modify the development of autoimmune diabetes. Specifically, diets containing partially digested proteins produce a lower rate of autoimmune diabetes than diets containing whole proteins, because whole proteins are more likely to result in the formation of antibodies against them. Next, some of these proteins actually cross-react with antigens on or within the beta cells of the pancreas. In humans, two proteins with the highest degree of incrimination are those found in milk (bovine serum albumin as well as bovine insulin) and wheat (gluten). For example, dietary bovine insulin differs from human insulin by only three amino acids—the building blocks of protein. If a person develops antibodies to bovine insulin, there is a very good chance that these antibodies will also attack their own insulin. In addition to causing antibody-mediated destruction of the beta cells, bovine insulin can activate T cells in those predisposed to diabetes in a manner that can also lead to beta cell destruction by direct attack by specialized T cells known appropriately as *T-killer cells* (see Figure 2.1).

There is very strong evidence implicating dietary factors such as cow's milk and gluten as important triggers of the autoimmune process that leads to type 1 diabetes. In contrast, breast-feeding has been identified as an important factor in establishing proper gut immune function

Figure 2.1. Theoretical Model for the Development of Type 1 Diabetes Due to Dietary Bovine (Cow's Milk–Derived) Insulin

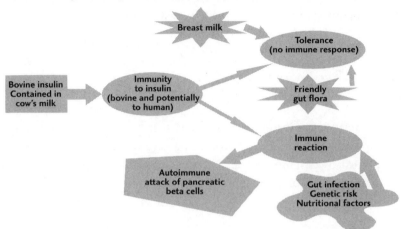

and reducing type 1 diabetes risk. It is well known that breast-feeding reduces the risk of food allergies and protects against both bacterial and viral intestinal infections. In case-controlled studies, patients with type 1 diabetes were more likely to have been breast-fed for less than 3 months and to have been exposed to cow's milk or solid foods before age 4 months. A critical review and analysis of all relevant citations in the medical literature indicates that early cow's-milk exposure may increase the risk by about 1.5 times.[7, 16] Also, while the risk of diabetes associated with exposure to cow's milk was first thought to relate only to intake during infancy, additional studies showed that ingestion at any age may increase the risk of type 1 diabetes.

Although the focus has been on cow's-milk proteins, other food proteins may be just as problematic.[17] In particular, there is considerable evidence that sensitivity to gluten—the major protein component of wheat, rye, and barley—may also play a role. Gluten sensitivity produces celiac disease, another autoimmune disorder. This disease is characterized by diarrhea and nutrient malabsorption and is associated with damaged small intestine structure. All of this is caused by the immune system's abnormal response to gluten. Celiac disease, like type 1 diabetes, is associated with gut immune function abnormalities. And, as with diabetes, breast-feeding appears to help prevent celiac disease, while early introduction of cow's milk is believed to be a major causative factor. The risk of developing type 1 diabetes is higher in children with celiac disease. Not surprisingly, the highest levels of antibodies to cow's-milk proteins are found in people with celiac disease.[18]

Factors That Set the Stage for Autoimmunity in Type 1 Diabetes

Only a relative few people develop type 1 diabetes, even though many are exposed to bovine insulin orally at a very young age. The immune system usually develops tolerance to this protein because it is so close to human insulin. Tolerance means that the immune system does not

---

Canker Sores Are Associated with Milk and Gluten Sensitivity

Canker sores are single or clustered shallow, painful ulcers found anywhere in the oral cavity. Recurrent canker sores (*aphthous stomatitis* is the medical term) are a common condition that affects about 20 percent of the U.S. population. Although not a serious medical condition, recurrent canker sores are quite bothersome.

Based on studies of initiating factors, many cases of recurrent canker sores appear to be related to food sensitivities, especially to milk and gluten.[19] The mouth is, obviously, the first site of contact for ingested allergens. The simple measure of eliminating gluten from the diet results in complete remission of recurrent canker sores in many patients. Given the known association of milk and gluten with initiating factors in type 1 diabetes, we would like to see research demonstrating how common recurrent canker sores are in patients with type 1 diabetes. From our clinical experience, it appears to be more common than in our general patient population. If you often suffer from canker sores it may indicate that your immune system is sensitive to gluten.

overreact to the presence of the antigen (bovine insulin) when it is presented in cow's milk to the gut immune cells. Several important factors contribute to developing tolerance to foods that might otherwise lead to autoimmune reactions if antibodies were to be formed against those food antigens: the type of gut microflora, the protection offered by breast-feeding, absence of infections of the gastrointestinal tract, and, of course, nutritional status.

In researching the scientific literature we were shocked that we could not find a single research study that has tried to determine the status of intestinal microflora in type 1 diabetics. It shocks us because of the growing awareness and the tremendous importance of gut microflora in human health—especially as it relates to the establishment of healthy gut immune function. There are actually at least ten times more bacterial cells in our intestinal tract than there are cells that make up the entire human body. In fact, there are more bacterial cells in our gut than there are stars in the known universe—and that is a whole lot of stars! The proper gut microflora is absolutely critical in establishing proper gut immune function, including the prevention of food sensitivities and gastrointestinal infections—two factors implicated in the development of type 1 diabetes.

Enteroviruses and Type 1 Diabetes

Recent population-based studies as well as experimental evidence have strengthened the notion that type 1 diabetes can be the result of viral infection, particularly viral infections of the gastrointestinal tract.[20] Gastrointestinal infections due to enteroviruses (polioviruses, coxsackieviruses, and echoviruses are all types of enteroviruses) and rotaviruses are quite common, especially in children. All of these viruses replicate in the gut and stimulate the gut immune system, which may activate the insulin-specific immune cells to seek out and destroy beta cells. These viruses and others can also infect pancreatic beta cells, causing the white blood cells to attack and destroy the beta cells in an attempt to kill the virus. Gastrointestinal virus infections may also increase the gut permeability and enhance the antibody response to dietary bovine insulin as a result of increased absorption of the intact protein. Remember that in animal experiments, intact proteins were more likely to create type 1 diabetes than partially digested proteins. The severe "leaky gut" or increased small intestinal permeability that occurs during and for some time following rotavirus infections (one of the most common causes of acute diarrheal illness in children) certainly exposes the gut immune cells to very large quantities of intact protein.

Vitamin D Deficiency

Cod-liver oil is an age-old remedy that may offer significant protection against developing diabetes because of its high vitamin D content. The use of cod-liver oil became quite popular during the 1890s to treat rickets, a vitamin A deficiency disease characterized by an inability to calcify the bone matrix, resulting in softened skull bones, bowed legs, spinal curvature, and an increased size of the joints. Beginning in the 1930s, vitamin D was added to milk at a level of 400 IU per quart. As a result, rickets is now uncommon in most developed countries.

There is emerging evidence that vitamin D supplementation from cod-liver oil and other sources during early childhood can prevent not only rickets but also type 1 diabetes.[21] Interestingly, vitamin D fortification in cow's milk may offset some of the milk's "diabetogenic" effect—but not by much, as the level shown to be protective was about 2000 IU per day, much higher than the amount typically ingested from vitamin D–fortified milk consumption.

In the most extensive of studies looking at vitamin D and type 1 diabetes, all pregnant women in northern Finland who were due to give birth in 1966 were enrolled (more than 12,000 women) and their children were monitored until December 1997.[22] Final analysis of 10,366 demonstrated that children who regularly took vitamin D primarily from cod-liver oil had an 80 percent reduced risk of developing type 1 diabetes, while those who had vitamin D deficiency actually had a 300 percent increased risk of developing the disease. In other words, if a child was given cod-liver oil, their risk of developing type 1 diabetes was extremely low (⅕ the risk) compared to a child not given cod liver oil. If a child had vitamin D deficiency and they were not given cod-liver oil, they were three times more likely to develop diabetes compared to a child who was not given cod-liver oil but who also was not deficient in vitamin D. One study even found that women who took vitamin D in cod-liver oil during pregnancy significantly reduced the frequency of type 1 diabetes in their children.[23] Furthermore, studies show that people who have been newly diagnosed with type 1 diabetes have much lower vitamin D levels in the blood than do healthy control subjects. Since vitamin D can be produced in our bodies by the action of sunlight on the skin, lack of sun exposure during childhood may also partially explain the higher type 1 diabetes rates in northern countries.

The bottom line from this research is that adequate vitamin D supplementation during pregnancy and early childhood may reduce the risk of type 1 diabetes. Vitamin D is important for normal immune system development. In addition, research has shown that vitamin D inhibits some of the autoimmune reactions that target the beta cells of the pancreas.

Omega-3 Fatty Acid Deficiency

In addition to the strong case that can be made for vitamin D as a protective factor, an equally strong case exists for the benefits of the omega-3 fatty acids in cod-liver oil and other fish oils. More than sixty different health conditions have been shown to be either prevented or improved by diets providing higher amounts of omega-3 fatty acids. These fatty acids have beneficial effects once they have been incorporated into cell membranes. Omega-3 fatty acids play a major role in helping cell membranes achieve a fluidlike nature necessary for proper cell function. An alteration in cell membrane function is the main cause of cell injury and death. Without a healthy membrane, cells lose their ability to hold water, vital nutrients, and electrolytes. As a result, they become extremely susceptible to free radical damage.

Omega-3 fatty acids are also very important in producing biochemical substances that reduce inflammation and excessive immune system responses throughout the body. Omega-3 fatty acids are the body's most important anti-inflammatory biochemicals. Given the importance of omega-3 fatty acids, other than the previously mentioned studies with cod-liver oil we are surprised that only one recent investigation looks at a possible role of omega-3 fatty acids may have in preventing type 1 diabetes.

In animal models of type 1 diabetes, beta cells are destroyed by administering compounds that generate free radicals (such as nitrosamines and alloxan, a drug often used to create diabetes in experimental animals because of its free-radical-damaging effects on beta cells). Recently, researchers decided to see what would happen if they gave the animals fish oil before receiving the diabetes-inducing drug alloxan. They discovered that the fish oils prevented chemically induced type 1 diabetes. The mechanisms responsible for this effect are related to improved cell membrane function leading to enhanced antioxidant status and suppression of the formation of inflammatory compounds known as cytokines.[24]

Nitrates

Clear links between increased levels of nitrate from dietary sources and water and an increased risk for type 1 diabetes has been established. Nitrates are produced by agricultural runoff from fertilizers and are also found in cured or smoked meats such as ham, hot dogs, bacon, and jerky to keep the food from spoiling. Nitrates react within the body to form compounds known as nitrosamines. Nitrates and nitrosamines are known to cause diabetes in animals. Infants and young children are believed to be particularly vulnerable to the harmful effects of nitrate exposure.

One of the most alarming features of type 1 diabetes is the fact that it is becoming much more prevalent, with a current growth rate of 3 percent per year worldwide.[3] Some areas are hit particularly hard, such as Finland, Great Britain, Canada, and the United States. Increased nitrate exposure may be a key factor, as the nitrate levels in ground and surface waters of agricultural regions have increased over the past forty years as a result of increases in the use of nitrogen fertilizers. Nitrate contamination occurs in geographic patterns related to the amount of nitrogen contributed by fertilizers, manure, and airborne sources, such as automobile and industrial emissions. Nitrate exposure may explain why some geographical pockets have a substantially higher rate of type 1 diabetes.[25, 26]

Circumstantial evidence from population-based studies also suggests that a higher dietary intake of nitrate consumption from smoked/cured meats is associated with a significantly higher risk for type 1 diabetes. It should be clear that these foods severely stress body defense mechanisms and need to be avoided. The habit of feeding children hot dogs, cold cuts, and ham is a good one for every parent to break. Health food stores now carry nitrate-free alternatives to these rather toxic food choices. Investing in a high-quality water purifier is also good insurance against ingesting nitrate-contaminated drinking water.

Next Steps

We have tried to paint the picture of what triggers the development of type 1 diabetes in a detailed manner so that you will appreciate the comprehensive program given in the next chapter. Because of the multitude of potential causative factors, it only makes sense that the best chance for prevention involves following an extremely comprehensive program that takes into consideration all of these issues.

Preventing Type 1 Diabetes

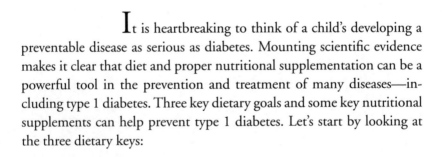

It is heartbreaking to think of a child's developing a preventable disease as serious as diabetes. Mounting scientific evidence makes it clear that diet and proper nutritional supplementation can be a powerful tool in the prevention and treatment of many diseases—including type 1 diabetes. Three key dietary goals and some key nutritional supplements can help prevent type 1 diabetes. Let's start by looking at the three dietary keys:

1. Proper early nutrition
2. Reduced intake of nitrates
3. Avoidance of food allergies

Proper Early Nutrition

Numerous population-based studies have shown that breast-feeding offers considerable protection against the development of type 1 diabetes as well as many other diseases. This protective effect against type 1 diabetes is probably related to two factors: the important role that breast milk plays in the formation of a healthy gut immune system, and the delayed introduction of cow's milk or infant formulas containing cow's-milk proteins to the infant.

The immunological benefits of breast-feeding are enormous to the developing child—which is why virtually every medical institution in the world is working diligently to increase the number of women who breast-feed. Unfortunately, due to many factors, only 29 percent of all mothers and 19 percent of black mothers in the United States breast-feed until the recommended age of 6 months. Breast-feeding not only can help prevent the development of food allergies, it also is vitally important in protecting against enterovirus and rotavirus infections and promotes the proper gut microflora.

Breast-feeding makes incredibly good sense as breast-fed babies are healthier, suffer fewer illnesses, and have higher IQs as their brains seem to develop faster. Mothers benefit, too, shedding pregnancy pounds faster. Long-term breast-feeding may lower some women's risk of getting breast cancer.

Ideally, a child should be breast-fed for at least 6 months. We recommend getting a breast pump and storing as much breast milk in plastic bags in the freezer as possible as a way to extend the breast-feeding period. When it's time for the baby to begin to eat solid food, parents should introduce foods slowly (no more than one new food every 2 days) to ensure that the baby can tolerate the food. Parents can find commercial baby food containing just about anything, or puree anything from pizza to steak in a blender or food processor. But it is important to give the baby the proper nutritious foods that are appropriate for his or her age.

The list of foods in Table 3.1 is from Dr. Janice Joneja, head of the Allergy Nutrition Clinic at Vancouver General Hospital and UBC Health Sciences Center. These foods are usually enjoyed and tolerated

Table 3.1. Sequence of Adding Solid Foods for Infants[1]

TIME OF INTRODUCTION	GRAINS AND CEREALS	VEGETABLES	FRUITS
6–9 months	Rice Millet	**All cooked:** Yams Sweet potatoes Squash (all types) Carrots Beets Broccoli Potatoes Green beans Cabbage	**All cooked:** Pears Peaches Bananas Apricots Nectarines Blueberries
9–12 months	Barley Rye Oats	Asparagus Avocado Cauliflower Brussels sprouts	Plums Prunes Pineapple Grapes Apples (cooked) Cranberries Raisins

12–24 months	Corn
	Wheat
	Other grains
		Green peas
		Spinach
		Tomatoes
		Celery
		Cucumbers
		Lettuce
		Onions
		Garlic
		Lima beans
		Broad beans
		Other legumes,
		  including soy
		Any raw
		  vegetables
			Citrus fruits:
			Oranges
			Grapefruits
			Lemons
			Limes
			Berries:
			Strawberries
			Raspberries
			Other:
			Melons
			Mangoes
			Figs
			Dates
			Cherries
			Any raw fruits

After 2 years	All	All	All

well by almost all infants and toddlers. You will notice that we do not feature some of the real staples of the American diet, such as milk, soy, wheat products, potatoes, nuts, orange juice, and eggs. The longer a parent can hold off from introducing the foods, the less likely the child will be to develop allergies to these foods. We also recommend intro-

MEATS AND ALTERNATIVES	MILK AND DAIRY	NUTS, SEEDS, OTHER

Lamb
Turkey
	Breast milk
	If absolutely necessary,
	  casein hydrolysate
	  or whey-based formulas
		None

Chicken
Veal
Beef
	Breast milk or
	  casein hydrolysate or
	  whey-based formulas
		None except
		  vegetable oils
		  in formula

Pork Fish Eggs	Yogurt (plain) Milk (whole) White cheese Cottage cheese	**Seed oils:** Canola Safflower Sunflower
Shellfish	All others, including ice cream	Peanuts Nuts Chocolate Seeds

ducing vegetables before fruits. The idea is to attempt to condition the tastebuds at an early age to enjoy vegetables. Another good rule of thumb is not to introduce fish until at least 12 months of age, and to offer only lamb or turkey before 9 months.

As children start getting older it is often difficult to encourage

Summary of Proper Infant Nutrition

- Breast milk until 6 months of age.
- Introduce only one new food at a time and no more than one new food every 2 days; closely follow the suggestions in Table 3.1.
- Give very small amounts of any new food: one or two teaspoonful.
- Use a very thin consistency when starting solid foods. Introduce foods that are gradually more solid as the infant learns how to use his or her tongue to propel the food back.
- Never force an infant to eat more of a food than he or she takes willingly.
- Check that the temperature of the food is neither too hot nor too cold.
- Don't be afraid to retry a food that the baby has previously shown a dislike to.
- Try to vary the diet, not only to encourage the baby to experience different tastes, but also to reduce the likelihood of food allergy.

healthful eating habits. Children appear to be very sensitive to the marketing messages of fast-food, candy, and soft-drink manufacturers. The basic dietary guidelines for children are essentially the same as those that we recommend for adults. Here are some things that we have found useful in helping kids eat better:

- Encourage healthy snacks of fruits and vegetables (carrot and celery sticks are very popular).
- Try to have at least one fresh piece of fruit or vegetable with each main meal.
- Choose healthier versions of fruit drinks and snacks—read labels carefully.
- Take the kids with you to shop at the natural food store—they will be more likely to try new foods if they choose them.

Learning Factors Daily Nutrient Boost Smoothie Mix

Dr. Lyon, with the help of Natural Factors, developed an innovative and delicious way to get kids of all ages (even adults) to enjoy high-quality nutrition. Learning Factors Daily Nutrient Boost Smoothie Mix provides a combination of thirty-five selected nutrients at optimal concentrations that support the brain, gastrointestinal tract, and immune system. This powdered, low-allergy-potential formula serves as the foundation for delicious blender smoothies. Learning Factors provides a quick and satisfying meal replacement or snack. Here is how to make a super-nutritious snack: Mix two scoops of the Smoothie Mix powder with one half cup frozen fruit (such as strawberries, cherries, blueberries, raspberries, and peaches) and one half to 1 cup water, rice milk, almond milk, or soy milk. If no frozen fruit is available, mix two scoops of powder with one half cup fresh fruit, one half to 1 cup water, and four ice cubes in a blender and blend until ice cubes are completely crushed. This low-allergy-potential food can be introduced by 9 months of age if weaning has begun.

To provide even higher-quality nutrition, add 1 teaspoon Learning Factors Liquid Essential Fatty Acids and 1 teaspoon Natural Factors Enriching Greens powder.

Reduced Intake of Nitrates

The nitrates found in many vegetables, especially beneficial green leafy vegetables like spinach, kale, and lettuce, do not form damaging nitrosamines because of the various protective antioxidants in the food such as vitamin C and flavonoids. Reducing your intake of nitrates means making sure your drinking water does not contain nitrates as well as avoiding smoked or cured meats.

State and federal laws set the maximum allowable level of nitrate-nitrogen in public drinking water at 10 mg/L (10 ppm). If you are on a public water supply, ask your local water department for a printout of the latest testing. If you have well water, have the water tested by a local water testing company. A nitrate test is recommended for all newly constructed private wells and wells that have not been tested during the past 2 years. Testing is especially recommended for wells used by pregnant women and is essential for wells that serve infants under 6 months of age. Wells with nitrate-nitrogen levels below 5 mg/L should be retested every 2 years. If the levels are between 5 and 10 mg/L, owners should consider testing more often to check for seasonal changes. Additional testing may also be useful if there are any known sources of nitrate or if high nitrate levels are detected in nearby wells.

In addition to being linked to diabetes, the intake of nitrates from water or from cured or smoked meats is also linked to a significantly increased risk of cancers, especially the major childhood cancers (leukemias, lymphomas, and brain cancers).[2] Here are some eye-opening statistics:

- Children who eat twelve hot dogs per month have nearly ten times the risk of developing leukemia compared with children who do not eat hot dogs.
- Children who eat hot dogs once a week double their chances of brain tumors; eating them twice a week triples the risk.
- Pregnant women who eat two servings per day of any cured meat have more than double the risk of bearing children who have brain cancer.
- Kids who eat the most ham, bacon, and sausage have three times the risk of lymphoma.
- Kids who eat ground meat once a week have twice the risk of acute lymphocytic leukemia compared with those who eat none; eating two or more hamburgers weekly triples the risk.

Fortunately, vegetarian alternatives to these standard components of the American diet are now widely available, and many of them actually taste quite good. Consumers can find soy hot dogs, soy sausage, soy bacon, and even soy pastrami at their local health food store as well as in many mainstream grocery stores. When our kids have had their friends over and we have served them "Smart Dogs" or "Tofu Pups," they did not even notice a difference. If you are really stuck on meat, then we would recommend using nitrate- and nitrite-free products, such as those from Applegate Farms. They can be found in most health food stores across the United States.

Avoidance of Food Allergies

Food allergies are an underlying factor in disturbing gut immune function and may contribute to the developing antibodies that cross-react with the beta cells. If you are allergic to a food, your body reacts to it as if it were a dangerous invader. The white blood cells migrate in large numbers to the mucous membranes and the lining of the intestinal tract. There they release allergic and inflammatory compounds in an attempt to kill the false invader. All this inflammation causes the intestinal tract to become more permeable. Increased intestinal permeability—or a "leaky gut"—can allow large food molecules to be absorbed into the bloodstream. The immune system rightfully recognizes these large molecules as foreign and develops antibodies against them. The result of this immune response can be asthma, eczema, psoriasis, and chronic ear infections; food allergies can even play a role in severe inflammatory conditions such as rheumatoid arthritis (see Table 3.2).

Many nutritionally oriented physicians perform blood tests to diagnose food allergies. However, in most cases such tests are not really necessary. For patients who have to pay for such tests out of pocket, the tests can be expensive. We often recommend that patients try a simple elimination diet first to see if their symptoms improve. If there is only partial improvement and we still think food allergy is a significant factor, then we will perform a blood test to identify food allergies. We recommend that you start by eliminating the most common allergens, especially milk products and wheat:

- Milk and all dairy products
- Wheat
- Corn

Table 3.2. What Symptoms Have Been Associated with Food Allergies and Other Adverse Reactions to Foods?

The following is a partial list of some of the most common symptoms or medical disorders that have been associated with food allergies or other adverse reactions to food. Symptoms recognized by most allergy specialists to be potential symptoms of true or fixed food allergies (immediate hypersensitivity reactions) are marked by an asterisk(*).

RESPIRATORY SYSTEM	SKIN
Non-seasonal runny nose, nasal congestion	Eczema*
Allergic rhinitis (hay fever)	Hives*
Allergic conjunctivitis (red, itchy eyes)	Swelling of mouth, eyelids, and lips (angioedema)*
Recurrent serous otitis media* (inflammation and fluid in the middle ear)	Itching skin*
Asthma/wheezing*	Flushed face or ears after eating
Throat swelling (in serious anaphylactic reactions)*	

BRAIN AND NERVOUS SYSTEM	DIGESTIVE SYSTEM
Dizziness	Diarrhea*
Irritability or aggression	Belly pain/cramping*
Hyperactivity, agitation, or anxiety	Constipation*
Poor concentration	Nausea and/or vomiting*
Mental exhaustion	Bloating*
Insomnia	Burping*
Migraine headache	Flatulence*
	Upset stomach or indigestion*

MUSCULOSKELETAL SYSTEM	MISCELLANEOUS
Muscle pain	Persistent or recurring fatigue
Muscular tension	Dark circles under eyes
Twitching muscles	Paleness
Muscular weakness	Excessive sweating or slight fever
Joint aches	Rapid heartbeat
Joint stiffness	Bed wetting
	Frequent urination and excessive thirst

Note: Symptoms may occur immediately after eating certain foods or may take up to 24 hours or more to manifest. Symptoms may occur occasionally or may be constantly present, depending upon many factors, including the following:

• Whether the adverse reaction is immediate (true allergy) or delayed (hypersensitivity or intolerance)
• The amount and frequency of food eaten
• The nutritional status of the individual
• The state of the individual's gastrointestinal health
• Other health problems such as chronic infection, accumulated environmental toxins, lack of exercise, or emotional stress

- Soy
- Citrus
- Peanuts and peanut butter
- Eggs
- Processed foods containing artificial food coloring

If your (or your child's) symptoms disappear or you notice an improvement in your mood or energy levels, you know that you're on the right track. By slowly reintroducing the various foods back into the diet (for example, trying one "new" food every three days), and paying attention to which ones cause symptoms to return, you can identify the real culprit.

Will you be able to eat that food again? That depends on whether the allergy is cyclic or fixed. *Cyclic* allergies develop slowly and result from repeatedly eating a certain food, especially if a leaky gut is present. In cyclic food allergies, after the allergenic food is avoided for a period of time (typically 3 to 4 months), it may be reintroduced. Usually the food won't cause symptoms again unless you eat it too frequently or in high amounts. Cyclic allergies account for roughly 80 to 90 percent of adverse food reactions. In the strictest sense, cyclic food allergies are not true food allergies (immediate reactions resulting in hives, swelling of the lips, or other symptoms), as identified with an asterisk (*) in Table 3.2, but they are certainly harmful to the health and are much more common than true or fixed allergies. *Fixed* allergies occur whenever a food is eaten, no matter how much time has passed. If you have a fixed allergy, you will likely remain allergic to the food for life. The exception to this is certain fixed food allergies in infants and young children. It isn't uncommon for children to eventually outgrow their fixed food allergies.

Nutritional Supplements to Prevent Type 1 Diabetes

In this age of processed foods and fast-paced, stressful lifestyles, we believe it is impossible for you to nourish your body completely through diet alone. That's especially true if you want to give yourself the best chance to prevent diabetes and other chronic diseases. We recommend five key supplements to prevent type 1 diabetes:

1. A high-potency multiple vitamin and mineral formula
2. Fish oil supplements
   a. Children: cod-liver oil (starting at 6 months of age)
   b. Adults: high-quality supplement (wild-caught salmon oil, DHA/EPA concentrate, or cod-liver oil)
3. Flavonoids (grapeseed extract is one of our favorites)
4. Probiotics (friendly bacteria)

A High-Potency Multiple Vitamin and Mineral Formula

Your body needs essential vitamins and minerals—each in the right amount—for your tissues to do their jobs. Every one of your billions of cells must have the right building blocks in order to function properly. One of the most crucial functions of vitamins and minerals is in the manufacture of enzymes—molecules that trigger and control chemical reactions. Most enzymes in the body have both a vitamin portion and a mineral portion. That's why we recommend taking a high-quality product—one that provides adequate levels of all (or most) of these essential vitamins and minerals. Our guidelines for selecting the right multiple vitamin and mineral formula are given in Appendix H.

Fish Oil Supplements

We recommend that children and adults take a high-quality fish oil product. For children, we recommend cod-liver oil—1 to 2 teaspoons daily. For adults, we recommend a high-quality fish oil product to provide a daily intake of 200 to 600 mg of total omega-3 fatty acids. When selecting a fish oil supplement, it is essential to use a brand that you trust. Quality control is an absolute must to ensure that the product is free from heavy metals, especially mercury, damaged fats (lipid peroxides), PCBs, and dioxins and other contaminants. Some brands that we recommend are Natural Factors, Carlson, and Nordic Naturals. These brands are widely available at your local health food store. For children, we particularly like the Carlson brand flavored cod-liver oil or the one made by Nordic Naturals.

The additional benefits of fish oils in diabetes are discussed in more detail later in the book. We want to focus some additional attention here on cod-liver oil. In studies showing the protective effect of vitamin D supplementation, the dosage used was much higher (about 2,000 IU per day) than the recommended dietary allowance (RDA) of 200 IU per day. The official U.S. and Canadian recommendations for daily vitamin D intake are as follows:

Infants age 0–12 months, 200 IU (5 mcg)
Males and females age 1–50 years, 200 IU (5 mcg)
Age 51–70, 400 IU (10 mcg)
Age 71 and older, 600 IU (15 mcg)
Pregnant women, 200 IU (5 mcg)
Nursing women, 200 IU (5 mcg)

When taken at recommended dosages, vitamin D appears to be safe. However, when used at considerable excess, vitamin D can build up in the body and cause toxic symptoms. Vitamin D toxicity is characterized by increased blood concentration of calcium (a potentially serious situation), deposition of calcium into internal organs, and kidney stones. The precise dosage at which intake becomes toxic is a matter of dispute, but tolerable upper limits for daily vitamin D intake have been set as follows:

Infants age 0–12 months, 1,000 IU (25 mcg)
Males and females age 1 year and older, 2,000 IU (50 mcg)
Pregnant and nursing women, 2,000 IU (50 mcg)

Very little vitamin D is found naturally in the foods we eat (see Table 3.3; the best sources are cold-water fish). In many countries, vitamin D is added to milk and breakfast cereals to ensure that needs are being met.

Table 3.3. Selected Food Sources of Vitamin D

FOOD	INTERNATIONAL UNITS
Cod-liver oil, 1 teaspoon	440 IU
Salmon, cooked, 3½ ounces	360 IU
Milk, 1 cup	100 IU
Dry cereal, vitamin D fortified	40 IU

Flavonoids

A group of plant pigments known as flavonoids exert antioxidant activity that is generally more potent and effective against a broader range of oxidants than the traditional antioxidant nutrients vitamin C, vitamin E, beta-carotene, selenium, and zinc. Flavonoids are sometimes considered "semi-essential" nutrients, but in our view they are as important to human nutrition as the so-called essential nutrients. Besides lending color to fruits and flowers, flavonoids are responsible for many of the medicinal properties of foods, juices, herbs, and bee pollen. More than 8,000 flavonoid compounds have been characterized and classified according to their chemical structure. Flavonoids are sometimes called "nature's biological response modifiers" because of their anti-inflammatory, antiallergic, antiviral, and anticancer properties.[3]

The most commonly used flavonoid supplements are citrus bioflavonoids (including rutin and hesperidin), quercetin, grapeseed and pine bark extracts, and green tea extracts. For prevention of diabetes we would list these flavonoids in the opposite order. Citrus bioflavonoids are the most widely used and least expensive flavonoid sources. However, they are also the least active. One of the most beneficial groups of flavonoids is the proanthocyanidins (also referred to as procyanidins). These molecules are found in high concentrations (up to 95 percent) in grapeseed and pine bark extracts. They exert significant antioxidant effects (as much as 50 to 200 times greater than vitamin C and E) and are particularly helpful in protecting against the form of free radical (hydroxyl) linked to causing the damage to insulin-producing beta cells. Even more powerful protection is provided by green tea.

Both green tea and black tea are derived from the same plant, *Camellia sinensis*. Of the nearly 2.5 million tons of dried tea produced each year, only 20 percent is green tea. In other words, four times as much black tea is produced and consumed as green tea. But green tea is healthier for you because it contains compounds called polyphenols that have high levels of therapeutic activity, including anticancer activity.

The difference between green and black teas results from the manufacturing process. To produce black tea, the leaves are allowed to oxidize. During oxidation, enzymes present in the tea convert polyphenols into substances with much less biological activity. In contrast, green tea is produced by lightly steaming the fresh-cut leaf. Steaming prevents the enzymes from converting polyphenols, so oxidation does not take place.

The major polyphenols in green tea are flavonoids, the most active of which is epigallocatechin gallate (EGCG). In addition to serving as direct antioxidants, green tea polyphenols may increase the activity of antioxidant enzymes in the small intestine, liver, and lungs. Experiments conducted in animal models have shown that green tea polyphenols inhibit cancer by blocking the formation of cancer-causing compounds such as nitrosamines (also an important action in blocking type 1 diabetes), suppressing the activation of carcinogens, and detoxifying or trapping cancer-causing agents. The forms of cancer that appear to be best prevented by green tea are cancers of the gastrointestinal tract, including cancers of the pancreas, stomach, small intestine, and colon; and lung, breast, and prostate cancer.[4]

Green tea can be consumed as a beverage made from either loose green tea leaves or tea bags. However, you must be aware that drinking three cups of green tea provides about the same dose of caffeine as one cup of coffee. Drinking green tea or taking caffeine-containing extract may be overstimulating, leading to such symptoms as nervousness, anxiety, insomnia, and irritability. Fortunately, decaffeinated green teas and decaffeinated green tea extracts are now widely available.

Ancient Ayurvedic Remedy Has Merit

Bark from the Malabar kino tree (*Pterocarpus marsupium*) has a long history of use in India as a treatment for diabetes. There appears to be some basis for this use, since a flavonoid, epicatechin, extracted from the bark has been shown to prevent beta cell damage in rats. Further, both epicatechin and a crude alcohol extract of *Pterocarpus marsupium* have been shown to actually regenerate functional pancreatic beta cells in diabetic animals.[5] In other words, in animal experiments this flavonoid has actually reversed the animal model for type 1 diabetes.

We believe that green tea, and specifically green tea polyphenol extracts, are a better choice than extracts of *Pterocarpus marsupium* in the prevention (and treatment) of type 1 diabetes, for several reasons. First, the epicatechin content in a high-quality green tea extract is actually higher than the level found in extracts of *Pterocarpus marsupium*. Second, green tea extract exerts a broader range of beneficial effects. Third, green tea polyphenols exhibit significant antiviral activity against rotavirus and enterovirus—two viruses implicated as a suspected cause of type 1 diabetes.[6] Finally, it is hard to find *Pterocarpus marsupium* in your local health food store.

Daily Dosage Recommendations for Flavonoids

Children under age 6
    Rutin, hesperidin, and citrus bioflavonoids: 200 to 500 mg
    Quercetin: 100 to 200 mg
    Grapeseed or green tea extract: 50 to 100 mg
Children age 6 to 12
    Rutin, hesperidin, and citrus bioflavonoids: 500 to 1000 mg
    Quercetin: 200 to 300 mg
    Grapeseed or green tea extract: 100 to 150 mg
Children age 12 and older and adults
    Rutin, hesperidin, and citrus bioflavonoids: 1,000 to 2,000 mg
    Quercetin: 200 to 400 mg
    Grapeseed or green tea extract: 100 to 200 mg

Probiotics

The term *probiotics* literally means "for life." Probiotics are friendly microflora (bacteria and other organisms) that are vital to our health. Normally at least 400 different species of these little critters colonize the human gastrointestinal tract. The most important healthful bacteria are *Lactobacillus acidophilus* and *Bifidobacterium bifidum*. These bacteria play a central role in gut immune function. Since they have such an important and positive effect on the gut immune system, we suspect that low levels of these beneficial bacteria are associated with an increased risk for type 1 diabetes.

Bifidobacteria are especially important in protecting against enterovirus, coxsackievirus, and rotavirus infection. Bifidobacteria are first introduced through breast-feeding to the sterile gut of the infant, after which large numbers are soon observed in the feces. Some of the protective effects of breast-feeding against type 1 diabetes may be the result of preventing gastrointestinal viral infection. Although breast-fed infants get the same rate of viral gastrointestinal infections, their infections are considerably milder than those of their bottle-fed counterparts.

It is very important that children on formula receive Bifidobacteria, but we also recommend giving Bifidobacteria to breast-fed infants as well. One study was conducted specifically to test the ability of probiotic supplementation in children on formula to protect against rotavirus. The presence of rotavirus-specific antibodies was used as an indicator of rotavirus infection.[7] The results indicated that while 30 percent of the control group (children receiving milk-based formula alone) had at least a fourfold increase in their antibody levels, indicating a rotavirus infection, not a single child receiving the Bifidobacteria had evidence of even a mild case of rotavirus infection. Subsequent studies have shown that Bifidobacteria enhance the ability of the gut immune system to fight rotavirus via several immune-enhancing mechanisms.[8]

Probiotic preparations are available in powder, liquid, capsule, and tablet form. The dosage is based upon the number of live organisms. The ingestion of 4 to 10 billion viable Lactobacillus and Bifidobacteria cells daily is a sufficient dosage for most people; infants and children up to age 6 usually need only 2 to 4 billion cells, and children age 6 to 12 usually need 4 to 6 billion cells. Amounts exceeding those recommended may induce mild gastrointestinal disturbances, while smaller amounts may not be able to colonize the gastrointestinal tract. Proper manufacturing, packaging, and storing of the product is necessary to ensure viability, the right amount of moisture, and freedom from contamination.

The best products for preventing gastrointestinal virus infection may be those containing *Bifidobacteria longum* BB536. This special strain of Bifidobacteria was originally isolated from the intestinal tract of a healthy infant and developed in Japan by the Morinaga Milk Industry Company. Detailed studies have shown it to colonize the human gas-

Rotavirus—a Major Cause of GI Infection

Rotavirus infection accounts for about 45 percent of severe diarrheal diseases in infants and young children in both developed and developing nations. In the United States, rotavirus causes approximately 20 to 40 deaths, 55,000 hospitalizations, and 500,000 physician visits that cost in excess of $1 billion annually. The outcome of infection is more devastating in developing countries, where an estimated 600,000 deaths occur annually, and surviving children may fail to thrive. Medical researchers are trying to develop a vaccine, but unfortunately the first rotavirus vaccine licensed was later withdrawn from the market because of an association with intussusception (a bowel obstruction in which one segment of bowel becomes enfolded within another segment). Until an effective and safe vaccine is developed, parents should attempt to prevent rotavirus infection by ensuring high levels of protective probiotics, particularly Bifidobacteria.

trointestinal tract, enhance immune responses, and suppress the growth of disease-causing microorganisms. What also sets this strain apart is its incredible stability. Most probiotic supplements are extremely fragile and lose much of their potency with time, heat, or too much or too little moisture. BB536, on the other hand, is so stable that it is even added to various food products around the world. Companies currently offering this strain in the United States are Natural Factors and Jarrow.

A relatively new probiotic product called Innersync may prove even more beneficial than other probiotics in boosting Bifidobacteria levels. Innersync provides the bacterium *Propionibacterium freudenrichii,* historically used in the production of Emmenthal Swiss cheese. This bacterium has been shown to dramatically increase the growth of beneficial Bifidobacteria by up to 900 percent as well as exert some beneficial actions of its own, including enhanced immune function and protection against colon cancer.[9] The dosage for Innersync is one to two capsules

(5 to 10 billion organisms) daily—equal to approximately 100 to 200 grams (3.5 to 7 ounces) of Emmenthal Swiss cheese, but without the fat and calories.

When to Take Your Supplements

- Multiple vitamin and mineral supplements are best taken with meals. Whether you take it at the beginning or end of a meal is up to you. If you are taking more than a couple of pills, you may find that taking them at the beginning of a meal is more comfortable. Taking a handful of pills on a full stomach may cause a little stomach upset.
- Fish oil supplements are best taken at or near the beginning of a meal to avoid any fishy aftertaste.
- Flavonoid extracts can be taken at any time.
- Probiotics should be taken with meals if they are enteric-coated for maximum benefit. If the product is not enteric-coated, it should be taken at least 5 minutes before or 1 hour after a meal, or at bedtime.

Chapter Four

A Closer Look at Risk Factors for Type 2 Diabetes

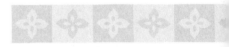

Let's start out with a straightforward—nonsugar-coated—statement: The major risk factor for type 2 diabetes (see Table 4.1) is obesity—or more precisely, excess body fat. Approximately 80 to 90 percent of individuals with type 2 diabetes are obese (20 percent or more above their recommended weight). If these people were not obese, they would not have developed diabetes. That is the bottom line. Therefore, the major focus of this chapter will be factors that are associated with increased body fat as well as type 2 diabetes.

How does excess body fat contribute to diabetes? When fat cells, particularly those around the abdomen, become full of fat they secrete a number of biological products (such as resistin, leptin, tumor necrosis factor, and free fatty acids) that dampen the effect of insulin, impair

Table 4.1. Risk Factors for Type 2 Diabetes

- Family history of diabetes (parent or sibling with type 2 diabetes)
- Obesity
- Increased waist/hip ratio
- Age—increasing age is associated with increased risk, beginning at age 45
- Race/ethnicity (for example, high-risk races include African American, Hispanic American, Native American/Canadian, Native Australian or New Zealander, Asian American, Pacific Islander)
- Previously identified IFG (impaired fasting glucose) or IGT (impaired glucose tolerance)
- History of gestational diabetes (diabetes during pregnancy) or delivery of baby over 9 lb
- Hypertension (blood pressure > 140/90)
- Triglyceride level > 250 mg/dL
- Low adiponectin levels, elevated fasting insulin levels
- Polycystic ovary syndrome (possible in any adult woman who is overweight with acne and infertility)

glucose utilization in skeletal muscle, promote glucose production by the liver, and impair insulin release by pancreatic beta cells. Also important is that the increase in the number and size of fat cells leads to reduced secretion of compounds that promote insulin action, including a novel protein produced by fat cells known as *adiponectin*. Adiponectin not only is associated with improved insulin sensitivity, it also has anti-inflammatory activity, lowers triglycerides, and blocks the development of atherosclerosis (hardening of the arteries). The net effect of all of these actions by fat cells is that they severely stress blood sugar control mechanisms and lead to the development of the major complication of diabetes—atherosclerosis. Because all of these newly discovered hormones are secreted by fat cells, many experts now consider adipose tissue (fat cells) a member of the endocrine system—like the pituitary, adrenals, thyroid, and so on.[1, 2] Measuring blood levels of adiponectin or other hormones secreted by fat cells may turn out to be the most meaningful predictor of the likelihood of developing type 2 diabetes.[3, 4]

In the early stages of the increased metabolic stress produced by the various secretions of fat cells and the lack of adiponectin, blood sugar levels remain normal despite the insulin resistance because the pancreatic beta cells compensate by increasing insulin output. As the metabolic stress increases and insulin resistance becomes more significant, eventually the pancreas is not able to compensate and elevations in blood sugar levels develop. As the disease progresses from insulin resistance to full-blown diabetes, the pancreas starts to "burn out" and produces less insulin. Ultimately complete failure to output insulin may ensue.

Fortunately, as long as the pancreas is still producing adequate amounts of insulin, there is hope that all of the metabolic stress on blood sugar control can be reversed. How does this reversal occur? Through elimination of the metabolic stress by achieving normal body weight— or better yet, ideal body fat levels. Weight loss is associated with restoration of normal levels of fat cell–derived regulating compounds, such as adiponectin and resistin, that lead to increased insulin sensitivity.

Body Fat vs. Body Weight

When you jump on the scales, you are looking at your total weight, not the relationship of fat to muscle or body composition. While being overweight is a risk factor for type 2 diabetes, it is not the critical risk factor. Correctly stated, increased body *fat* is associated with type 2 diabetes, not increased body *weight*. While there is a strong correlation between body weight and body fat content, people of normal body weight can develop type 2 diabetes if they have an increased body fat percentage, especially if that excess fat is collecting around the waist or gut. That spare-tire accumulation of fat can lead to what is referred to as *metabolic obesity*.

To more accurately determine body composition, we recommend a scale that uses a safe, low-level amount of electricity, known as bioelectrical impedance, to determine body fat percentage. Since fat does not conduct much bioelectricity, a higher degree of impedance is associated with higher body fat percentage. The most popular scales of this sort are manufactured by Tanita (see www.tanita.com) and range in cost from $55 to $200 depending on desired features. Ideally, women should strive to keep their body fat percentage below 25 percent and men should aim for 20 percent (see Table 4.2).

Table 4.2. Body Fat Rating Chart for Use with a Body Fat Measuring Scale

Male

AGE	RISKY	EXCELLENT	GOOD	FAIR	POOR
19–24	< 6%	10.8%	14.9%	19.0%	23.3%
25–29	< 6%	12.8%	16.5%	20.3%	24.4%
30–34	< 6%	14.5%	18.0%	21.5%	25.2%
35–39	< 6%	16.1%	19.4%	22.6%	26.1%
40–44	< 6%	17.5%	20.5%	23.6%	26.9%
45–49	< 6%	18.6%	21.5%	24.5%	27.6%
50–54	< 6%	19.8%	22.7%	25.6%	28.7%
55–59	< 6%	20.2%	23.2%	26.2%	29.3%
60+	< 6%	20.3%	23.5%	26.7%	29.8%

Female

AGE	RISKY	EXCELLENT	GOOD	FAIR	POOR
19–24	< 9%	18.9%	22.1%	25.0%	29.6%
25–29	< 9%	18.9%	22.0%	25.4%	29.8%
30–34	< 9%	19.7%	22.7%	26.4%	30.5%
35–39	< 9%	21.0%	24.0%	27.7%	31.5%
40–44	< 9%	22.6%	25.6%	29.3%	32.8%
45–49	< 9%	24.3%	27.3%	30.9%	34.1%
50–54	< 9%	26.6%	29.7%	33.1%	36.2%
55–59	< 9%	27.4%	30.7%	34.0%	37.3%
60+	< 9%	27.6%	31.0%	34.4%	38.0%

You will need to perform one more measurement to assess your risk for metabolic obesity, a measurement of your waist and hips called the *waist/hip ratio*. An increased waist/hip ratio carries a more serious metabolic connotation. In addition to the association with diabetes, this fat distribution pattern is associated with a significant increased risk for heart disease. The reason? The fat cells in the abdomen are more active in secreting regulating compounds that either improve or dampen insulin sensitivity.

You can easily determine your waist/hip ratio. To do this, measure the circumference of your waist about ½ inch above the navel and measure the circumference of your hips at the greatest protrusion of the buttocks. Divide the waist circumference by the hip circumference. A waist/hip ratio above 1.0 for men and above 0.8 for women increases the risk of developing type 2 diabetes, high blood pressure, coronary heart disease, stroke, and gout.

Genetics of Type 2 Diabetes and Obesity

In the discussion of the role of genetics in type 1 diabetes, we described how twin studies are used to assess the role of genetic factors on risk for a particular disease. In diseases that are due primarily to genetic defects, both identical twins will develop the disease in most cases. If one identical twin develops the disease, but in most cases the second twin does not, then environmental and dietary factors are usually responsible. In studies of identical twins, the concordance rate was between 70 and 90 percent for type 2 diabetes. This high concordance points to a very strong genetic relationship. Data from family studies provide additional support; children with one parent with type 2 diabetes have an increased risk of diabetes in their lifetime; if both parents have the disease, the risk in offspring is nearly 40 percent.[5]

So, are we saying that type 2 diabetes is a genetic disease? Not exactly, but genetics are a major factor, and a family history is of major significance. Many of the genetic and family history links are related to the fact that there is also a very strong relationship between genes and obesity.

The Case of the Pima Indians

The Pima Indians of Arizona have the highest rate of type 2 diabetes and obesity anywhere in the world. Research has demonstrated a strong genetic predisposition, but even with this strong tendency it is extremely clear that the high rate of type 2 diabetes in this group is clearly related to diet and lifestyle. First, all we have to do is compare the rate of diabetes and obesity of Pima Indians living in Arizona to those living in Mexico that still cultivate corn, beans, and potatoes as their main staples plus a limited amount of seasonal vegetables and fruits such as zucchini squash, tomatoes, garlic, green peppers, peaches, and apples. The Pimas of Mexico also make heavy use of wild and medicinal plants in their diet. They also work hard, have no electricity or running water in their homes, and walk long distances to bring in drinking water or to wash their clothes. They use no modern household devices; consequently, food preparation and household chores require extra effort by the women. In contrast, the Pima Indians of Arizona are largely sedentary and follow the dietary practices of typical Americans. The results are astounding. While roughly 22 percent of Arizona Pimas have type 2 diabetes and 70 percent are obese, type 2 diabetes is a rarity in the Mexican Pimas and only about 10 percent could be classified as obese. The average difference in body weight between the Arizona and Mexican Pima men and women was more than 60 pounds![6]

Further evidence that diet and lifestyle appear to be able to overcome even the strongest genetic predisposition comes from intervention studies of the Pima Indians. When they were placed on a more traditional diet along with physical exercise, their blood sugar levels improved dramatically and weight loss occurred. The focus right now by various medical organizations such as the National Institutes of Health for dealing with the epidemic of diabetes and obesity in the Pima Indians is to educate children on the importance of exercise and dietary choices to reduce diabetes risk.

Other Genetic and Racial Factors

Other racial and ethnic groups besides the Pima Indians that have a higher tendency for type 2 diabetes include other Native Americans, African Americans, Hispanic Americans, Asian Americans, Australian Aborigines, and Pacific Islanders. In all of these higher-risk groups, it is again important to point out that when they follow the traditional dietary and lifestyle practices of their original culture, the rate of diabetes is extremely low. It appears that these groups are simply very sensitive to the Western diet and lifestyle.

A Personal Note from Dr. Lyon

Back in the mid-1980s I had a chance to gain some firsthand experience working with Native Americans while working as a resident physician at one of the largest Native American hospitals in the U.S. public health system in Oklahoma. Over the three years of my residency I spent many months and uncountable 100-plus-hour workweeks serving the delightful people of the surrounding Native American communities. As a struggling resident I could not justify the expense of driving my car 35 miles each day to work, and so I rode my bicycle back and forth along the hot and hilly roads of eastern Oklahoma. During the many months of my 70-mile-per-day bike treks, I ate as much as I could hold and I still lost weight and felt fantastic. This was a real bonus for a kid who had grown up quite overweight and with a very strong family history of diabetes. At that point in my life, my obesity- and diabetes-prone genes were in complete harmony with my athletic lifestyle, and I looked and felt better than ever before, even though I probably packed away more than 5,000 calories per day or more (all wholesome food) just to fuel my big commute! I still exercise almost every day, but because I don't have the time or the inclination to ride a bike 70 miles per day, I have to watch my diet very closely or the "thrifty genes" take over and I gain weight at the drop of a hat.

I saw a stark contrast to my lifestyle in most of the patients who came to the hospital (more than 500 new patient visits per day between about fifteen to twenty doctors!). It soon became clear to me that in whatever department I had to work, obesity and diabetes were the primary concern. Sedentary lifestyles and fast food were a great curse to these great people. In pediatrics, we spent a great amount of time counseling parents of overweight kids to keep their kids active and to get the junk food out of their diets. In obstetrics, gestational diabetes was almost the rule and seriously complicated pregnancies and deliveries were commonplace. In internal medicine, managing poorly controlled diabetes, premature heart disease, blindness, and end-stage kidney disease were routine. Sadly, in surgery, I became quite adept at performing amputations on so many diabetics who lost toes, feet, or legs to gangrene. All in all, this was a moving experience in many ways and it motivated me to take lifestyle counseling, early diabetes detection, and aggressive diabetes management very seriously in all of my overweight patients. I am quite sure that I (now in my mid forties) would be a diabetic by now if I had let my "bad" genes dictate my fate, but I have avoided this by always paying close attention to my way of life and what goes into my mouth. Since my residency experiences were so vividly etched in my mind I have been motivated to coach, exhort, counsel, and encourage hundreds of others to change the course of their lives and to spoil the dark plans that diabetes has for them. I now know with certainty that when it comes to diabetes, it is not just "all in the genes."

The Western Diet and Diabetes

One of the most famous books detailing the link between diet and chronic conditions such as diabetes and heart disease is *Western Diseases: Their Emergence and Prevention* by Denis Burkitt, M.D., and Hugh Trowell, M.D. This landmark book, first published in 1981, was based upon extensive studies examining the rate of diseases in various populations (epidemiological data) and Burkitt and Trowell's own observations of primitive cultures. These pioneers formulated the following sequence of events:

First stage: In cultures consuming a traditional diet consisting of whole, unprocessed foods, the rate of chronic conditions such as heart disease, diabetes, and cancer is quite low.

Second stage: Commencing with eating a more Western diet, there is a sharp rise in the number of individuals with obesity and diabetes.

Third stage: As more and more people abandon their traditional diet, conditions that were once quite rare become extremely common. Examples include constipation, hemorrhoids, varicose veins, and appendicitis.

Fourth stage: Finally, with full westernization of the diet, other chronic degenerative or potentially lethal conditions such as heart disease, cancer, osteoarthritis, rheumatoid arthritis, and gout become extremely common.

Since Burkitt and Trowell's pioneering research, a virtual landslide of data has continually verified the role of the Western diet as the key factor in virtually every chronic disease, but especially in obesity and diabetes.

Risk Factors for Obesity

Weight gain is the result of a simple equation—more calories are being consumed than are being burned off. While that equation is quite easy to understand, what is considerably more complex is trying to comprehend why obesity is such a rampant problem in developed countries despite growing awareness of the health consequences. Currently, about 79 percent of all Americans are overweight (see Table 4.3). As mentioned earlier, being even a few pounds overweight (especially if it represents increased body fat) carries a significantly increased risk for type 2 diabetes, but the greater the fat accumulation the greater the likelihood of developing type 2 diabetes.

In 1983, only 15 percent of adults met the definition of obesity. By 1990 this number had not changed significantly, but by 1995 it had reached 22 percent and in 2000 it was up to 32 percent, more than double the proportion of adults who were obese 17 years earlier. In other words, approximately **65 million adult Americans are now obese—** more than the total population of Great Britain, France, or Italy. The percentage of children who are obese is also rising at an alarming rate and will undoubtedly contribute to an enormous rise in the rates of diabetes in the future.

Table 4.3. The Dramatic Increase in the Percentage of
American Adults Who Are Overweight

YEAR	% AMERICANS WHO WERE OVERWEIGHT	% AMERICANS WHO WERE OBESE (20% OR MORE OVERWEIGHT)
1983	58	15
1984	56	N/A
1985	62	15
1986	59	N/A
1987	59	15
1988	64	18
1989	61	17
1990	64	16
1991	63	15
1992	66	N/A
1994	69	N/A
1995	71	22
1996	74	24
1997	72	27
1998	76	28
1999	74	27
2000	79	32

What are the contributing factors to this epidemic of obesity? They are the same factors that are contributing to the other epidemics of our generation—heart disease, cancer, and, of course, diabetes. The factors we are referring to are the Western diet and modern lifestyle. That is no startling revelation, as the risk for diabetes in individuals consuming the Western diet is quite clear. To illustrate this link, let's look at results from the famous Physicians Health Study conducted by Harvard researchers with more than 42,000 male physicians. When these doctors were divided into two major dietary patterns—one labeled "prudent," as it was characterized by higher consumption of vegetables, fruit, fish, poultry, and whole grains, and the other labeled "Western," as it was characterized by higher consumption of red meat, processed meat, french fries, high-fat dairy products, refined grains, and sweets and desserts. The Western diet alone carried with it a 50 percent increased risk of developing type 2 diabetes. When the Western dietary pattern

---

Diet, Exercise, Lifestyle, and Diabetes Risk

Findings from the U.S. government's Third National Health and Nutrition Examination Survey (NHANES III) make it quite clear that diabetes is a disease of diet and lifestyle. Of individuals with type 2 diabetes, 69 percent did not exercise at all or did not engage in regular exercise; 62 percent ate fewer than five servings of fruits and vegetables per day; 65 percent consumed more than 30 percent of their daily calories from fat and more than 10 percent of total calories from saturated fat; and 82 percent were either overweight or obese.[7]

---

was combined with low physical activity, the risk for type 2 diabetes nearly doubled. And if obesity was present, the risk jumped 1,100 percent (eleven times more likely to develop the disease).[8]

Our Successful Program

In this book we offer a successful plan to achieving long-term ideal body weight through a comprehensive program designed to address the major reasons why people overeat—from both a psychological and physiological perspective. Our program for achieving or maintaining ideal body weight is consistent with the basic foundations of good health—a positive mental attitude, a healthy lifestyle (a regular exercise program is especially important in battling obesity and type 2 diabetes), a health-promoting diet, and supplementary measures. All of these components are interrelated, creating a situation where no single component is more important than the other. Improvement in one facet may be enough to result in some positive changes, but improving all components yields the greatest results. Our program works because it incorporates strategies that reduce appetite by increasing the feeling of satiety; it improves metabolism; and it increases the sensitivity of body cells to insulin.

The Amish Lifestyle and Diabetes

Insights into the independent role of the modern lifestyle versus diet and obesity in the development of type 2 diabetes can be gleaned from the Old Order Amish. These 30,000 or so individuals, whose ancestors arrived on U.S. shores in the eighteenth century, maintain religious and cultural beliefs that preclude regular use of modern conveniences such as electrical appliances, telephones, and cars, and they have a physically active lifestyle. By comparison, the 200 million typical Americans living alongside them have, over the past 250 years, willingly adopted advances of modern technology, making life less physically demanding.

While the typical Amish diet and rate of obesity do not differ from those of typical Americans, the rate of diabetes is considerably less—about 50 percent lower. While the percentage of Amish with impaired glucose tolerance (prediabetes) is about the same as in other Caucasians living in America, apparently not as many Amish go on to develop diabetes. This occurrence suggests that physical activity has a protective effect against type 2 diabetes, independent of obesity or body fat percentage.[9, 10]

Results from other studies corroborate this hypothesis. Lifestyle changes alone are associated with a 58 percent reduced risk of developing diabetes in people at high risk due to evidence of impaired glucose tolerance based upon the results from the Diabetes Prevention Program—a large intervention trial of more than 1,000 subjects. The two major goals of the program were a minimum of 7 percent weight loss/weight maintenance and a minimum of 150 minutes per week of physical activity similar in intensity to brisk walking.[11]

We want to highlight some of the important dietary risk factors for both obesity and type 2 diabetes. These risk factors will be eliminated by the dietary recommendations given in Chapter 5. To keep things simple, we are going to focus here on the four key dietary factors that promote obesity and type 2 diabetes:

1. Eating more calories (in any form) than are used by the body.
2. Eating refined carbohydrates instead of high-fiber sources.
3. Eating the wrong type of fats.
4. Eating an insufficient intake of antioxidant nutrients.

Typically in people consuming a Western diet, all four factors come into play. Not surprisingly, for people who cannot seem to lose weight, failure to address these four key factors is one of the primary reasons why most diets fail.

Eating Refined Carbohydrates vs. High-Fiber Sources

Dietary carbohydrates play a central role in the cause, prevention, and treatment of type 2 diabetes. Carbohydrates are required to provide us with the energy we need for body functions. There are two groups of carbohydrates, simple and complex. Simple carbohydrates, or sugars, are quickly absorbed by the body for a ready source of energy. It is thought by many that the assortment of natural simple sugars in fruits and vegetables have an advantage over sucrose (white sugar) and other refined sugars in that they are balanced by fiber and a wide range of nutrients that aid in the use of the sugars. Problems with carbohydrates begin when they are refined and stripped of these nutrients. Virtually all of the fiber, phytochemical, vitamin, and trace element content has been removed from white sugar, white breads and pastries, and many breakfast cereals.

As stated earlier, when low-fiber, high-starch, or high-sugar foods are eaten alone, blood sugar levels rise quickly, producing a strain on blood sugar control. Eating foods high in simple sugars can be harmful to blood sugar control—especially if you are insulin resistant, experience reactive hypoglycemia, or are diabetic. Read food labels carefully for clues on sugar content. If the words *sucrose, glucose, maltose, lactose, fructose, corn syrup,* or *white grape juice concentrate* appear on the label, extra sugar has been added. Currently, more than half of the carbohydrates being consumed are in the form of sugars being added to foods as sweetening agents.

Complex carbohydrates, or starches, are composed of many simple sugars joined together by chemical bonds. As long as they are present in high-fiber foods, the body breaks down complex carbohydrates into simple sugars more gradually, which leads to better blood sugar control. More and more research is indicating that high-fiber, complex carbohydrates should form a major part of the diet. Vegetables, legumes, and whole grains are excellent sources of high-fiber complex carbohydrates.

A QUICK LOOK AT SUGARS | Simple sugars are either monosaccharides composed of one sugar molecule or disaccharides composed of two sugar molecules. The principal monosaccharides that occur in foods are glucose and fructose. The major disaccharides are sucrose (white sugar), which is composed of one molecule of glucose and one molecule of fructose; maltose (glucose and glucose); and lactose (glucose and galactose).

Glucose is not particularly sweet tasting compared to fructose and sucrose. It is found in abundant amounts in fruits, honey, sweet corn, and most root vegetables. Glucose is also the primary repeating sugar unit of most complex carbohydrates (starches).

Fructose or fruit sugar is the primary carbohydrate in many fruits, maple syrup, and honey. Fructose is very sweet and is roughly 1½ times sweeter than sucrose (white sugar). Although fructose has the same chemical formula as glucose ($C_6H_{12}O_6$), its structure (shape) is quite different (see Figure 4.1). In order to be used by the body, fructose must be converted to glucose within the liver.

Many physicians have recommended that individuals with diabetes or hypoglycemia avoid fruits and fructose. However, recent research challenges this recommendation. Fructose does not cause a rapid rise in

Figure 4.1. Chemical Structures of Fructose and Glucose

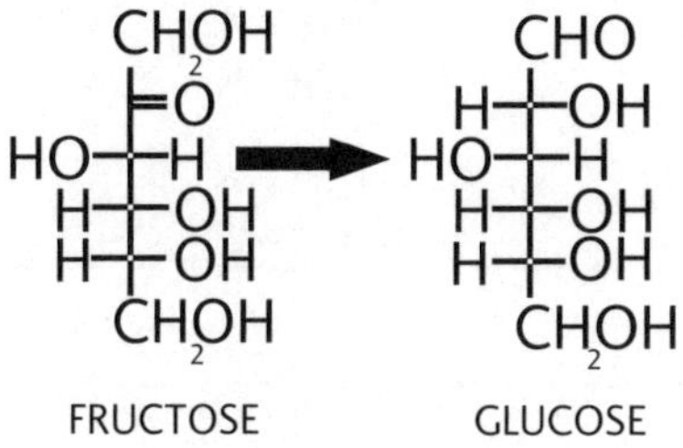

FRUCTOSE   GLUCOSE

blood sugar levels and has been shown to actually improve insulin action.[12] Because fructose must be changed to glucose in the liver in order to be used by the body, the result is that blood glucose levels do not rise as rapidly after fructose consumption compared to other simple sugars like sucrose, maltose (rice syrup and malt), glucose (dextrose), and honey. In fact, fructose has a more gentle effect on the blood sugar of a diabetic than that of low-fiber, white-flour products such as wheat pasta.

THE GLYCEMIC INDEX | More important than labeling a sugar a complex or simple carbohydrate is the *glycemic index* (GI). This numerical value expresses the rise of blood glucose after eating a particular food. The standard value of 100 is based on the rise seen with the ingestion of glucose. The glycemic index ranges from about 20 for fructose and whole barley to about 98 for a baked potato. The insulin response to carbohydrate-containing foods is similar to the rise in blood sugar.

The glycemic index is often used as a guideline for dietary recommendations for people with either diabetes or hypoglycemia. In addition, eating foods with a lower glycemic index is associated with a reduced risk for obesity and diabetes.[13, 14] Basically, we recommended avoiding foods with high values and choosing carbohydrate-containing foods with lower values. In general, as illustrated in Figure 4.2, the more that a food is processed, the higher the glycemic index.

Because of the harmful effects of carbohydrates on blood sugar con-

Figure 4.2. Blood Sugar Response/Glycemic Index of One Food (Wheat) in Different Forms

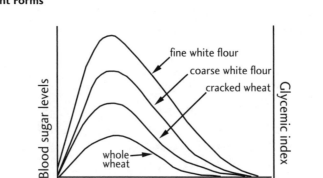

Determining the Glycemic Index of a Food

To determine a food's GI rating, measured portions of the food containing 50 grams of carbohydrate are fed to at least ten healthy people after an overnight fast. For example, to test boiled spaghetti, the scientists give their subjects 200 grams of spaghetti, which according to standard food composition tables provides 50 grams of available carbohydrate. Blood glucose samples are taken at 15- to 30-minute intervals over the next 2 hours. Rather than measuring a single point, the blood samples are used to construct a blood sugar response curve for the 2-hour period. The area under the curve (AUC) is calculated and reflects the total rise in blood sugar (glucose) levels after eating the test food. The scientists compare this response with the volunteer's response to a reference food, which may be either glucose or white bread. The GI rating of the test food is calculated by dividing the AUC for the test food by the AUC for the reference food (white bread or glucose) and multiplying by 100. The average of the GI ratings from all ten subjects is published as the GI of that food. First described by Dr. David Jenkins at the University of Toronto, the glycemic index is now a concept accepted and researched at universities around the world. To date, the most detailed program to determine the GI of foods has been conducted by a team of researchers at the University of Sydney in Australia.

trol, some popular diets have led people to believe that the best way to eat is to avoid carbohydrates almost entirely. We don't agree with this approach. The best approach is to focus on carbohydrate sources with a low to moderate rating on the glycemic index and avoid those with higher ratings. In fact, based on results from short-term clinical trials as well as from large population-based studies, diets that have a higher intake of low-glycemic-index carbohydrates are consistently associated with lower diabetes risk.[15] In diabetic patients, evidence from clinical studies also shows that replacing high-glycemic-index carbohydrates with low-glycemic-index carbohydrate will improve blood sugar control. The same is true for people with impaired glucose tolerance (prediabetes) even if they eat a high-carbohydrate diet.[16] Simply replacing products made with potatoes and white flour with whole-grain, minimally refined products can have dramatic impact on improving blood sugar levels and is associated with a lower risk for both diabetes and cardiovascular disease. One of the key reasons may be that whole-grain foods are rich in magnesium, while this vital nutrient has been stripped away in refined flour. In one analysis, the protective effect of whole-grain consumption was lost when the relative risk was adjusted for magnesium intake.[17]

To provide some general guidelines, Table 4.4 lists various foods and their glycemic index classification. To view the specific values of these foods, see Appendix I on page 328.

THE GLYCEMIC LOAD | One of the shortcomings of the glycemic index is that it tells us only about the quality of the carbohydrates, not the quantity. Obviously, quantity matters too, but the measurement of the glycemic index of a food is not related to portion size. That is where the *glycemic load* (GL) comes into play. The GL is a relatively new way to assess the impact of carbohydrate consumption that takes the glycemic index into account, but provides much more accurate information than the glycemic index alone. A GI value tells you only how rapidly a particular carbohydrate source turns into blood sugar. It doesn't tell you how much of that carbohydrate is in a serving of a particular food. You need to know both things to understand a food's effect on blood sugar. For instance, watermelon has a GI of 72 compared to glucose, but the amount of carbohydrate in ½ cup is only 6 grams. The GL is calculated by multiplying the amount of carbohydrate in a serving of food by that food's GI (as compared to glucose) as a decimal. Therefore, to calculate the GL for a ½-cup serving of watermelon we would multiply 6 times 72 to equal a GL of 4.3. Compare this to ½ cup of Grape-Nuts, which has a GI of 71 but provides 47 grams of carbohydrate, yielding a whopping GL of 33; 1 cup of white rice also has a GI of 72, but provides 36 grams of carbohydrate so its GL is 26. So while the GI is important, it is not as critical as the GL. A GL of 20 or more is regarded as high, a GL of 11 to 19 is medium, and a GL of 10 or less is low. The higher the GL, the greater the stress on insulin (see Table 4.5). In Appendix I we provide the GI and GL for many common foods.

Table 4.4. Classification of Foods by Glycemic Index Scores

Fruits and Vegetables			
VERY HIGH	**HIGH**	**MEDIUM**	**LOW**
None	Bananas	Cantaloupes	Apples
	Beets	Grapes	Apricots
	Raisins	Oranges	Asparagus
		Orange juice	Broccoli
		Peaches	Brussels sprouts
		Pineapple	Cauliflower
		Watermelon	Celery
			Cherries
			Cucumbers
			Grapefruit
			Green beans
			Green peppers
			Lettuce
			Mushrooms
			Onions
			Plums
			Spinach
			Strawberries
			Tomatoes
			Zucchini
Grains, Nuts, Legumes			
VERY HIGH	**HIGH**	**MEDIUM**	**LOW**
Refined sugar	Bagel	Oatmeal	Lentils
Most cold cereals	Bread (white flour)	Pasta	Nuts
(Grape-Nuts,	Carrots	Peas	Seeds
Corn Flakes, Raisin	Corn	Pita bread	
Bran, etc.)	Granola bar	Pinto beans	
Rice cakes	Kidney beans	Rye bread	
Granola	Muffin (bran)	Whole-grain	
	Potatoes	breads	
	Pretzels	Yams	
	Rice		
	Tortillas		

In another method used to measure glycemic load, the amount of carbohydrate in a typical serving of the food is used in a calculation along with glycemic index. (Glycemic load = glycemic index divided by $100 \times$ the available carbohydrate content (carbohydrates minus fiber) in grams of a typical identified serving of the food.) In this case, as long as modest portions of the low glycemic-load food are eaten, its impact on

Table 4.5. GI, GL, and Insulin Stress Scores of Selected Foods

FOOD	GI	GL	INSULIN STRESS
Carrots, cooked, ½ cup	49	1.5	Low
Peach, fresh, 1 large	42	3	Low
Watermelon, ½ cup	72	4	Low
Whole-wheat bread, 1 slice	69	9.6	Low
Baked potato, medium	93	14	Medium
Brown rice, cooked, 1 cup	50	16	Medium
Banana, raw, 1 medium	55	17.6	Medium
Spaghetti, white, cooked, 1 cup	41	23	High
White rice, cooked, 1 cup	72	26	High
Grape-Nuts, ½ cup	71	33	Very high
Soft drinks, 375 mL	68	34.7	Very high

blood sugar should still be acceptable even if the food is higher on the glycemic index scale.

Research studies are just starting to use the GL as a more sensitive marker for the role of diet in chronic conditions such as diabetes and heart disease. The preliminary results are showing an even stronger link in predicting diabetes than the one shown for the GI.[18] Researchers are also showing that a high-GL diet is associated with an increased risk for heart disease. For example, when researchers from the Nurses Health Study used GL measures to assess the impact of carbohydrate consumption on women, they found that high-GL diets (and, by extension, high-GI foods and greater total carbohydrate intake), correlated with even more significantly greater risk for heart disease than high GI-Diets because of lower levels of protective HDL cholesterol and higher triglyceride levels.[19] Increased risk for diabetes and heart disease started, on average, at a daily GL of 161. Therefore, we recommend using the information in Appendix I to help keep your total daily GL below 150 at the very highest. Keep in mind that the GL is based on the stated serving size; the larger the serving size, the greater the GL.

Eating the Wrong Type of Fats

Dietary fat also plays a central role in the likelihood of developing type 2 diabetes. Large controlled trials have shown that a reduction of fat in-

The Importance of Dietary Fiber in Modifying Glycemic Index/Glycemic Load

Population studies, as well as clinical and experimental data, show diabetes to be one of the diseases most clearly related to inadequate dietary fiber intake. The term *dietary fiber* refers to the components of the plant cell wall as well as the indigestible residues from plant foods. Different types of fibers possess different actions. The type of fiber that exerts the most beneficial effects on blood sugar control is the water-soluble forms. Included in this class are hemicelluloses, mucilages, gums, and pectin substances. Foods that have these sorts of fibers, or are combined with supplements containing these types of fibers, typically have a lower glycemic index. This is because these types of fibers are capable of slowing down the digestion and absorption of carbohydrates, thereby preventing rapid rises in blood sugar. These types of fibers are also associated with increasing the sensitivity of tissues to insulin and improving the uptake of glucose by the muscles, the liver, and other tissues, thereby preventing a sustained elevation of blood sugar.[20, 21]

Particularly good sources of water-soluble fiber are legumes (beans), oat bran, nuts, seeds, psyllium seed husks, pears, apples, and most vegetables. The important thing is to consume a large amount of plant foods to obtain adequate levels of dietary fiber. Although even the simple change from white-flour products to whole-grain versions is associated with a reduced risk for type 2 diabetes,[22, 23] our recommendation is to consume at least 35 grams of fiber a day from a variety of food sources, especially vegetables. To help you achieve this goal, we have provided a list of foods and their fiber content in Appendix I along with their GI and GL values. Keep a diet diary for a few days to calculate your daily fiber intake. Although we encourage everyone to eat a high-fiber diet, supplements can be taken to achieve even greater effects in lowering the glycemic index. PGX™, a mixture of highly soluble polysaccharide fibers based on research at the University of Toronto, is the most effective way to lower the glycemic index of foods. If taken prior to meals, PGX™ curbs the appetite and slows the absorption of sugars.

Some warning is necessary if you are not used to eating a high-fiber diet. You can have too much of a good thing. Increasing your fiber intake can increase the amount of intestinal gas (flatulence) and can result in more frequent bowel movements or even transient diarrhea. Don't worry; these side effects will diminish and will not be a problem after your body has had a chance to adjust. We suggest that you increase the amount of dietary fiber gradually. Start with small amounts and build up to the recommended level over the course of a few weeks. You'll know you're overdoing it if you experience excessive gas or other abdominal symptoms. Cut back until the symptoms resolve, and then proceed more slowly until you reach a level you can tolerate.

take as part of a healthy lifestyle combined with weight reduction and exercise reduces the risk of type 2 diabetes. However, more important than the amount of fat in the diet is the *type* of fat consumed.[24] To reduce the risk of type 2 diabetes as well as heart disease and cancer, the goal is to *decrease* your total fat intake (especially intake of saturated fats and margarine) while *increasing* your intake of omega-3 fatty acids and monounsaturated (omega-9) fatty acids. Some of these terms can be confusing. To help you understand, here's a quick chemistry lesson.

Fat molecules are made of atoms of carbon, hydrogen, and oxygen. Each atom attaches to the others only in certain predetermined ways. The backbone of a fat is a chain of carbon atoms (C):

$$| \quad | \quad | \quad |$$
$$- C - C - C - C -$$
$$| \quad | \quad | \quad |$$

Hydrogen (H) and oxygen (O) atoms can then attach to the carbons. A *saturated fat* is a fat molecule in which all of the available binding sites are occupied with another atom. In other words, the carbons are *saturated* with all of the atoms they can hold:

```
   H   H   H   H

   |   |   |   |

H – C – C – C – C – O

   |   |   |   |

   H   H   H   H
```

An *unsaturated fat* has one or more bonding sites left unoccupied; the two neighboring carbon atoms will take up the slack by forming a double bond:

```
   H               H

   |               |

H – C – C = C – C – O

   |   |   |   |

   H   H   H   H
```

A fat molecule with one double bond is called a monounsaturated fat. Molecules with more than one double bond are called polyunsaturated fats. *Mono-* means "one"; *poly-* means "many." When an unsaturated fat contains the first double bond at the third carbon, it is referred to as an omega-3 fatty acid. If the first double bond is at the sixth carbon, it is an omega-6 fatty acid; if the first double bond occurs at the ninth carbon, it is an omega-9 fatty acid.

Most Americans eat way too much saturated fat found in meats and the omega-6 oils found in most vegetable oils. Because of this, they suffer from a relative deficiency of monounsaturated fats from olive oil and nuts and even more so the omega-3 fats found in fish and flaxseed oil—a situation that is associated with an increased risk for diabetes and about sixty other conditions including heart disease, stroke, high blood pressure, skin diseases, and cancer. Particularly important to good health are the longer-chain omega-3 fatty acids such as eicosapentaenoic acid (EPA) and docosahexaenoic acid (DHA) found in fish, especially cold-water fish such as salmon, mackerel, herring, and halibut. Although the body can convert alpha-linolenic acid from flaxseed and other vegetable sources, it is much more efficient to get these fatty acids from the diet.

WHAT ABOUT MARGARINE? | Margarine and shortening are manufactured from vegetable oils through *hydrogenation*. This means that a hydrogen molecule is added to the natural unsaturated fatty acid molecules of the vegetable oil to make it more saturated. Hydrogenation, the adding of hydrogen molecules, results in changing the structure of the natural fatty acid to many "unnatural" fatty acid forms as well as from the *cis* to the *trans* configuration (see Figure 4.3). The result is that the vegetable oil is now solid or semisolid, but that structural change carries with it significant health risks.

WHAT MAKES SATURATED FATS AND MOST MARGARINES "BAD" AND MONOUNSATURATED AND OMEGA-3 FATTY ACIDS "GOOD?" | The answer has to do with the function of fats in cellular membranes. Membranes are made mostly of fatty acids. What determines the type of fatty acid present in the cell membrane is the type of fat you consume. A diet composed mostly of saturated fat, animal fatty acids, and trans

Figure 4.3. Cis vs. Trans Configuration

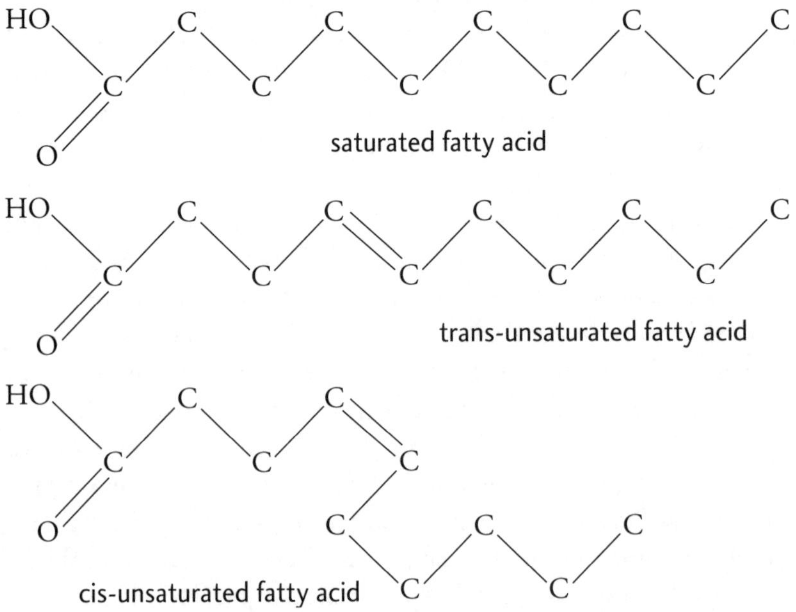

saturated fatty acid

trans-unsaturated fatty acid

cis-unsaturated fatty acid

fatty acids (from margarine, shortening, and other sources of hydrogenated vegetable oils) and high in cholesterol results in membranes that are much less fluid in nature than the membranes in a person who consumes optimum levels of unsaturated fatty acids.

According to modern pathology, or the study of disease processes, an alteration in cell membrane function is the central factor in the development of virtually every disease. As it relates to diabetes, abnormal cell membrane structure due to eating the wrong types of fats leads to impaired action of insulin.

Without a healthy membrane, cells lose their ability to hold water, vital nutrients, and electrolytes. They also lose their ability to communicate with other cells and be controlled by regulating hormones including insulin. Without the right type of fats in cell membranes, cells simply do not function properly. Considerable evidence indicates that cell membrane dysfunction is a critical factor in the development of diabetes.

The type of dietary fat profile linked to type 2 diabetes is an abundance of saturated fat and trans fatty acids (hydrogenated vegetable oils) along with a relative insufficiency of monounsaturated and omega-3 fatty acids. One of the key reasons appears to be the fact that since dietary fat determines cell membrane composition, such a dietary pattern leads to reduced membrane fluidity, which in turn causes reduced insulin binding to receptors on cellular membranes and/or reduced insulin action. Particularly harmful to cell membrane function are margarine, vegetable oil shortening, and other foods containing trans fatty acids and partially hydrogenated oils. These "unnatural" forms of fatty acids interfere with the body's ability to use important essential fatty acids. One study estimated that substituting polyunsaturated vegetable oils for (hydrogenated-vegetable-oil-containing) margarine would reduce the likelihood of developing type 2 diabetes by a whopping 40 percent.[25]

In contrast to the dampening of insulin sensitivity caused by margarine and saturated fats, clinical studies have shown that monounsaturated fats and omega-3 oils improve insulin action.[26] Adding further support is the fact that population studies have also indicated that frequent consumption of monounsaturated fats such as olive oil, nuts, and nut oils and omega-3 fatty acids from fish protect against the development of type 2 diabetes. All of this evidence clearly indicates that altered cell membrane composition and fluidity play a critical role in the development of type 2 diabetes.

Nut Consumption Reduces the Risk for Type 2 Diabetes

Many people shy away from eating nuts because they are high in calories. While that is true, studies have shown that people who frequently consume nuts actually have less of a problem with obesity than people who do not eat nuts. A recent study in women has also shown that consumption of nuts was inversely associated with risk of type 2 diabetes, independent of known risk factors for type 2 diabetes, including age, obesity, family history of diabetes, physical activity, smoking, and other dietary factors. *Inversely associated* means that the higher the intake of nuts, the less likely a woman was to develop type 2 diabetes. What was really amazing was that this relationship was seen even in women who were obese.[27]

In addition to providing beneficial monounsaturated and polyunsaturated fats that improve insulin sensitivity, nuts are also rich in fiber and magnesium and have a low glycemic index. Higher intakes of fiber and magnesium and foods with a low glycemic index have been associated with reduced risk of type 2 diabetes in several population-based studies.

Since nuts are very high in calories (most have about 1,000 calories per cup), we still advocate moderation (frequent small servings) when it comes to nuts in order to promote optimal body weight. We also advocate the use of mostly raw or lightly roasted fresh nuts and seeds rather than commercially roasted and salted nuts and seeds.

Low Intake of Antioxidant Nutrients

Having the right type of fatty acids in our cell membranes is only one factor in developing healthy cell membranes. Equally important is having adequate levels of antioxidants. The cell membranes of the human body are constantly under attack by free radicals and pro-oxidants. Strictly speaking, a free radical is a molecule that contains a highly reactive unpaired electron, while a *pro-oxidant* is a molecule that can promote oxidative damage. These highly reactive molecules can bind to and destroy cell membranes as well as other cell components. Just as iron is oxidized to rust or an apple cut in half turns brown with time, the cells in our body also suffer oxidative or free radical damage.

Free radicals assault us from all directions. Some come from our environment, in pollutants such as chemicals or cigarette smoke, or from our diet in the form of fats damaged by frying or the presence of nitrates in smoked or cured meats. But most free radicals result from normal metabolic processes such as energy production, detoxification reactions, and immune defense mechanisms.

Free radicals severely damage cell membranes, tearing gaping holes and putting the cell at risk. A free radical can also damage other cell compounds, including our DNA.

Cumulative free radical damage leads to cellular aging and is a major factor contributing to type 2 diabetes as well as many other chronic degenerative diseases including heart disease, cancer, arthritis, macular degeneration, and cataracts. Fortunately, nature offsets most of the free radicals formed and the oxidation they cause within the body by neutralizing them with other molecules known as *antioxidants*. These quench the unpaired electron of a free radical by donating one of their own electrons, effectively "calming down" the free radical. Because they mop up free radicals, antioxidants are powerful weapons in the fight against diabetes and other degenerative diseases. Because they protect cell integrity, antioxidants slow down the aging process, enhance immune function, reduce inflammation, and fight allergies.

Since fruits and vegetables are the major sources of dietary antioxidants, we would expect to see a reduced risk of diabetes in people who consume higher levels of these foods. Has research verified this assumption? Absolutely, as several large population-based studies have shown that the higher the intake of fruit and vegetables, the better blood glucose levels are controlled and the lower the risk for type 2 diabetes.[28] Other factors may explain this inverse correlation; for example, fruit and vegetable intake may be associated with reduced stress on blood sugar control due to the fiber or nutrient content. A higher level of antioxidant status is also thought to be a major factor. Even something as simple as regular salad consumption is associated with a reduced risk for type 2 diabetes.[29]

Studies looking at levels of individualized antioxidants have also shown similar inverse correlations—the higher the level of vitamin C, vitamin E, or carotenes, for example, the lower this risk for type 2 diabetes.[30, 31, 32] Likewise, low levels of antioxidants and higher levels of fats damaged by free radicals (lipid peroxides) increase the risk for developing type 2 diabetes.[33] In one study, 944 men age 42 to 60 were followed closely for 4 years. None of these men had diabetes at the beginning of the study. At the end of this time, 45 men had developed diabetes. Researchers found that a low vitamin E concentration was associated with a 390 percent increase in the risk of incidence of type 2 diabetes in the study subjects.[34]

HOW DOES FREE RADICAL DAMAGE LEAD TO DIABETES? | One of the hallmarks of type 2 diabetes is the presence of higher levels of free radicals and pro-oxidants.[35] In particular is the presence of an increased production of reactive oxygen species (ROS) and reactive nitrogen species (RNS).[36] These compounds greatly stress antioxidant mechanisms, as they directly oxidize and damage cell components such as DNA, proteins, and cell membrane fatty acids. In addition to their ability to directly inflict damage on these structures, ROS and RNS indirectly induce damage to tissues by activating a number of inflammatory compounds, such as nuclear factor-kappa B, that ultimately lead to both insulin resistance and impaired insulin secretion. These same compounds are also activated by high blood glucose and elevated saturated fat levels.

Final Comment—Lifestyle vs. Drugs to Prevent Type 2 Diabetes

Several well-designed, large trials have shown that lifestyle and dietary modifications (such as what we will be presenting in Chapter 5 more thoroughly) can be used to effectively prevent type 2 diabetes. That fact has not dissuaded drug companies from sponsoring studies attempting to prevent diabetes with their drugs. However, the degree of prevention with drugs pales in comparison to the effectiveness of diet and lifestyle. For example, in one of the most celebrated studies, 3,234 subjects with impaired glucose tolerance (prediabetes) were randomly assigned to (1) a group receiving a placebo, (2) a group receiving the blood-sugar-lowering drug metformin (850 mg twice daily), or (3) a lifestyle-modification program with goals of at least a 7 percent weight loss and at least 150 minutes of physical activity per week. The average follow-up was 2.8 years. The incidence of diabetes was 11.0, 7.8, and 4.8 cases per 100 person-years in the placebo, metformin, and lifestyle groups, respectively. The lifestyle intervention reduced the incidence of diabetes by 58 percent and metformin by 31 percent, as compared with placebo. Clearly the lifestyle intervention was significantly more effective than metformin—a drug with sometimes serious side effects.[37]

Preventing Type 2 Diabetes

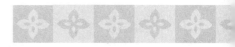

Prevention of type 2 diabetes is actually quite straight-forward. It consists of reducing the risk factors given in the previous chapter via a three-pronged approach:

1. Achieving and maintaining ideal body weight
2. Maximizing the sensitivity of cells to insulin
3. Preventing oxidative and metabolic stress

Being successful in these goals also consists of focusing on three areas: lifestyle, diet, and proper nutritional supplementation. The fourth cornerstone for good health is a positive mental attitude; this factor is discussed thoroughly in Chapter 10.

We have previously described the growing epidemic of type 2 diabetes worldwide and stressed its strong link to the Western diet and a sedentary lifestyle. We have also pointed out that although genetics plays a role, type 2 diabetes is clearly an entirely preventable disease in the overwhelmingly majority of cases. Because of the enormity of the problem, it may seem naïve to offer what on the surface may seem like simple solutions. But the bottom line is that based on our experience as well as the results from numerous large-scale studies, the solutions are simple.

If the solutions are so simple, then why are so many Americans suffering from obesity and type 2 diabetes? The answer is that while the solutions are indeed simple, successful application of the necessary dietary and lifestyle changes is often difficult. It is clear that most people would rather take the easy way out and rely on a pill—either natural or synthetic—than commit to the lifestyle and dietary choices that promote health. Don't be one of these people; choose health and make a commitment to leading a lifestyle and following a diet that will reduce your risk not only for diabetes, but also heart disease, strokes, cancer, cataracts, and other chronic degenerative diseases.

A Health-Promoting Lifestyle

We have already stated that a healthier lifestyle lowered the risk for progressing to type 2 diabetes by 58 percent in people already showing signs of impaired glucose tolerance. The key components of a healthy lifestyle are to not smoke or drink excessive amounts of alcohol; get enough sleep each night; and engage in regular physical activity and relaxation exercises.

Exercise and Type 2 Diabetes Prevention

Regular physical exercise is obviously a major key to good health, and its ability to prevent cardiovascular disease is well-known, but can it prevent diabetes? Yes! As mentioned previously, there is considerable evidence that increased physical activity, whether from structured exercise or physical labor, offers protection against the development of type 2 diabetes.[1] The benefits of regular exercise in the battle against diabetes can be attributed to its ability to improve sensitivity to insulin as well as its ability to promote a leaner body mass (that is, to burn fat). Exercise is a critical component of any weight loss or weight maintenance program:

- When weight loss is achieved by dieting without exercise, a substantial portion of the total weight loss comes from the lean tissue, primarily as water loss.
- When exercise is included in a weight loss program, body composition usually improves due to a gain in lean body weight because of an increase in muscle mass and an accompanying decrease in body fat.
- Exercise helps to counter the reduction in basal metabolic rate that usually accompanies calorie restriction alone.
- Exercise increases the basal metabolic rate for an extended period of time following the exercise session. Thus extra calories are consumed for many hours after each exercise session.
- Moderate to intense exercise may have an appetite suppressant effect.
- Individuals who exercise during and after weight reduction are better able to maintain the weight loss than those who do not exercise.
- Exercise helps diminish anxiety and reduces depression—two major factors that drive people to the refrigerator in their search for comfort.

While the immediate effect of exercise is stress on the body, with regular exercise the body adapts; it becomes stronger, functions more efficiently, and has greater endurance. The entire body benefits from regular exercise (see Table 5.1), largely as a result of improved cardiovascular and respiratory function. Exercise enhances the transport of oxygen and nutrients into cells. At the same time, exercise enhances the transport of carbon dioxide and waste products from the tissues of the body to the bloodstream and ultimately to the eliminative organs. As a result, regular exercise increases stamina and energy levels.

CREATE A REGULAR EXERCISE ROUTINE | Even though everyone agrees that exercise is vital to good health, less than 20 percent of Americans exercise on a regular basis. It is absolutely essential that you motivate

Table 5.1. The Benefits of Regular Exercise

Musculoskeletal system
  Increases muscle strength and muscle mass
  Increases flexibility of muscles and range of joint motion
  Produces stronger bones, ligaments, and tendons
  Lessens chance of injury
  Enhances posture, poise, and physique
  Prevents osteoporosis

Heart and blood vessels
  Lowers resting heart rate
  Strengthens heart function
  Lowers blood pressure
  Improves oxygen delivery throughout the body
  Increases blood supply to muscles
  Enlarges the arteries that provide blood to the heart muscle
  Reduces the risk of coronary heart disease
  Helps lower blood cholesterol and triglyceride levels
  Raises levels of HDL, the "good" cholesterol

Bodily processes
  Improves immune function
  Aids digestion and elimination
  Increases endurance and energy levels
  Promotes lean body mass; burns fat

Mental processes
  Provides a natural release from pent-up feelings
  Helps reduce tension and anxiety
  Improves mental outlook and self-esteem
  Helps relieve moderate depression
  Improves the ability to handle stress
  Stimulates improved mental function
  Induces relaxation and improves sleep
  Increases self-esteem
  Improves sexual function in both men and women

yourself to overcome any excuse not to exercise. Create the time, energy, and motivation that you need to make exercise a part of your daily routine. If you kept your dietary intake the same as it is now and simply exercised for 25 to 30 minutes a day at a moderate intensity level, over the course of a year you would lose 20 to 25 pounds. By combining exercise with the dietary and lifestyle guidelines given in this chapter as well as those in Chapters 7 and 10, the pounds will come off!

Exercise is clearly one of the most powerful medicines available. The time you spend exercising is a valuable investment in your good health.

TURN OFF THE TV TO LOSE WEIGHT | Television watching has been shown to produce a dose-related effect on body weight especially in children—the more TV that is watched, the greater the risk for obesity. Several physiological effects of watching television promote obesity, such as reducing physical activity and the actual lowering of resting (basal) metabolic rate to a level similar to that experienced during trancelike states.

Food is also the most frequently advertised product category on children's TV, with the overwhelming majority of these ads featuring fast-food restaurants or highly sweetened products. Controlled studies on children's food choices have consistently shown that children exposed to advertising choose advertised food products at significantly higher rates than do those not exposed. Greater TV use has been associated with higher intakes of total calories, fat, sweet and salty snacks, and soft drinks, and lower intakes of fruit and vegetables. Is it any wonder that several large studies have documented a clear association between number of hours of TV watched and the rate of obesity?[2]

To lose weight, we recommend turning off the TV and tuning into your own life. If you are a parent, limiting the time your child watches TV can significantly reduce the risk for obesity and type 2 diabetes.

The Importance of Sleep

No one would argue that sleep is absolutely critical to human health; after all, sleep is when the body and mind are recharged. But does sleep *quality* have anything to do with the likelihood of developing type 2 diabetes? Well, according to recent scientific studies, the answer is a dramatic yes. It now appears that in addition to causing daytime drowsiness, cardiovascular disease, mood and memory disturbances, impotence, and car wrecks, sleep disorders also promote insulin resistance.[3]

Sleep plays a prominent role in hormone regulation, including the hormones that regulate blood sugar levels. Sleep deprivation has been shown to lead to impaired insulin action and multiple metabolic disturbances consistent with type 2 diabetes. According to surveys, more than 60 percent of adults in the United States report having sleep problems a few nights a week or more. In addition, more than 40 percent of adults experience daytime sleepiness severe enough to interfere with their daily activities at least a few days each month—with 20 percent reporting problem sleepiness a few days a week or more. At least 40 million Americans suffer from sleep disorders, yet more than 60 percent of adults have never been asked about the quality of their sleep by a physician and less than 20 percent ever initiated a discussion.

Sleep disorders that are especially stressful to blood sugar control mechanisms are those associated with sleep-disordered breathing, but even snoring is linked to poor glucose regulation. In an analysis of data from 70,000 female nurses followed for 10 years, occasional snoring was associated with a 41 percent increase and regular snoring was associated with a 100 percent increase in the frequency of developing type 2 diabetes. This increased risk occurred irrespective of body weight, indicating that snoring is an independent risk factor for type 2 diabetes.[4]

Nasal Strips and Throat Sprays to Relieve Snoring

If you have watched a professional football game since the mid-1990s you probably noticed that many of the players are wearing nasal strips. These adhesive strips mechanically open the nasal passages. The most popular brand is Breathe Right. These nasal strips were invented by Bruce Johnson in 1991. Bruce had always had trouble breathing through his nose, especially at night. Besides suffering from an array of allergies, Bruce has a deviated septum, a structural abnormality of the nose that constricts airflow through one nostril. This combination left his nose chronically congested and made sleeping through the night quite difficult. Lying in bed one night in 1988, he wondered, "Why not try opening the nasal passages mechanically from the outside of the nose?" His answer, after three years of development, took the form of a spring-loaded adhesive strip that he placed across the bridge of his nose to open it up. The device relieved his congestion and improved his sleep quality dramatically. He soon received a patent for his invention and brought it to market in 1992.

Since that time, several clinical studies have validated what Bruce experienced himself—dilating the nasal passages can dramatically improve sleep quality and relieve snoring.[5-8] However, it is not a cure-all. A variety of factors can contribute to snoring—weight, alcohol, smoking, sleeping on your back, age, climate, and allergies—but the most common causes are related to airflow disruption through the nose, throat, or both.

In the clinical studies, about half of the subjects experienced significant benefit while the other half did not. These results led to the development of Snore Relief Throat Spray. This product is designed to help people who snore not as a result of impaired nasal airflow, but rather because of loose tissue in the throat. This natural product contains a blend of wintergreen, peppermint, anise, and clove oil that tightens the throat tissue and reduces irritation, which seems to help many snorers sleep better. Some people experience best results when they use both products.

For more information on these products, see www.breatheright.com.

Even more problematic than snoring is *sleep apnea,* the most common example of sleep-disordered breathing. First described in 1965, sleep apnea is a breathing disorder characterized by brief interruptions of breathing during sleep. It owes its name to the Greek word *apnea,* meaning "want of breath." These breathing pauses are almost always accompanied by snoring between apnea episodes, although not everyone who snores has this condition. Sleep apnea can also be characterized by choking sensations. The frequent interruptions of deep, restorative sleep often lead to excessive daytime sleepiness and may be associated with an early morning headache. Approximately 18 million Americans are thought to suffer from sleep apnea.

Early recognition and treatment of sleep apnea is important because it is associated not only with an increased risk for type 2 diabetes, but also with marked daytime fatigue, irregular heartbeat, high blood pressure, heart attack, stroke, and loss of memory function and other intellectual capabilities. For many people with sleep apnea, their bed partners or family members are the first ones to suspect that something is wrong, usually from their heavy snoring and apparent struggle to breathe. Co-workers or friends may notice that the individual falls asleep during the day at inappropriate times (such as while driving a car, working, or talking). The person usually does not know he or she has a problem and may not believe it when told. It is important that the person see a doctor if he or she snores heavily or if a sleep partner has noticed periods of interrupted breathing during sleep. Sleep apnea should also be considered in anyone with significant daytime drowsiness or changes in intellectual function. Sleep apnea can be properly diagnosed only through the services of a sleep disorder specialist and usually in a sleep laboratory. Home testing equipment may also be provided through a sleep disorder specialist. The American Academy of Sleep Medicine (www.aasmnet.org) certifies specialists and sleep laboratories; the person's physician can provide a referral to one of these centers.

Sleep apnea is most often caused when an excess amount of fatty tissue accumulates in the airway and narrows it. With a narrowed airway, the person continues his or her efforts to breathe, but air cannot easily flow into or out of the nose or mouth. This results in heavy snoring, periods of no breathing, and frequent arousals (causing abrupt changes from deep sleep to light sleep). Ingestion of alcohol and sleeping pills increases the frequency and duration of breathing pauses in people with sleep apnea. In some cases sleep apnea occurs even if no airway obstruction or snoring is present. This form of sleep apnea, called *central sleep apnea,* is caused by a loss of perfect control over breathing by the brain. In both obstructive and central sleep apnea, obesity is the major risk factor and weight loss is the most important aspect of long-term management. People with sleep apnea experience periods of anoxia (oxygen deprivation of the brain) with each episode, which ends in arousal and a reinitiation of breathing. Seldom does the sufferer awaken enough to be aware of the problem. However, the combination of frequent periods of oxygen deprivation (twenty to several hundreds of times per night) and the greatly disturbed sleep can greatly diminish the quality of life and lead to some very serious problems, including diabetes. Sleep apnea needs to be taken seriously and it should always be treated.

The most common treatment of sleep apnea is the use of nasal continuous positive airway pressure (CPAP). In this procedure, the patient wears a mask over the nose during sleep, and pressure from an air blower forces air through the nasal passages. The air pressure is adjusted so that it is just enough to prevent the throat from collapsing during sleep. The pressure is constant and continuous. Nasal CPAP prevents airway closure while in use, but apnea episodes return when CPAP is stopped or is used improperly. CPAP equipment is readily available and can be obtained by a doctor's prescription. It takes quite a while to get used to CPAP, but it usually works well and we highly recommend this over surgery. Weight loss is also a critical part of the successful management of sleep apnea. Surgery for reducing soft tissue in the throat/soft palate should be used only as a last resort because it often does not work or makes things worse. Laser-assisted uvulopalatoplasty is a highly promoted surgical option. In this procedure, doctors use lasers to surgically remove excessive soft tissue from the back of the throat and from the palate (the roof of the mouth, which separates the mouth from the nasal cavity). This procedure works well initially in about 90 percent of sleep apnea sufferers, but within one year many people are the same or even worse than before because of scar tissue that invariably forms.

From Our Patient Files

Tom once prided himself on his quick wit and his ease at remembering the details of things that others would just forget. Tom was a sharp businessman, and his innovative ideas had brought him a great deal of financial success and the respect of his small community. However, the long hours and high stresses required to run a small business had made it easy to neglect his health and now he was in my office looking for help. "I just seem exhausted all the time and I can't seem to remember things the way I used to," he said. "Yesterday, I almost drove my pickup off the road because I fell asleep at the wheel. Hey, it was 3 P.M.; that's just not right."

Tom was seriously overweight, he smoked, and his blood pressure was 150/100. Tom looked like a setup for diabetes—really, he was a setup for disaster. His marriage was also under a great deal of stress. "My wife and I have been sleeping in separate bedrooms for

2 years because I snore so loud that she can't get to sleep. Needless to say, that has put quite a damper on our sex life and the tension around the house is so great you can almost see it."

Tom was showing signs of both impaired glucose tolerance (prediabetes) and sleep apnea, so he was sent in for a sleep study. As suspected, he had sleep apnea. Tom began to use CPAP and set a goal to quit smoking and to lose weight through diet and exercise. He embarked on his new lifestyle with the same passion that brought him success in business, and 6 months later he was like a new man. He had lost 25 pounds, his energy level had returned to what it was decades before, his memory and mental sharpness were restored, and he was sharing a bedroom once again with his wife. His marriage was back on track and his business actually grew even though his workweek was much less than before. Tom had brought balance back into his life, and the renewed energy, enthusiasm, and creativity that he now possessed more than made up for decreased hours at work. Since he was no longer being asphyxiated thirty or forty times per night, thanks to CPAP and weight loss, his brain, heart, and blood sugars were much healthier. When I rechecked his blood, he no longer showed any signs of impaired glucose tolerance. Tom had stopped diabetes in its tracks. It was encouraging to know that I had helped send Tom down a new direction in his life when, before, he was heading straight to the edge of a cliff.

Improving sleep quality is an important goal for most people. Table 5.2 provides some suggestions for better sleep.

Key Dietary Principles to Prevent Type 2 Diabetes

The importance of diet in the development of type 2 diabetes was highlighted in the previous chapter. What we want to do in this section is clearly define the key dietary principles that will help you reduce the risk for type 2 diabetes. Without question, a good diet is essential for good health. Mounting scientific evidence makes it clear that poor dietary

Table 5.2. Tips for a Good Night's Sleep

1. Avoid sleep inhibitors, including caffeine and alcohol.
2. If you eat bedtime snacks, eat very light and choose low-glycemic-index whole-grain cereals or breads that will keep blood sugar levels steady throughout the night and increase serotonin levels within the brain.
3. Get regular exercise, but avoid exercising (other than stretching) 2 hours or less before bed.
4. Use an eye mask to block out excessive light, and foam earplugs or a white-noise generator to block out excessive sound.
5. Don't use your bed for anything but sleep and sex.
6. Learn stress management techniques (see Chapter 10, page 213).
7. Consider nutritional and supplemental strategies to improve sleep: • Melatonin is a hormone that regulates sleep and wakefulness. Try taking a melatonin supplement ($\frac{1}{2}$ to 3 mg at bedtime). If that does not work, give 5-hydroytryptophan (5-HTP) a try (50 to 100 mg at bedtime). • Some people benefit by taking plant products known to promote sleep, such as passionflower (300 to 450 mg of dry powdered extract) or valerian (150 to 300 mg of dry powdered extract), 45 minutes before bedtime. • If you have muscle cramps or "restless legs" that disturb sleep, try taking magnesium (250 mg at night) and vitamin E (400 to 800 IU per day).
8. To reduce snoring, use Breathe Right Nasal Strips and/or Snore Relief Throat Spray (for more information, see www.breatheright.com). If you snore, or if your sleep partner has noticed that you stop breathing periodically while asleep, be sure to get a referral for a sleep study to rule out sleep apnea.

habits cause or contribute toward many diseases, including diabetes. By the same token, a nourishing diet can minimize the risk of developing type 2 diabetes. By following some important guidelines, you'll give your body its best chance of avoiding not just diabetes but a range of other chronic diseases as well.

A Critical Look at Food Pyramids

In an attempt to create a new model in nutrition education, the U.S. Department of Agriculture first published the Food Guide Pyramid in 1992 (see Figure 5.1). Since that time it has received harsh criticisms from numerous experts and other organizations. One big question con-

Figure 5.1. USDA Food Guide Pyramid

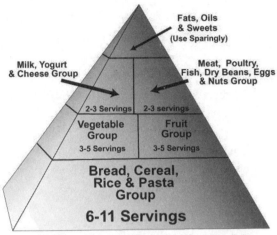

USDA Food Guide Pyramid

sumers may want to ask is, "Is it appropriate to have the USDA making these recommendations?" After all, the USDA serves two somewhat conflicting roles: (1) It represents the food industry and (2) it is in charge of educating consumers about nutrition. Many people believe that the pyramid was weighted toward dairy products, red meat, and breads due to influence of the dairy, beef, and grain farming and processing industries. In other words, the pyramid was not designed as a way to improve the health of Americans but rather to promote the USDA agenda of supporting multinational agrafoods giants.

One of the main criticisms of the Food Guide Pyramid is that it does not stress strongly enough the importance of quality food choices. For example, the bottom of the pyramid represents the foods that the USDA thinks should make up the bulk of your diet: the Bread, Cereal, Rice, and Pasta Group. At six to eleven servings a day from this group, you are supposedly on your way to a healthier life. What the pyramid doesn't tell you, though, is that you are setting yourself up for insulin resistance, obesity, and adult-onset diabetes if you consistently make poor choices in this important category.

The Food Guide Pyramid does not take into consideration the glycemic index (GI) of foods. This term, introduced in Chapter 4, refers to how quickly blood sugar levels will rise after eating a certain type of food. There are two versions of the GI. One uses glucose scored as 100, while the other uses white bread; the foods are then tested against the results of the selected standard. Foods with a lower glycemic index will create a slower rise in blood sugar, and foods with a higher glycemic index will create a faster rise in blood sugar.

If we take a quick look at the glycemic indices of some of the foods that the pyramid directs Americans to eat more of, it is easy to see the problem. Virtually any cold cereal, even those perceived as healthful, typically have a glycemic index of 100 or higher; rice cakes have a GI of 116; a bagel or bran muffin has a GI of 105; and a couple of servings of bread have a GI of 90 to 100. Blood sugar control would be stressed for most people who choose these foods.

Glycemic Load—a More Intelligent Measure

As described on page 78, the glycemic load (GL) is a relatively new way to assess the impact of carbohydrate consumption that takes the glycemic index into account but gives a fuller picture than does glycemic index alone, because it also factors in the amount of carbohydrate. The carbohydrate in beet root, for example, has a high GI. But there isn't a lot of carbohydrate in it, so a typical serving of cooked beet root has a glycemic load that is relatively low (about 5). (A GL of 20 or more is high, a GL of 11 to 19 is medium, and a GL of 10 or less is low.) Thus, as long as a diabetic eats a reasonable portion of a low-glycemic-load food, the impact on blood sugar is acceptable, even if the food has a high GI. For example, if you are a diabetic, enjoy some watermelon (GI of 72) but keep the serving size reasonable (120 g has a glycemic load of only 4) rather than joining in on the watermelon-eating contest!

In essence, foods that are mostly water (such as apple or watermelon), fiber (such as beet root or carrot), or air (such as popcorn) will not cause a steep rise in your blood sugar, even if their glycemic index is high, as long as you exercise moderation in portion sizes.

Figure 5.2. The Optimal Health Food Pyramid

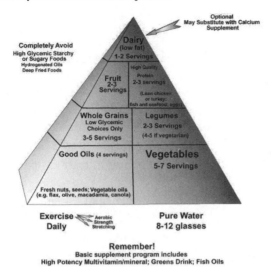

Our Version of a Food Guide Pyramid

Most experts in human nutrition agree that the USDA Food Guide Pyramid is wrong. In fact, some believe that it has been proven a dangerous and misleading dietary guide that has contributed greatly to the growing problems of obesity and type 2 diabetes. We like the concept of graphically illustrating what constitutes a healthful diet, so we are offering our version of a Food Guide Pyramid—the Optimal Health Food Pyramid (see Figure 5.2).

If you compare our version to the USDA's you will notice some clear differences. Our version incorporates the best from two of the most healthful diets ever studied—the traditional Mediterranean diet and the traditional Asian diet. These diets have also been shown to protect against heart disease and cancer. Our pyramid is also quite similar to the new Healthy Eating Pyramid developed by the Harvard School of Public Health. The difference is that we more clearly define what are healthy vegetable oils that should be included in the diet, and we believe that regular fish consumption should be a part of a healthful diet. The four key principles of our diet program are to avoid high-calorie, low-nutrient foods such as junk foods, candy, and soft drinks; eat a "rainbow" of fruits and vegetables; reduce the intake of meat and animal products; and eat the right types of fats.

Avoid High-Calorie, Low-Nutrient Foods

It probably is not necessary for us to make the following statement, but we still need to say it: Don't eat "junk foods." High-sugar junk food diets definitely lead to poor blood sugar regulation, obesity, and ultimately type 2 diabetes. According to the third National Health and Nutrition Examination Survey, which studied eating habits among 15,000 American adults, one-third of the average diet in this country is made up of unhealthy foods, including potato chips, crackers, salted snack foods, candy, gum, fried fast food, and soft drinks. These items offer little in terms of protein, vitamins, or minerals. What they do have, though, is lots of "empty calories" in the form of sugar and fat. These empty calories are exactly what is leading to the epidemic of obesity and diabetes.

Here are some guidelines for making healthier eating choices:

- Read labels carefully. If sugar, fat, or salt is one of the first three ingredients listed, it is probably not a good option.
- Be aware that words such as *sucrose, glucose, maltose, lactose, fructose, corn syrup,* and *white grape juice concentrate* on the label mean that sugar has been added.
- Look not just at the percentage calories from fat, but also the number of grams of fat. For every 5 grams of fat in a serving, you are eating the equivalent of 1 teaspoon of fat.
- Avoid saturated fats and hydrogenated or partially hydrogenated oils.
- If a snack doesn't provide at least 2 grams of fiber, it's not a good choice.

Eat a "Rainbow" of Fruits and Vegetables

A diet rich in fruits and vegetables is your best bet for achieving your dietary fiber intake as well as maximizing antioxidant protection. By "rainbow," we simply mean that by selecting foods of multiple colors—red, orange, yellow, green, blue, and purple—you'll be giving your body the full spectrum of antioxidant compounds as well as the nutrients it needs for optimal function and protection against disease.

We feel that fruits and vegetables should constitute a major portion of the human diet, based upon our anatomy and the way humans evolved. We are omnivorous, which means we can digest foods from both plant and animal sources. In prehistoric times, our survival as a species depended on our ability to gather food both by hunting other animals and by gathering fruits and vegetables.

Still, anthropologists tell us that our bodies are built primarily to process foods from plant sources. They base that conclusion on the shape and arrangement of our teeth, the way our jaws move, and the length of our digestive tract (our intestines are more than 20 feet long, while most carnivores have intestines only a few feet in length). The point is that the human body is designed to function efficiently by getting most of its energy and nutrition from plant sources.

In fact, some experts have said—and we believe—that diseases such as diabetes and cancer are the result of a "maladaptation" over time to a reduced intake of fruits and vegetables. For the earliest humans, eating animal foods was possible—perhaps even a luxury—but was not absolutely crucial for survival. But over the millennia, the balance in the human diet shifted to include more foods from animal sources and fewer fruits and vegetables. The digestive system does the best it can with what we provide it, but without the important vitamins and minerals available in plant foods, the chances of cell damage increases. And that raises the risk of degenerative diseases such as diabetes.

A vast number of substances found in fruits and vegetables are known to promote health. Such substances include antioxidant nutrients such as vitamin C and folic acid and a group of other compounds known as *phytochemicals*. Phytochemicals include pigments such as carotenes, chlorophyll, and flavonoids; dietary fiber; enzymes; vitamin-like compounds; and other minor dietary constituents. Although phytochemicals work in harmony with antioxidants such as vitamin C, vitamin E, and selenium, phytochemicals provide considerably greater protection against free radical damage compared to these simple nutrients.

A CLOSER LOOK AT PLANT PIGMENTS | Among the most important groups of phytochemicals are the pigments. As you might have guessed, pigments give foods their color. Color contributes to food's "eye appeal." Equally important for survival, color helps us recognize when a food has spoiled. But pigments do more than just make food look pretty or rotten. They are powerful chemicals that contribute to your body's metabolic activity.

The carotenes are the best-known pigments and the ones found most widely in foods. These are the red and yellow pigments found in vegetables such as carrots, peppers, yams, and tomatoes, and in fruits such as apricots, watermelons, and cherries. Carotenes are also found in green leafy vegetables, such as spinach, and in legumes, grains, and seeds. More than 600 carotenes exist in nature, including perhaps fifty that the body can transform into vitamin A. Beta-carotene is often considered the most active of the carotenes because more of it is converted to vitamin A, but several other carotenes such as lutein and lycopene exert greater antioxidant and anticancer effects. Some evidence shows that a wide range of carotenes protect against diabetes. The leading sources of carotenes are the dark green leafy vegetables: kale, collards, and spinach. The deeper the green color, the greater the concentration of carotenes. Regular consumption of carrots and/or pumpkin appears to offer the greatest degree of protection against diabetes.[9] If you are a Zone Diet follower, this should come as good news, since carrots are considered "out of the zone" because of their glycemic index. However, since carrots have such a low glycemic load, they are a perfectly acceptable food for diabetics; since they are such a rich source of carotene, all diabetics should consume them regularly.

Perhaps even more important for diabetics than carotenes are another group of plant pigments known as flavonoids. These are sometimes called "nature's biological response modifiers" because of their anti-inflammatory, antiallergic, antiviral, and anticancer properties. They also appear to offer some protection against the development of diabetes.[10] Good dietary sources of flavonoids include citrus fruits, berries, onions, parsley, legumes, green tea, and red wine. Flavonoids are extremely important in the prevention of chronic conditions such as cancer and heart disease. They are also very important in preventing some of the complications of diabetes.

HOW TO EAT A RAINBOW OF FRUITS AND VEGETABLES | To reach your daily quota of vegetables (3 to 4 servings) and fruit (2 to 3 servings) you first need to know what constitutes a serving. A serving equals

Table 5.3. The Rainbow of Fruits and Vegetables

RED	DARK GREEN	YELLOW AND LIGHT GREEN	ORANGE	PURPLE
Apples (red)	Artichokes	Apples	Apricots	Beets
Bell peppers	Asparagus	(green or	Bell peppers	Blueberries
(red)	Bell peppers	yellow)	(orange)	Blackberries
Cherries	(green)	Avocado	Butternut	Currants
Cranberries	Broccoli	Banana	squash	Cabbage
Grapefruit	Brussels	Bell peppers	Cantaloupe	(purple)
Grapes (red)	sprouts	(yellow)	Carrots	Cherries
Radishes	Chard	Bok choy	Mangoes	Eggplant
Raspberries	Collard	Cabbage	Oranges	Onions
Plums (red)	greens	Cauliflower	Papaya	(red)
Strawberries	Cucumbers	Celery	Pumpkin	Grapes
Tomatoes	Green beans	Fennel	Sweet	(purple)
Watermelon	Grapes	Kiwi fruit	potatoes	Pears
	(green)	Lemons	Yams	(red)
	Honeydew	Lettuce		Plums
	melons	(light green		(purple)
	Kale	types)		Radishes
	Leeks	Limes		
	Lettuce	Onions		
	(dark green	Pears		
	types)	(green or		
	Mustard	yellow)		
	greens	Pineapple		
	Peas	Squash		
	Spinach	(yellow)		
	Turnip	Zucchini		
	greens	(yellow)		

1 cup raw leafy vegetables (such as lettuce or spinach); ½ cup raw non-leafy or cooked vegetables; ½ cup cooked green beans or peas; 1 medium fruit or ½ cup small or cut-up fruit; ½ cup 100 percent juice; or ¼ cup dried fruit. Next, choose at least one food per day from each of the five key color groups—red, dark green, yellow and light green, orange, and purple (see Table 5.3).

WHICH IS BETTER—RAW OR COOKED? | On one level, the answer to this question is: It doesn't matter! What's important is to make sure you're eating enough fruits and vegetables, in whatever form. In Table 5.4, we provide some useful tips to reach the five-a-day goal.

Grapefruit—Not Such a Great Fruit?

Citrus fruits are an important part of a cancer-fighting diet because they provide vitamin C, other essential nutrients, and important phytochemicals. But grapefruit contains high levels of a flavonoid (plant compound) called naringin that can be a problem if people are taking certain drugs. Naringin reduces the activity of CYP3A enzymes, part of the P450 enzyme family. Your body uses these enzymes to break down certain drugs, such as calcium channel blockers (used in the treatment of high blood pressure), cholesterol-lowering "statin" drugs, sedatives (for example, midazolam), and cyclosporin (an immune suppressant given to people who have received organ transplants). If the drugs are not metabolized, they remain in the body in higher concentrations. This increases the risk of unwanted toxic effects.

If you are taking a prescription medication, ask your doctor if you should avoid eating grapefruit or drinking grapefruit juice. Some drugs, such as Neoral (oral cyclosporin), already carry a warning. For a complete list of drugs currently known to be affected by grapefruit, see www.Drug-Interactions.com.

Fortunately for citrus lovers, there are plenty of other choices. Oranges, tangerines, and tangelos do not contain significant amounts of naringin but have lots of other important nutrients and flavonoids.

As a rule, we recommend eating at least two of the servings of fruit or vegetables in their raw, fresh state. However, we must note that some carotenes (such as lycopene and lutein) are better absorbed from cooked foods. In addition, it may not be wise to consume more than four servings per week of raw cabbage-family vegetables (including broccoli, cauliflower, and kale) because these foods in their raw state contain compounds that can interfere with thyroid hormone production. When you cook vegetables, we recommend lightly steaming them or stir-frying them in olive oil.

Table 5.4. Tips to Reach Your Five-a-Day Goal

- Buy many kinds of fruits and vegetables when you shop, so you have plenty of choices.
- Stock up on frozen vegetables for easy cooking so that you always have a vegetable dish with every dinner.
- Use the fruits and vegetables that go bad easily (peaches, asparagus) first. Save hardier varieties (apples, acorn squash) or frozen goods for later in the week.
- Keep fruits and vegetables where you can see them. The more often you see them, the more likely you are to eat them.
- Keep a bowl of cut-up vegetables on the top shelf of the refrigerator.
- Keep a fruit bowl on your kitchen counter, table, or desk at work.
- Pack a piece of fruit or some cut-up vegetables in your briefcase or backpack; carry moist towelettes for easy cleanup.
- Add fruits and vegetables to lunch by having them in soup, in salad, or cut up raw.
- At dinner, serve microwaved or steamed vegetables.
- Increase portion sizes when you serve vegetables.
- Choose fresh fruit for dessert. For a special dessert, try a fruit parfait with low-fat yogurt or sherbet topped with lots of berries.
- Add extra varieties of vegetables when you prepare soups, sauces, and casseroles (for example, add grated carrots and zucchini to spaghetti sauce).
- Take advantage of salad bars, which offer ready-to-eat raw vegetables and fruits and prepared salads made with fruits and vegetables.
- Use vegetable-based sauces such as marinara sauce and juices such as low-sodium V8 or tomato juice.

Reduce the Intake of Meat and Other Animal Foods

Study after study confirms one basic truth: The higher your intake of meat and other animal products, the higher your risk of every major chronic degenerative condition, including diabetes, cancer, and heart disease. There are many reasons for this association. Meat lacks the antioxidants and phytochemicals that protect us from cancer. At the same time, it contains lots of saturated fat and other potentially harmful compounds—including pesticide residues, heterocyclic amines, and polycyclic aromatic hydrocarbons, which form when meat is grilled, fried, or broiled. The more well-done the meat, the higher level of amines it contains.

Some proponents of a diet high in meats claim that we should eat the way our cave-dwelling ancestors did. That argument doesn't really hold up. The first thing to consider is that anthropologists tell us that primitive

peoples who lived primarily on meat probably had a life expectancy between 30 and 40 years—not exactly a goal to aspire toward. As well, the
meat of wild animals that early humans consumed was much different
from the industrially produced, shrink-wrapped meat we find in supermarkets today. The demand for tender meat has led to the breeding of cattle
whose meat contains 25 to 30 percent fat, or more. In contrast, meat from
free-living animals and wild game has a fat content of less than 4 percent.

It's not just the amount of fat. The composition is also different. Do-
mestic beef contains primarily saturated fats and virtually no beneficial
omega-3 fatty acids (discussed shortly), while the fat of wild animals
contains more than five times the polyunsaturated fat per gram and has
substantial amounts (about 4 percent) of omega-3 fatty acids.

Range-fed animals also contain ten times as much conjugated
linoleic acid (CLA) as grain-fed animals. CLA is a slightly altered form
of the essential fatty acid linoleic acid. It occurs naturally in meat and
dairy products. CLA was discovered in 1978 when researchers at the
University of Wisconsin were looking for cancer-causing compounds
that result from cooking. Instead, they found CLA, which appears to be
an anticancer compound. Preliminary animal and test tube studies
show that CLA might reduce the risk of cancers at several sites, including the breast, prostate, colon, rectum, lung, skin, and stomach. In addition to its cancer-fighting effects, CLA is also showing some hope for
prevention of diabetes and heart disease as well. In animal and preliminary human studies CLA normalizes impaired glucose tolerance in non-
insulin-dependent diabetes. CLA has also been shown to help promote
maintenance of weight loss.[11]

If you choose to eat red meat, use the following guidelines:

- Ideally, limit red meat to twice per month.
- Limit your intake to no more than 3 or 4 ounces daily—about the
  size of a deck of playing cards—and choose the leanest cuts available (it is important to point out that the USDA allows the meat
  and dairy industries to label fat content by weight rather than by
  percent of calories).
- Avoid consuming well-done, charbroiled, and fat-laden meats.
- Don't eat cured meats (bacon, hot dogs, and so on), especially if
  you are pregnant; this also applies to children under age 12.
- Consider buying free-range meats or wild game.

Table 5.5. Healthier Food Choices

TO REDUCE INTAKE OF:	SUBSTITUTE:
Red meat	Fish and white meat or poultry
Hamburgers and hot dogs	Soy-based or vegetarian alternatives
Eggs	Egg Beaters and similar reduced-cholesterol products, tofu
High-fat dairy products	Low-fat or nonfat products
Butter, lard, other saturated fats	Olive oil, macadamia nut oil, coconut oil
Ice cream, pies, cake, cookies, etc.	Fruits
Fried foods, fatty snacks	Vegetables, fresh salads
Salt and salty foods	Low-sodium foods, light salt
Coffee, soft drinks	Herbal tea, green tea, fresh fruit and vegetable juices
Margarine, shortening, and other source of trans fatty acids or partially hydrogenated oil	Olive oil, macadamia nut oil, coconut oil, canola oil, vegetable spreads that contain no trans fatty acids (available at most health food stores)

STAY AWAY FROM SMOKED AND CURED MEATS | Just as in type 1 diabetes and cancer, the most problematic meats are cured or smoked meats such as ham, hot dogs, bacon, and jerky, which contain sodium nitrate and/or sodium nitrites—compounds that keep the food from spoiling but dramatically increase the risk for cancer and also have been linked to a higher risk for type 2 diabetes.[12] Fortunately, vegetarian alternatives to these standard components of the American diet are now widely available, and many of them actually taste quite good. Consumers can find soy hot dogs, soy sausage, soy bacon, and even soy pastrami at their local health food store as well as in many mainstream grocery stores. Table 5.5 provides additional examples of Healthier Food Choices.

Eat the Right Type of Fats

In Chapter 4, we stressed how important it is to insulin function to have the right types of fat in the diet. The key goal as it relates to dietary fat is to decrease your total fat intake (especially intake of saturated fats) while increasing your intake of omega-3 fatty acids and monounsaturated fatty acids. Let's talk about the importance of monounsaturated fats first. The best sources of these compounds are olive oil, nuts, nut oils, and canola oil. Although monounsaturated fats are not as unsaturated as polyunsaturated, they still contribute to healthier cell membranes because they are more fluid than saturated fats. And because they only have one unsaturated bond, they are more stable and provide better protection against oxidative damage to cell membranes than the polyunsaturated oils.

Olive oil consists not only of the monounsaturated fatty acid oleic acid, it also contains several antioxidant agents that may also account for some of the health benefits. Olive oil is the chief source of fat in the traditional *Mediterranean diet*. This term has a specific meaning. It reflects food patterns typical of some Mediterranean regions in the early 1960s, such as Crete, parts of the rest of Greece, and southern Italy. The traditional Mediterranean diet has shown tremendous benefit in fighting heart disease and cancer, as well as diabetes. It has the following characteristics:

- Olive oil is the principal source of fat.
- It focuses on an abundance of plant food (fruit, vegetables, breads, pasta, potatoes, beans, nuts, and seeds).
- Foods are minimally processed and there is a focus on seasonally fresh and locally grown foods.
- Fresh fruit is the typical daily dessert, with sweets containing concentrated sugars or honey consumed a few times per week at the most.
- Dairy products (principally cheese and yogurt) are consumed daily in low to moderate amounts.
- Fish is consumed on a regular basis.
- Poultry and eggs are consumed in moderate amounts (one to four times weekly) or not at all.
- Red meat is consumed in low amounts.
- Wine is consumed in low to moderate amounts, normally with meals.

Olive oil is particularly valued for its protection against heart disease. It lowers the harmful LDL cholesterol and increases the level of protec-

Macadamia Nut Oil

The best oils to cook with in baking recipes, stir-fries, and sautés are the monounsaturated oils and coconut oil. While olive oil and canola oil are by far the most popular monounsaturated fats in use, macadamia nut oil is superior for cooking because of its lower level of polyunsaturated oil (3 percent for macadamia nut oil versus 8 percent for olive and 23 percent for canola). As a result, while olive oil and canola oil can form lipid peroxides (rancid by-products created through oxidation) at relatively low cooking temperatures, macadamia nut oil is stable at much higher temperatures (more than twice as stable as olive oil and four times as stable as canola). Macadamia nut oil, like olive oil, is also very high in natural antioxidants. In fact it contains more than 4.5 times the amount of vitamin E in olive oil. For more information on macadamia nut oil, visit www.macnutoil.com.

tive HDL cholesterol. It also protects against free radical damage and has been proven to contribute to better control of the elevated blood triglyceride levels that are so common in diabetes.[13] Some of these effects may be related to the ability of monounsaturated olive oil to improve insulin sensitivity. This effect has been seen not only in diabetics, but also in volunteers without diabetes, including teens and adults of both sexes.[14,15]

Olive oil is extremely versatile. It enriches the taste of fish, pasta, and vegetables; it is often used as the base of salad dressings and as a dip to give bread great flavor. An alternative to olive oil is macadamia nut oil (see box above). We recommend that you avoid the omega-6 vegetable oils such as sunflower, grapeseed, soy, corn, and safflower.

Even more stable for cooking than monounsaturated fats are saturated fats from coconut oil. These saturated fats are different from the ones found in animal products—they are shorter. Coconut oil contains what are referred to as short- and medium-chain triglycerides, while the saturated fats in animal products are long-chain triglycerides. Being shorter, short- and medium-chain triglycerides are handled by the body differently. In fact, these fats actually have been shown to promote weight loss by increasing the burning of calories (thermogenesis), and they lower cholesterol as well.[16]

Another important aspect to getting the right type of oils in your diet is to eat fish rich in the omega-3 fatty acids, such as salmon, mackerel, herring, and halibut, or take pharmaceutical-grade fish oil supplements (discussed on page 116). Omega-3 fatty acids from fish offer significant protection against not only diabetes, but also heart disease and major cancers such as lung, colon, breast, and prostate.[17,18] While we encourage you to eat more fish, we need to give you some guidelines. Nearly all fish contains trace amounts of methyl mercury. In most cases this is of little concern because the level is so low. The fish most likely to have the lowest level of methyl mercury are salmon (usually nondetectable levels), cod, mackerel, cold-water tuna, farm-raised catfish, and herring. But certain seafood, particularly swordfish, shark, and some other large predatory fish, may contain high levels of methyl mercury. Fish absorb methyl mercury from water and aquatic plants. Larger predatory fish also absorb mercury from their prey. Methyl mercury binds tightly to the proteins in fish tissue, including muscle; cooking does not reduce the mercury content significantly. Methyl mercury levels have also been rising dramatically in freshwater fish worldwide. As a general rule, freshwater fish should be assumed to be mercury laden unless specifically proven otherwise.

We suggest limiting fish intake to no more than about 2 pounds per week. That translates to four 8-ounce servings per week maximum. Limit your intake of swordfish, shark, and warm-water tuna to very occasional only and all freshwater fish to no more than once a week (women of childbearing age who might get pregnant and children should avoid all of these fish these completely); and eat most of your fish baked or steamed and avoid fried, grilled, or barbecued fish.

Key Supplements to Prevent Type 2 Diabetes

In this age of processed foods and fast-paced, stressful lifestyles, it can be very hard—if not actually impossible—for you to nourish your body completely through diet alone. That's especially true if you want to give yourself the best chance to prevent diabetes and other chronic diseases. If you're like most people, you may need a little help in the form of nutritional supplements. We recommend three key dietary supplements to promote health and prevent disease:

1. A multiple vitamin and mineral supplement
2. A green drink
3. A pharmaceutical-grade fish oil supplement

Multiple Vitamin and Mineral Supplements

A high-potency multiple vitamin and mineral formula, especially one that provides sufficient levels of antioxidant nutrients, provides extra insurance that you are giving your body all of the essential vitamins and minerals it needs. A deficiency of any one of several key nutrients required for the proper manufacture and function of insulin can lead to impaired sugar metabolism. Especially important are the B vitamins and the minerals magnesium, chromium, zinc, and manganese. The use of multiple vitamin and mineral supplements is associated with at least a 30 percent reduction of diabetes risk in men and a 16 percent reduction in risk for women; however, the supplements used in these studies are in our opinion far from ideal.[19] In Appendix H on pages 325–327 we provide our recommendations for selecting a high-quality formula, while a more in-depth discussion of the role of individual nutrients helpful in fighting diabetes is provided in Chapter 7.

Multiple vitamin and mineral supplements are best taken with meals. Whether you take them at the beginning or end of a meal is up to you. If you are taking more than a couple of pills, you may find that taking them at the beginning of a meal is more comfortable. Taking a handful of pills on a full stomach may cause a little stomach upset.

Green Drinks

The term *green drinks* refers to green tea and a number of commercially available products containing dehydrated barley grass, wheat grass, or algae sources such as chlorella or spirulina. Such formulas are rehydrated

Warning—Green Tea

Green tea, green drinks, green leafy vegetables, and other natural sources of vitamin K can interfere with the blood thinner coumadin (Warfarin). This drug blocks blood clotting in part by interfering with the actions of vitamin K. However, coumadin can effectively be used even if you consume vitamin K–containing foods, as long as the quantities you intake remain constant from day to day. The standard blood tests done when you are taking coumadin allows your doctor to simply adjust the coumadin dose to compensate for any increase in vitamin K intake.

by mixing with water or juice. Some of the more popular brands are Enriching Greens, Green Magma, Kyo-Green, Greens +, Barlean's Greens, and ProGreens. These products—packed full of phytochemicals, especially carotenes and chlorophyll—are more convenient than trying to sprout and grow your own source of greens. An added advantage is that they tend to taste better than, for example, straight wheatgrass juice.

Green foods such as young barley grass, wheat grass, spirulina, and chlorella are exceptionally high in nutritional value. Using any of the popular brands listed previously results in a more concentrated and convenient source of phytochemicals than eating two to four cups of a well-rounded salad. We recommend drinking one to two servings daily in addition to eating a diet rich in phytochemicals. Try to consume these drinks 20 minutes before or 2 hours after a meal.

Pharmaceutical-Grade Fish Oil Supplements

Adding a fish oil supplement to your daily routine provides extra insurance that you are getting sufficient levels of these important oils. Using a high-quality fish oil supplement is the perfect solution to people wanting the health benefits of fish oils without the mercury, PCBs, dioxins, and other contaminants often found in fish.

We prefer fish oils to flaxseed oil, because although the body can convert alpha-linolenic acid from flaxseed oil into the more potent molecules of EPA and DHA, it is much more efficient to use fish oils. All told, about sixty different health conditions have been benefited by fish oil supplementation, including not only diabetes, but also cancer, heart disease, rheumatoid arthritis and other autoimmune diseases, psoriasis, eczema, asthma, attention deficit disorder, and depression. It is estimated that the use of fish oil supplements may reduce overall cardiovascular mortality by as much as 45 percent.[20]

We use the term *pharmaceutical-grade* to signify a high-potency fish oil product that is also free of heavy metals, environmental contaminants, lipid peroxides, and other harmful compounds. The specific product that we recommend is RxOmega-3 Factors from Natural Factors because we know firsthand the quality control steps employed to ensure that the product is free of contaminants. Each capsule provides 600 mg of long-chain omega-3 fatty acids (400 mg EPA and 200 mg DHA). We recommend one capsule daily for general health; if greater support is needed the dosage increases to two to three capsules daily.

Fish oil supplements are best taken at or near the beginning of a meal to avoid any fishy aftertaste—some people burp up a little of the oil if they take it at the end of the meal on a full stomach.

Final Comments

Type 2 diabetes is a progressive disease, but it can be stopped and even reversed. That should be obvious to you. Seize the opportunity for health while you still can. Diabetes, like most diseases, is easiest to reverse in the early stages. And, like most diseases, it is easier to prevent than it is to treat. The human body is one of the most remarkable creations in the world. It is the vessel of your soul, so take care of it and nourish it so that it serves you well.

Part Two

Treating Diabetes

with Natural Medicine

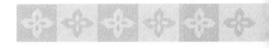

Chapter Six

Monitoring Diabetes

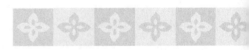

Knowledge and awareness are the greatest allies of people with diabetes. An individual with diabetes who makes a strong commitment to learning about his or her condition and who accepts the lead role in a carefully supervised monitoring program greatly improves the likelihood of leading a long and healthy life. On the other hand, individuals who remain blissfully ignorant about their disease and who refuse to undergo regular testing or self-monitoring are far more likely to face years of unnecessary suffering and, more often than not, catastrophic health problems.

Unless it is properly managed and supervised, diabetes can be viewed as a state of biochemical anarchy that will lead to organ injury and accelerated aging. Diabetes damages many of the complex control systems that faithfully govern and protect the body. To regain control, diabetics must learn how to maintain intimate awareness of their blood sugar, risk factors for atherosclerosis (hardening of the arteries), blood pressure, body mass index, level of fitness, and other factors that determine their risk of developing diabetic complications and experiencing an erosion of their quality of life.

Fortunately, diabetics who develop a keen awareness of these risk factors through regular testing and a properly supervised self-monitoring program are much more likely to benefit from changes in lifestyle, diet, supplements and, when necessary, medications. Making alterations in any of these areas without careful monitoring is like trying to repaint your house in the dark. Without accurate and regular feedback as to your progress, your efforts to improve your health will likely be largely unsuccessful.

Utilizing the dietary, supplementation, and lifestyle recommendations given in this book will lead to definite improvements in blood sugar control. These improvements will subsequently be demonstrated by changes in the results obtained with the different monitoring tools, but especially in self-monitored blood sugar levels. We have found that when patients start to see results with our program, it leads to even greater compliance. Use the available monitoring tests to make sure that you are on the right track.

Urine Glucose Monitoring

Until the mid-1970s the only option that diabetics had to monitor blood sugar was indirect monitoring through urine glucose testing. Normally, the kidneys are able to conserve all of the sugar in the blood that they have to constantly filter. However, if blood sugar gets too high, the kidneys are unable to conserve all of the sugar in the blood that it is filtering and sugar (glucose) will then begin appearing in the urine. Since the average diabetic's kidneys are able to completely conserve sugar until the blood glucose reaches about 180 mg/dL (10 mmol/L), a negative urine glucose reading indicates that the blood glucose since the time of previous voiding has been less than 180 mg/dL (10 mmol/L).

Unfortunately, urine glucose testing does not give any indication of blood sugar levels below 180 mg/dL (10 mmol/L). Therefore, it is only a crude measurement of blood sugar control and it is completely worthless in detecting dangerously low blood sugar (hypoglycemia).[1] As well, this method gives no indication when an individual is experiencing extremely high levels of blood sugar. Therefore, urine glucose monitoring is of very little value in determining the success of blood sugar control and does not provide adequate feedback when lifestyle, diet, or other treatments are adjusted. Nowadays, most diabetics can do away with urine glucose measurements as long as they are willing and able to follow a proper program of blood glucose monitoring.

Urine Ketone Testing

Glucose is a clean burning cellular fuel, generating only carbon dioxide (which you breathe off) and water. In any circumstance when the body must derive its primary source of energy from fat, a group of acidic substances called ketones will be produced as a by-product. If the level of ketone production is high enough, ketones will appear in the urine. Because of this, ketones will appear in the urine during starvation, during very-low-carbohydrate diets ("Atkins"-style diets), and during pregnancy when a woman is unable to eat due to nausea.

As well, in a diabetic, ketones will appear in the urine when there is a severe deficiency in the availability or the activity of insulin. This can occur if an insulin-dependent diabetic accidentally or purposefully forgets to take his or her insulin. It can also occur when a diabetic becomes ill, is injured, or is given high doses of cortisone-related drugs. All of these phenomena may result in a severe loss of insulin effectiveness, resulting in an inability of cells to take up and use glucose. In such circumstances, blood glucose will rise to very high levels, high amounts of fat will be used by cells that cannot take in glucose, and the blood will become polluted with toxic levels of acidic ketones. Severe dehydration also rapidly occurs because the kidneys are unable to conserve water in the presence of such extraordinary levels of blood sugar. This dangerous state, called *diabetic ketoacidosis,* must be treated as a medical emergency, usually necessitating intravenous insulin, high amounts of IV fluids, and careful monitoring, usually in an intensive-care unit. Ignoring ketoacidosis can rapidly lead to death.

Because of this, urine ketone testing remains an important part of monitoring, particularly (but not only) in patients with insulin-dependent diabetes. The presence of urine ketones (accompanied by high blood sugar readings) may indicate impending or even established ketoacidosis, thus requiring immediate medical attention. For this reason, all people with diabetes should frequently test their urine for ketones during acute illness or severe stress, especially when blood glucose levels are consistently elevated (> 300 mg/dL [16.7 mmol/L]); regularly during pregnancy; or when symptoms suggestive of ketoacidosis, such as nausea, vomiting, or abdominal pain, are present. Outside these circumstances, no specific schedule of urine ketone monitoring is recommended.

Self-Monitoring of Blood Glucose

In just a few years since its introduction, self-monitoring of blood glucose (SMBG) has revolutionized the treatment of diabetes.[2] Since the publication of the landmark Diabetes Control and Complications Trial[3] (which examined intensive glucose control in type 1 diabetics) and the United Kingdom Prospective Diabetes Study (UKPDS)[4] (which examined intensive glucose control in type 2 diabetics), it has been widely accepted that the most important factor in determining the long-term risk of serious diabetic complications in both type 1 and type 2 diabetics is blood sugar control. Diabetics who do not maintain vigilant awareness of their blood sugar and who do not make every effort to keep their blood sugar under tight control can expect a significant increase in their risk of serious health problems such as eye, kidney, and heart disease as well as a host of other problems such as depression, fatigue, impotence, and chronic infections. Self-monitoring of blood glucose is important for a variety of reasons:[5]

1. Modifications of treatment to achieve appropriate blood glucose control
2. Detection and diagnosis of hypoglycemia

Optimal Range for Self-Monitored
Blood Glucose*

Fasting or before meals—80 to 110 mg/dL (4.4 to 6.7 mmol/L)
2 hours after eating (postprandial)—under 140 mg/dL (7.8 mmol/L)
At bedtime—100 to 140 mg/dL (5.6 to 7.8 mmol/L)

Please note that these are whole-blood values that typically run 10 mg/dL (0.6 mmol/L) higher than the levels your doctor obtains based on serum values (serum is the fluid in blood minus blood cells). To avoid confusing numbers, some home glucose monitoring kits, even those using whole-blood samples, are now calibrating to serum levels. Check your glucose monitor documentation to find out if it is set up to determine whole-blood or serum glucose levels.

*Slightly higher values may be acceptable in elderly or young children because of higher risk of dangerous hypoglycemia.

---

3. Adjusting care in response to daily life circumstances (food intake, exercise, stress, illness)
4. Detection and treatment of severe hyperglycemia (high blood sugar)
5. Increasing compliance to therapy (helps to combat apathy and denial)
6. Improvement in motivation because of immediate positive and negative feedback

Type 1 Diabetes and Self-Monitoring of Blood Glucose

Without a doubt, all type 1 diabetics must monitor their blood sugar frequently if they want to achieve and maintain good health. In the ab-

Optimal Schedule for Self-Monitoring of Blood Glucose

1. Test upon awakening and just before each meal. Ideal blood sugar before meals is under 120 mg/dL (6.7 mmol/L).
2. Test 2 hours after each meal. Ideal blood sugar 2 hours after meals is under 140 mg/dL (7.7 mmol/L).
3. Test at bedtime. Ideal blood sugar at bedtime is under 140 mg/dL (7.7 mmol/L).

sence of diabetes, the pancreas monitors blood sugar continuously and adjusts its insulin output depending on the moment-by-moment changes in blood glucose. In order to achieve blood sugar levels that are consistently as close to normal as possible, type 1 diabetics must replicate this natural situation as closely as possible. This means that they need to monitor their blood sugar frequently, and they must learn to use this information to make ongoing adjustments to their insulin injections, diet, and exercise. Until the most recent past, type 1 diabetics were often prescribed combinations of short- and medium-action or long-action insulin one to two times per day, and many diabetics measured their blood infrequently— some less than once per day.

This trend is rapidly changing. Increasingly, diabetics are being trained to keep their blood sugar in an ideal range around the clock through a combination of intensive insulin therapy and frequent blood sugar monitoring. This is being made possible largely by a new category of rapid-acting and short-duration insulins. Intensive insulin therapy involves either frequent injections with these newer, very-short-duration insulins (Humalog [Insulin Lispro] or Novolog [Insulin Aspart]) or the use of an insulin pump (an electronic device that provides a continuous injection of very-short-acting insulins with extra "boluses" before meals).

Intensive insulin therapy allows a diabetic to achieve near-normal levels of blood glucose along with enjoying improved lifestyle flexibility.

With conventional, infrequent insulin injections, diabetics must structure their meals and other lifestyle aspects around their injections or face serious abnormalities of blood sugar. On the other hand, with intensive insulin therapy that relies upon very-rapid-acting, short-duration insulin, the timing and size of doses can be adjusted to suit the events of the day.[6] Even though it may involve multiple injections (usually before each meal and often at bedtime) and blood glucose measurements up to six times or more each day, intensive insulin therapy results in greater dietary and lifestyle freedom, a higher quality of life and well-being, and near-nondiabetic blood sugar control, which is vital for long term health.

Great strides are being made in developing easier ways to administer intensively (closer to the natural administration of insulin). Insulin pumps are currently the most exciting area of technology looking to meet this need, along with advancements toward pancreatic cell transplantation or even pancreatic regeneration. Remarkable advancements in blood glucose monitoring technology are also making more intensive monitoring easier than ever before.

Type 2 Diabetes and Self-Monitoring of Blood Glucose

Self-monitoring of blood glucose has an important place in the management of type 2 diabetes as well. Every type 2 diabetic will lie somewhere on a spectrum, with one end of the spectrum being mild glucose intolerance (accompanied by insulin resistance and higher than normal levels of insulin) and the other end being more advanced forms (with more severe insulin resistance, the potential for very high blood sugars, ketoacidosis, and partial or near-complete pancreatic failure with an accompanying lack of insulin). Depending upon the severity of the diabetic, SMBG will play a varying role. Every type 2 diabetic should own a blood glucose monitor and should become intimately familiar with its use. Even diabetics whose blood sugar is well controlled through diet, lifestyle, and supplements should measure their own blood sugar regularly.

Type 2 diabetics who are not on insulin and whose blood sugar is well controlled according to regularly scheduled laboratory testing (discussed later in this chapter) would still be wise to designate an intensive blood sugar measuring day every 1 to 3 weeks. On this day, the person should check his or her blood glucose before breakfast (fasting), just before meals, 2 hours after meals, and before bed and record these measurements, along with diet, exercise, and supplements in a journal. Doing this on a regular basis and any time there are significant changes in diet or lifestyle will help type 2 diabetics become more aware of the effects of various factors on their blood sugar. Type 2 diabetics whose blood sugar is poorly controlled should monitor their blood sugar intensively each day and should seek professional assistance to help regain optimal blood glucose control.

Numerous dietary factors, supplements, exercise, stress, and illness can all have a significant impact on blood sugar control. Becoming intimately aware of how all of these factors influence diabetes will help motivate type 2 diabetics to make positive changes and will provide immediate feedback as to the success of any changes that they have made.

Diabetics who have more advanced diabetes and who have diminished pancreatic insulin production may also benefit from efforts to establish consistently near-normal blood sugar control using intensive insulin therapy similar to that of type 1 diabetics.[7] A blood test of *C-peptide levels* can provide an estimate of how much insulin the type 2 diabetic is producing and is one way to help determine the appropriateness of using insulin. A diabetic on an intensive insulin therapy program must perform SMBG as frequently as type 1 diabetics on intensive insulin therapy (usually before and 2 hours after each meal).

Many advanced type 2 diabetics will have diminished insulin production (evidenced by less than normal C-peptide levels). A common trend to achieve optimal blood glucose in these individuals is to give one injection of a new, very-long-acting insulin, Lantus (insulin glargine), that provides a smooth, continual release of insulin for 24 hours in addition to diet and medication (Chapter 9 will describe natural products that may allow reduction or replacement of medications). Diabetics on this type of program will need to measure blood sugar frequently (usually before and 2 hours after each meal).

Do You Know Your C-Peptide Level?

It is very important to know whether the pancreas of a diabetic is making insulin and, if so, how much. This can have a great influence on treatment, especially in a diabetic hoping to avoid or cease using insulin. The level of pancreatic insulin production can also partially determine the type of medication or natural products that are more likely to be effective. Once it is known how well the pancreas is producing insulin, the focus may be shifted toward replacing deficiencies in insulin production, stimulating insulin production, preserving pancreatic function, reducing insulin resistance, or a combination of these therapeutic efforts.

So how can we determine how well the pancreas is making insulin? One way is to determine the level of a substance known as C-peptide. The pancreas manufactures a large protein called proinsulin first. A piece of this protein (called C-peptide) is then snipped off by enzymes and both C-peptide and the remaining insulin are released into the bloodstream (see Figure 6.1). Injected insulin has no C-peptide. Therefore, even in diabetics already on insulin, a measurement of C-peptide can help determine the degree of remaining pancreatic function. This is particularly important for type 2 diabetics with poor blood sugar control. High or normal C-peptide levels in a type 2 diabetic confirms that the pancreas is making insulin, and should direct attention to efforts that will reduce insulin resistance and improve insulin sensitivity. On the other hand, a poorly controlled type 2 diabetic with low C-peptide levels probably needs to be on insulin.

Note: Don't confuse C-peptide with C-reactive protein—an indicator of systemic inflammation and a marker for heart disease risk.

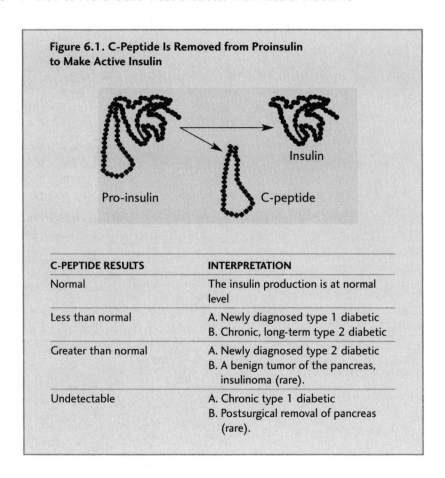

Figure 6.1. C-Peptide Is Removed from Proinsulin to Make Active Insulin

C-PEPTIDE RESULTS	INTERPRETATION
Normal	The insulin production is at normal level
Less than normal	A. Newly diagnosed type 1 diabetic B. Chronic, long-term type 2 diabetic
Greater than normal	A. Newly diagnosed type 2 diabetic B. A benign tumor of the pancreas, insulinoma (rare).
Undetectable	A. Chronic type 1 diabetic B. Postsurgical removal of pancreas (rare).

Self-Monitoring of Blood Glucose— a Rapidly Evolving Technology

There have been dramatic technological advancements in SMBG, beginning with the introduction of blood glucose monitoring strips. Until fairly recently, most diabetics checked their blood sugar at home by pricking their finger, placing a large drop of blood on the end of a blood glucose strip, wiping off the blood after a specific number of seconds, and then determining their blood sugar by comparing the color of the tip to color-coded boxes. Although this represented a great breakthrough in that it allowed diabetics to check their blood sugar at home, it required a fairly large drop of blood (which meant a rather deep and painful finger stick) and good vision (which some diabetics do not have).

In more recent years, tremendous strides have been made in the development of electronic devices that allow SMBG to be conducted with less pain, less time, greater simplicity, and greater accuracy. The best blood glucose monitoring devices are marvels of electronic technology and miniaturization, requiring very tiny amounts of blood. This means that finger pricks can be very superficial and seldom painful. As well, many of the newest devices allow tiny drops of blood to be taken from superficial, virtually painless pricks on the arms, allowing diabetics to give their fingers a break if they become sore from frequent testing. This means that diabetics can obtain more frequent blood sugar measurements with only minimal discomfort.

Most of the new machines are also extremely portable, fast, and very simple. A diabetic may prefer to choose one of the smallest and simplest machines that require very tiny amounts of blood (as little as ⅓ of a microliter of blood, which is the size of a pinhead) and have no buttons to push. Alternatively, technologically comfortable diabetics may choose devices that are more sophisticated and possess an ever-increasing range of features. Some of the more sophisticated features of these machines include the following:

- Many units allow the user to transfer blood glucose measurements to a computer for use in a variety of computer programs.
- Some units link to existing personal digital assistants (PDAs) such as Palm or Pocket PC devices and incorporate PDA blood glucose storage and diabetes management software.
- Some units have a built-in PDA that allows the user to track and plan exercise, meal composition, insulin or medication dosage, and blood sugar and lab test results.
- Some use cartridges containing multiple testing devices to avoid the need to load a new strip each time.
- Some use an audible voice system to guide the testing steps and to communicate the results.
- Some combine a blood glucose meter with an insulin injection system.

Certainly, the technology available for SMBG is advancing at an incredible pace. As it has become increasingly clear that frequent blood glucose monitoring is essential for the optimal control of blood sugar in many diabetics, the technology to make this possible is becoming better all the time.

GlucoWatch

Without a doubt, the greatest breakthrough in blood glucose monitoring is found in the device known as the GlucoWatch.[8] The GlucoWatch is worn much like a wristwatch. A small electrical current from the device works to extract a tiny amount of fluid through the skin. A thin plastic sensor on the back of the watch measures glucose levels using this fluid—instead of blood—every 20 minutes for 12 hours. The device sounds an alarm if the wearer's glucose reaches dangerously high or low levels.

Clinical studies conducted by the manufacturer indicated that GlucoWatch measurements generally were consistent with results from traditional finger-prick blood tests.[9] However, the results differed by more than 30 percent up to a quarter of the time. The GlucoWatch was less effective at detecting very low glucose levels (hypoglycemia) than it was at detecting very high levels (hyperglycemia). In addition, the device would not measure blood sugar at all if the wearer's arm was too sweaty. The device also caused mild to moderate skin irritation in at least 50 percent of those involved in the studies.

This type of device is a significant first step in a new direction in the monitoring of blood glucose levels. Continuous and extended monitoring of blood glucose levels allows physicians to see patterns that are unobtainable with single-test monitoring. Because of the potential for error, physicians and people with diabetes should never use a single GlucoWatch reading alone to make changes in insulin dosages. Instead, GlucoWatch results should be interpreted with several sequential readings over time and always checked against a device that uses a finger prick to determine blood sugar levels before taking action. Because of these limitations, most people would be wise to wait a while longer for this technology to mature before changing from a conventional

Figure 6.2. Glycosylated Hemoglobin

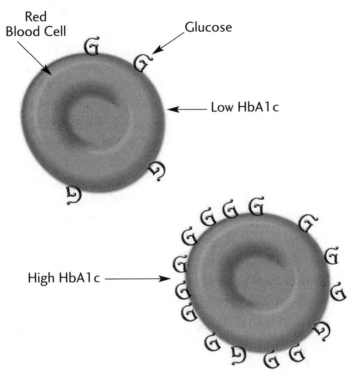

blood glucose monitor. With the advent of this device, there is now little doubt that the days of finger sticks will eventually be over for diabetics.

Physician Monitoring of Blood Glucose

Although diabetics must take charge of their condition and be very much in control of their diet, lifestyle, and glucose monitoring, they are unlikely to have success without professional guidance. Diabetes is one condition where medical doctors, naturopathic physicians, and certified diabetes educators should all play a significant role in education, coaching, and prescribing of care. Numerous studies have determined that physician monitoring through laboratory measurements of blood sugar control can have a major impact on a diabetic's long-term health.

HEMOGLOBIN A_1C—SUGAR-COATED BLOOD PROTEIN | On average, red blood cells live 120 days. During their life, if glucose is present in excessive amounts, components of the red blood cell (the red pigment, hemoglobin) will become glcosylated ("sugar coated") with glucose (see Figure 6.2). Measuring the percentage of hemoglobin that is sugar coated or glycosylated is the basis for the glycosylated hemoglobin A_1C test. Unlike direct measurements of blood glucose, which detect the level of blood sugar at the moment of testing, the A_1C test reflects the average level of blood sugar over the preceding 3 months. Studies have shown that the level of A_1C closely correlates to the level of risk for diabetic complications.[10] Having an A_1C level of 6 percent or less is ideal; it reflects that blood sugar levels have averaged in a range that is essentially nondiabetic. Having an A_1C less than 6 is ideal, but it might be unobtainable for many diabetics, and never being able to reach this goal can lead to discouragement. Fortunately, most studies suggest that an A_1C of less than 7 is still in keeping with a much lower risk of diabetic complications, and this is the goal of most diabetic teaching centers. Because of its great importance, all diabetics, type 1 and type 2, should have their A_1C measured every 2 to 4 months depending on the stability of their condition. This is usually done through a medical or naturopathic physician's office. A new portable A_1C testing device (see www.A1CNow.net) makes on-the-spot testing available in a physician's office or at home.

FRUCTOSAMINE—ANOTHER SUGAR-COATED PROTEIN | Besides hemoglobin, other proteins become "sugar coated" in the blood of diabetics. A variety of blood proteins last only 2 to 3 weeks, unlike the hemoglobin of red blood cells, which lasts 3 to 4 months.[11] Fructosamine is a test that looks at the shorter-duration blood proteins; it reflects the average blood sugar over the past 2 to 3 weeks. This test is primarily used when diabetes management is very complex and insulin needs to be adjusted quite frequently, such in a pregnant type 1 diabetic. Once portable fructosamine testing devices are available (one was available, but it has been discontinued because of technical problems) this test will probably be recommended strongly for certain applications. Particularly, type 2 diabetics who are generally well controlled enough that frequent self-monitoring of blood glucose is unnecessary would benefit from more frequent assessments of control than that provided by A_1C.

CONTINUOUS BLOOD GLUCOSE MONITORING SYSTEM | An interesting advancement is the availability of continuous glucose monitoring through a device that is worn on the belt for up to 3 days, attached to a tiny needle under the skin, that provides 288 glucose measurements every day. This system (known as the MiniMed Continuous Glucose Monitoring System [CGMS; MiniMed Inc., 800-440-7867])[12] is placed by a physician who wants to get a better look at a diabetic's blood sugar control around the clock. This is especially helpful in determining a better insulin, diet, and lifestyle regimen for type 1 diabetics with poor HgA_1C measurement and where self-monitoring of blood glucose does not provide clear guidance as to the needed changes.[13] It is also very helpful when changes to treatment must be made for type 1 diabetics who are experiencing frequent episodes of severe hypoglycemia.[14]

Physician Monitoring of Other Risk Factors

Although it is clear that optimal blood glucose control is critical to the health of the diabetic, there are several other risk factors that need to be carefully monitored in every diabetic. Early detection of problems through a program of regular screening and monitoring will allow preventive efforts and treatments to be put in place before serious complications or catastrophic problems occur.

Blood Pressure

Unfortunately, diabetics have a significant risk of developing cardiovascular problems such as stroke, heart attack, or blocked leg arteries. They are also at high risk of developing kidney disease related to damage to the microscopic vessels of the kidney. Normalizing blood sugar will indeed reduce these risks, but other factors play a leading role as well.

More than half of diabetics (both type 1 and type 2) have high blood pressure (hypertension). It has been shown that controlling hypertension is critically important in reducing the diabetic's risk of both cardiovascular and kidney disease.[15] Effective blood pressure control has also been shown to help maintain insulin sensitivity in the diabetic. Ideal treatment will maintain a diabetic's blood pressure consistently at less than 130/85. Achieving this goal is discussed in Chapter 11, pages 240–249.

In addition to having blood pressure checked when visiting the doctor, it is wise for all diabetics to own and regularly use an electronic home blood pressure monitor. The results of home blood pressure readings should be recorded and the machine should accompany the diabetic to physician visits, where the home readings can be examined and the home blood pressure monitor can be compared to the physician's monitor. We also recommend that all diabetics with a history of hypertension periodically (at least once per year) undergo ambulatory blood pressure monitoring.[16] This procedure involves wearing a special cuff and an accompanying electronic device that allows blood pressure readings to be taken every few minutes for 24 hours or more. Ambulatory blood pressure monitoring enables the physician to determine whether blood pressure is under ideal control around the clock and in a variety of circumstances.

Blood Lipids

Abnormalities in the level of blood lipids (cholesterol, HDL, LDL, VLDL, triglycerides) is very common in diabetics and is one of the first manifestations of insulin resistance, often years before the onset of type 2 diabetes. Numerous studies have demonstrated the importance of regular blood lipid testing in all diabetics and the effectiveness of treating lipid abnormalities.[17] Fortunately, diet, exercise, and several natural health products (discussed in Chapter 12, pages 252–263) are usually able to effectively normalize blood lipids and reduce their accompanying risks. Ideally, diabetics need to aim for the following levels: LDL, < 100 mg/dL; triglycerides, < 200 mg/dL; and HDL, > 45 mg/dL (55 mg/dL for females).

Kidney Function

Diabetes is the primary cause of kidney failure, dialysis, and kidney transplant.[18] Fortunately, early detection of kidney problems followed by careful treatment has been shown to greatly improve the odds that normal kidney function will be preserved. All diabetics should undergo regular monitoring for early kidney disease through measuring the level of small amounts of the protein albumin in the urine every 3 months when visiting the doctor for A_1C determination. The presence of small amounts of albumin leaking into the kidneys from the blood is the first sign of diabetic kidney disease (nephropathy).

Physical Examination

Diabetics should also be carefully followed by an eye specialist (ophthalmologist) who should perform a retinal eye exam (after pupils are dilated) at least once per year. It is also important for all diabetics to have a foot exam (usually every 3 months) to look for breaks or ulcers in the skin, damage to or abnormalities of the nails, and quality of circulation, and also sensory tests to rule out nerve damage (the ability to feel a standard thickness nylon monofilament should be determined every 3 months along with a visual foot inspection). Treadmill testing should be performed in diabetics before beginning or if contemplating changes in an exercise program. Treadmill testing is useful as a screen for coronary artery blockages as well as a general measure of aerobic fitness. Diabetics with a good level of aerobic fitness have a much-decreased risk of most diabetic complications. Body mass index (BMI) is an important measure of risk for a diabetic. Diabetics need to strive to maintain an ideal body weight as indicated by their BMI. This will be discussed in detail in Chapter 10.

Other Laboratory Tests

Since individuals with diabetes have two to three times the risk of dying prematurely of heart disease or stroke compared to nondiabetic individuals, and 55 percent of deaths in diabetes patients are caused by cardiovascular disease, we feel it is very important for diabetics to be regularly screened (at least once a year) for additional factors linked to atherosclerosis. For example, measurement of C-reactive protein is a good indication of the degree of inflammation in the body and has been shown to be a sensitive indicator of the risk of heart disease in diabetics.[19] Homocysteine, a toxic by-product of human biochemistry that can damage the lining of blood vessels, is another cardiovascular risk factor.[20] Fibrinogen is a marker of blood clotting that is often elevated in diabetes and is also associated with an increased risk of cardiovascular disease.[21]

In addition to being linked to death, atherosclerosis (hardening of the arteries) and other vascular lesions are the underlying factors in the development of many of the chronic complications of diabetes. Lesions to the microvascular system (small blood vessels) lead to reduced delivery of oxygen and nutrients to important tissue such as nerves, the eyes, and the kidneys. We recommend performing the tests given in Table 6.1 on an annual basis; if there is an abnormality, follow the recommendations given in Appendix B or C, for three months and repeat the test.

Table 6.1. A Complete Cardiovascular Assessment

Laboratory tests
Total cholesterol
LDL cholesterol
HDL cholesterol
Triglycerides
Lipoprotein (a)
C-reactive protein
Fibrinogen
Homocysteine
Ferritin (an iron-binding protein)
Lipid peroxides
Exercise stress test
Electrocardiogram (EKG)

Doctor Visit Checklist

In Appendix D on pages 306–307 we provide a doctor's visit checklist. Take this list to your doctor to discuss implementing it in the monitoring of your health. Diabetes is a disease you can live with, or it is one that can kill you. It is vital that you take responsibility for your health and do everything you can to achieve good metabolic control.

Chapter Seven

Diet Therapy in Managing Diabetes

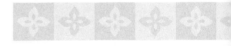

$\mathbf{D}$iet is fundamental to the successful treatment of diabetes, whether it be type 1 or 2. Over the years there has been quite a war of opinions as to the best diet for people with diabetes. One of the first dietary strategies was to completely restrict carbohydrates of all sorts in favor of high-protein and fatty foods. Unfortunately, this diet proved disastrous to the long-term health of diabetics, as it carried with it severe consequences to cardiovascular and kidney health. On the other end of the spectrum was the high-complex-carbohydrate, low-fat diet. This diet was also doomed because it did not differentiate the quality of carbohydrates. Furthermore, eating the right type of oils promotes proper insulin action. Any diet that severely restricts beneficial oils would ultimately fail. After reviewing every scientific article on the role of diet in diabetes treatment that we could find, we offer here an easy-to-follow program that will produce results based upon the evolutionary understanding of the optimal diet for people with diabetes. While it is currently not the diet that the American Diabetes Association (ADA) recommends, we believe that it soon will be, as it is based on a large body of positive clinical research.

Does this mean that if you have diabetes, we want you to disregard what your doctor is telling you about diet? Well, first of all, your doctor has most likely never talked to you at all about diet; if he or she has, it was likely only in general terms—stay away from sugar, cut down on the amount of saturated fat, try to eat more high-protein foods, and so on—or perhaps your doctor gave you a brochure on the Food Guide Pyramid. We are going to make very specific recommendations here to provide you with the absolute best diet to battle diabetes based on our Optimal Health Food Pyramid (see Chapter 5, page 103) as summarized in Table 7.1. If your doctor is telling you to follow the diet program endorsed by the ADA, please tell him or her that you are following our recommendations and provide a copy of our open letter to physicians (see Appendix D, page 306) and our dietary pyramid. We are sure that if your doctor looks at the scientific studies on diet and diabetes, he or she will endorse our program, as so many others have done. You will need to have a good working relationship with your doctor so that you can be monitored properly.

> PLEASE READ CHAPTERS 4 AND 5 BEFORE
> PROCEEDING ANY FURTHER IN THIS CHAPTER!

Our Daily Food Prescription

The optimal diet for the treatment of diabetes is virtually the same as the program that we presented in Chapter 5. The difference is that there often needs to be an even stricter avoidance of foods with a high glycemic load (above 19; see Appendix I, pages 328–336). How strict you will need to be with your intake of carbohydrates depends on your ability to get your blood sugar measurements and glycosylated hemo-globin (hemoglobin A_1C) levels under control and achieve/maintain ideal body weight. Obviously, the poorer the control, the more you will have to restrict carbohydrate intake. Initially, some people with dia-betes—especially those who have poorly controlled blood sugar levels—may need to avoid meals with a total glycemic load of more than 30 and space these meals at least three hours apart. Higher-glycemic-load meals can be consumed if one of the special natural products designed to slow gastric emptying and to blunt after-meal blood sugar levels is used (these compounds are discussed in Chapter 9).

In Appendices A, B, and C, we provide a daily plan for treating dia-betes with natural medicine that includes diet, lifestyle, and supple-mentation recommendations. Included in this appendix is a sample 4-day menu complete with recipes. In this chapter we present our daily food prescription based on a 2,000-calorie-a-day diet, followed by a brief description of the individual food groups, the clinical research on diet therapy in diabetes, and the importance of the three foundational supplements discussed in Chapter 5.

If you need to increase your caloric intake, try to get the extra calo-ries you need by increasing the number of servings of vegetables, nuts, and legumes, as these are the best foods for improving blood sugar con-trol. For athletes or people engaged in heavy physical labor or exercise, be sure to add another serving of seafood, meat, or poultry to your daily intake, or add a soy protein or whey protein smoothie providing an ad-ditional 25 to 30 grams of protein.

Foods to Avoid Entirely
- Refined white-flour products: pastas, cakes, muffins, pretzels, and so on
- Refined sugar-loaded cereals, candies, baked goods, and so on
- Processed foods packed full of empty calories (sugar and fat) or salt (soups, microwave or theater-style popcorn, chips, and so on)
- Margarine, butter, and shortening
- Smoked or cured meats: bacon, hot dogs, smoked luncheon meats, sausages, ham, SPAM, and so on
- Meats cooked at extremely high temperatures or cooked to well-done
- Heavily sweetened or artificially sweetened soft drinks, Kool-Aid, juice-flavored drinks, and so on

Table 7.1. Daily Food Group Recommendations

FOODS	DAILY SERVINGS (2,000-CALORIE DIET)
Vegetables, total servings	5 to 7
Green leafy and cruciferous vegetables	2 to 4
Low-glycemic-load vegetables	2 to 3
Other vegetables	1 to 2
Whole grains	3 to 5
Legumes	2 to 3 (4 to 5 if vegetarian)
Fruit	2 to 3
Good oils	
Total servings	4
Nuts and seeds	1
Olive, macadamia, flaxseed, or canola oil	2 to 3
Dairy	1 to 2 (optional)
High-quality protein	2 to 3

- Fried foods, including french fries, potato chips, corn chips, and doughnuts

Vegetables—5 to 7 Servings Daily

The Latin root of the word *vegetable* means "to enliven or animate." Vegetables give us life and should be the main focus of any health-promoting diet. Vegetables provide the broadest range of nutrients of any food class. They are rich sources of vitamins, minerals, carbohydrates, and protein. Vegetables also provide high quantities of anticancer phytochemicals.

It is very important not to overcook vegetables. Overcooking not only will result in loss of important nutrients; it will also alter the flavor of the vegetable. Light steaming, baking, and quick stir-frying are the best ways to cook vegetables. Do not boil vegetables unless you are making soup, as most of the nutrients are left in the water. If fresh vegetables are not available, frozen vegetables are preferred over their canned counterparts. The only exception is tomato products (such as soup, paste, and sauce) because these products actually provide more absorbable lycopene than raw tomatoes.

We have divided your vegetable intake into three categories: green leafy and cruciferous vegetables, low-glycemic-index vegetables, and starchy vegetables. This will encourage you to eat a variety of these life-giving foods, help you consume a rainbow of vegetables, and allow you to focus on low-glycemic-index items. One serving equals 1 cup of raw leafy vegetables (such as lettuce or spinach), ½ cup of raw nonleafy or cooked vegetables, or ½ cup of fresh vegetable juice.

Green Leafy and Cruciferous Vegetables— 2 to 4 Servings Daily

Alfalfa sprouts	Dandelion
Beet greens	Endive
Bok choy	Escarole
Broccoli	Kale
Brussels sprouts	Lettuce (the darker, the better)
Cabbage	Mustard greens
Cauliflower	Parsley
Chard	Spinach
Chinese cabbage	Turnip greens
Collard greens	Watercress

Low-Glycemic-Load Vegetables—2 to 3 Servings Daily

Artichoke (1 medium)	Onions
Asparagus	Peas (fresh or frozen)
Bean sprouts	Radishes
Bell peppers	Rhubarb
Carrots	String beans, green or yellow
Celery	Summer squash
Cucumber	Tomatoes, tomato paste,
Fennel	tomato sauce, tomato juice,
Mushrooms	vegetable juice cocktail
Okra	Zucchini

Starchy Vegetables—1 to 2 Servings Daily (Only if Blood Sugar Levels Are Well Controlled)

Beets	Potatoes
Parsnips	Pumpkin

Rhubarb
Rutabagas
Yams or sweet potatoes

Winter, acorn, or
butternut squash

Whole Grains—3 to 5 Servings Daily

It is very important to choose whole-grain products (whole-grain breads, whole-grain-flour products, brown rice, and so on) over their processed counterparts (white bread, white-flour products, white rice, and so on). Whole grains provide substantially more nutrients and health-promoting properties. Whole grains are a major source of complex carbohydrates, dietary fiber, magnesium and other minerals, and B vitamins. The protein content and quality of whole grains is also greater than that of refined grains. Diets rich in whole grains have been shown to be helpful in both prevention and treatment of diabetes, but they must have a low glycemic load (certainly below 20). See Appendix I, pages 328–336, for the specific values. To further improve blood sugar levels, we recommend taking PGX™—a special fiber mixture— or natural glucosidase inhibitors (both of these natural products will be discussed in Chapter 9) before a meal containing any complex carbohydrates, to slow down the absorption of the sugars.

One of the following equals one serving:

Bread	
Whole wheat, rye or other whole grain	1 slice
Cereals	
Whole-grain cereal	½ cup
Corn	
Cooked whole-kernel corn	½ cup
Corn on cob	1 small
Flour and flour products	
Whole-wheat flour (uncooked)	2½ tbsp
Whole-grain pasta (cooked)	½ cup
Whole grains (cooked)	
Rice, oats, wheat, barley, quinoa, spelt, etc.	½ cup

Legumes—2 to 3 Servings Daily

Beans are a mainstay in most diets of the world and are second only to grains in supplying calories and protein to the world's population. Compared to grains, they supply about the same number of total calories, but usually provide two to four times as much protein and are a richer source of the soluble fiber that lowers cholesterol and stabilizes blood sugar levels. While we do not recommend using canned vegetables or fruit, canned beans retain their fiber content and anticancer flavonoids. Plus, given the long preparation time for cooking beans, canned beans are extremely quick and convenient.

There are a variety of delicious beans to choose from:

Black-eyed peas	Lima beans
Chickpeas	Pinto beans
Kidney beans	Soybeans, including tofu
Lentils	Split peas

Fruit—3 to 4 Servings Daily

Fruits are a rich source of many beneficial nutrients, and regular fruit consumption has been shown to offer significant protection against diabetes and other chronic degenerative conditions, including cancer, heart disease, cataracts, and strokes. Fruits make excellent between-meal snacks and super desserts (fresh berries alone are fantastic). It is easy to get into the habit of eating only a few varieties of fruit. Again, we encourage you to eat a rainbow assortment of fruits over the course of a week. Since flavonoids are so important to the prevention of the complications of diabetes, we also encourage supplementing your diet with flavonoid-rich extracts (discussed in Chapter 11, pages 249-251).

A general rule of thumb is that one serving equals one medium fruit or ½ cup of small cut-up fruit, 4 oz. of 100 percent juice, or ¼ cup dried fruit.

Good Oils (Nuts, Seeds, and Oils)—4 Servings Daily

These foods provide the beneficial oils, especially the monounsaturated fats, and regular nut consumption has been shown to improve blood sugar regulation. Focus on raw nuts and seeds. Definitely avoid nuts and seeds roasted in oils or coated with sugar. Nuts and seeds are great to add to salads and sautéed greens. Try to mix it up a bit by eating a variety of nuts and seeds, such as almonds, brazil nuts, walnuts, pecans, flaxseeds, sunflower seeds, and pumpkin seeds.

Use olive, macadamia, flaxseed, or canola oil to replace the butter, margarine, and shortening that you use for cooking or as a salad dressing. We also recommend using flaxseed oil in homemade salad dressings, so we provide some recipes in Appendix A. Never cook with flaxseed oil; it is too rich in polyunsaturated fats that are easily damaged by heat. Macadamia nut oil is the best cooking oil, but olive oil is great for sautéed vegetables while canola oil is usually best for baked goods because it has the least "nutty" flavor. Coconut oil is also very stable in cooking and is fine to use in small quantities. It contains saturated fat, but it is metabolized differently from animal-derived saturated fats and it is safe to use in moderation.

We want you to have at least one serving of nuts or seeds (one serving equals ¼ cup) and 3 tablespoons of the healthy oils daily, along with taking a high-quality fish oil supplement.

Dairy—1 to 2 Servings Daily (Optional)

We have found that many people are allergic to milk or lack the necessary enzymes to digest dairy products. Even for people who do tolerate dairy foods, milk consumption should be limited to no more than one or two servings per day. Use nonfat or reduced-fat dairy products over whole-milk varieties. Also, fermented dairy products such as yogurt, kefir, and acidophilus-fortified milk are preferred over regular milk. If you haven't tried some of the soy milk alternatives to cow's milk, they are delicious, especially the flavored varieties such as vanilla and chocolate. One serving equals 1 cup of milk, yogurt, or cottage cheese or 1 ounce of hard cheese. If you do not consume dairy products, we recommend that you take a high-potency multiple vitamin and mineral formula that provides sufficient levels of calcium (see Appendix H, page 327).

High-Quality Protein—2 to 3 Servings Daily

We have continually stressed the detriment of saturated fat and the importance of the omega-3 fatty acids in fish in the battle against developing diabetes, so our recommendation in this category should be no surprise. We want you to consume fish at least three, but no more than six, times per week. Fish is an excellent source of high-quality protein. Chicken and turkey can also provide excellent protein with very little fat, especially if you eat only the white meat (breast) and do not eat the skin. Eggs are also a very good source of high-quality protein. An egg has 5.5 grams of protein (11.1 percent of the daily value for protein) and only 68 calories. Although some people are concerned about the cholesterol content of eggs, studies have now shown that most people can eat one or two eggs a day without measurable changes in their blood cholesterol levels. If you are concerned about the cholesterol, use only the egg whites or choose one of the several egg-white products on the market, such as Egg Beaters.

In perhaps one of the most important recommendations, we want you to keep your intake of red meat (beef, veal, or lamb) to no more than two servings per month; choose the leanest cuts possible, keep the portion size limited to about the size of a deck of cards, and do not char-broil or cook the meat to overdone (which increases the formation of cancer-causing compounds). Also, consider alternatives to beef such as buffalo, venison, elk, rabbit, ostrich, and emu. These emerging beef alternatives are lower in saturated fat and provide higher levels of omega-3 fatty acids.

One serving equals about the size of a deck of cards. That translates to roughly 4 ounces.

Clinical Studies with Diet Therapy in Type 1 Diabetes

In Chapter 6, we stressed the importance of monitoring blood sugar levels in both type 1 and type 2 diabetes. In type 1 diabetes it is an absolute necessity. Achieving optimal daily blood glucose measurements and hemoglobin A_1C levels ensures a longer, healthier life for people with type 1 diabetes. In that goal, diet is also critical, but so is intensified insulin therapy as described in Chapter 8.[1] Numerous clinical studies have shown impressive results in improving blood sugar control for people on diets high in fiber and low in glycemic load. This fact holds true in both adults and children, and in both type 1 and type 2 diabetes.

In regards to studies in children, let's take a look at a study conducted in children age 8 to 13 in Melbourne, Australia.[2] The subjects were divided into one group that followed the ADA's exchange program diet and another group that was instructed to eat low-glycemic-index foods. While there was no change in A_1C in the exchange diet, that is, it stayed at 8.6 percent, the group eating the low-glycemic-index foods dropped the A_1C from 8.6 percent to 8.0 percent—an acceptable value in children. Rates of excessive blood sugar levels were 66 percent for the exchange diet versus 35 percent for those eating low-GI foods. While these results are great, the study really highlighted the impact of eating a low-GI diet on the quality of life. There were significantly fewer family conflicts, limitations placed on family activities, and difficulties in meal selections. Furthermore, parents and children alike showed a clear preference for the low GI diet.

Similar results have been seen in adults with type 1 diabetes, including pregnant women with type 1 diabetes, following a high-fiber, low-GI diet.[3-6] These studies and others indicate that a low-GI, low-GL diet is emerging as the most scientifically proven dietary support for type 1 diabetes. We have taken the proven diet to a much higher level by also considering the role of fats on insulin action.

Clinical Studies with Diet Therapy in Type 2 Diabetes

Diet is a key therapeutic area in type 2 diabetes. In fact, diet alone can often be effective as the sole factor in treating and reversing type 2 diabetes. Of course, we are recommending more than diet alone, as lifestyle and supplements are also important. Our point is that treatment of type 2 diabetes really begins with diet. And, just as in type 1 diabetes, there is considerable evidence from clinical trials that the diet we recommend is emerging as the most scientifically proven approach, especially when considering not only its effect on blood glucose levels but also its effects in reducing conditions resulting from diabetes such as high cholesterol levels, heart disease, high blood pressure, and other complications.[7]

From Our Patient Files

Susan was 24 when I began to see her for regular diabetic care. Already a type 1 diabetic for 10 years, Susan was frustrated with her "brittle" diabetes. Although she wanted to achieve better blood sugar control—her hemoglobin A₁C was usually over 9.5 percent and her daily blood sugars were often over 250 mg/dL (14 mmol/L)—if she tried to keep her blood sugars lower with increased insulin dosages, she would often become hypoglycemic. Over the past year, she had had to visit the emergency department three times with severe insulin reactions (hypoglycemia) and she was afraid that she would never get her driver's license back again. On the other hand, she didn't feel well much of the time and she knew that a hemoglobin A₁C of 9.5 put her at high risk for serious diabetic complications. On top of this, her insulin requirements had increased about 30 percent over the past 5 years. This and her elevated triglyceride level suggested that she was becoming insulin resistant. In essence, although she was a type 1 diabetic, she was developing signs of type 2 diabetes as well (insulin resistance, elevated triglycerides, and increased body fat).

Susan had a body mass index (BMI) of 27 (155 lb and 5'4") and she didn't exercise much. She was very carefully following the ADA diet plan that was taught at the hospital diabetic education center. However, even though she was eating the 1,800 calorie diet as prescribed, she had gained more than 10 pounds over the past 5 years. Susan was very good about avoiding sugar but she loved (white) bread and pasta. She used exchanges almost every meal to increase the servings of bread and pasta without increasing her daily calories. Her appetite was often ravenous before meals and she found it hard not to eat more than her diet allowed. When I talked to her about the importance of glycemic index and glycemic load, she was surprised that no one had ever mentioned these concepts or even had her consider the fiber in her diet. When I reviewed a diet diary she completed over 3 days, it was clear that the total glycemic load (GL) of her diet was far higher than ideal and she probably ate less than 10 grams of fiber on most days. She didn't eat enough protein and when she did, it was usually ground beef or cheese. She ate too much saturated fat, not enough omega-9 and omega-3 fatty acids, insufficient antioxidant phytochemicals, and far too little fiber. I was glad to learn about all of this because there were so many positive things she could do to improve her health!

The first thing I did was get Susan to commit to a regular exercise program. To start with, she agreed to walk for ½ hour on most days. I estimated that she could burn an extra 200 calories per day during her walk and increase her metabolic activity. If she kept her calories the same she would be able to burn an extra 1,200 to 1,400 calories per week. By this calculation alone, she would be able to lose about 2 pounds per month or 24 pounds per year. I had her aim for a 10 percent reduction in weight. This modest weight loss would promote a restoration of insulin sensitivity and allow for a lower total daily insulin dose, which would help counteract the weight-promoting effects of excessive insulin. As well, I gave her a table showing the glycemic index and glycemic load of foods. She agreed to select the low-GI foods as much as possible and to keep her total glycemic load below 150 per day. Instead of using exchanges to increase her starch intake, she began to eat a lot more fresh vegetables and fruits (along with a green drink daily), and she also began to eat fish and chicken instead of ground beef and cheese. She ate moderate servings of whole-grain products and I had her take a water-soluble fiber supplement before each meal, fish oil capsules, and a high-potency multivitamin.

Within a few days of beginning this program, Susan began to notice that her insulin requirements were less. As well, her appetite decreased significantly on the higher-protein, higher-fiber, and low-glycemic-index/glycemic-load diet. She started feeling so good from her walks that she ended up walking 1 hour most days and she also began going to a gym twice per week to lift weights (instead of walking on those days). Within 3 months she had lost 18 pounds (more than the 10 percent weight loss goal) and her insulin requirements were down one-third from when we started. Her hemoglobin A_1C was just under 8 and her triglycerides were normal. At this point, I referred her for training to begin intensive insulin therapy with a goal to get her on an insulin pump and to get her blood sugars under even better control. Overall, she felt better than she had in years and she hadn't had a significant hypoglycemic episode since she began her dietary and lifestyle changes.

One of the key goals is to get the total fiber intake from foods to at least 50 grams. In one study the effects of two diets on blood sugar levels were compared.[8] One diet contained 24 grams of dietary fiber (8 g of soluble fiber and 16 g of insoluble fiber) based upon the recommendations of the ADA, while the other provided a total of 50 grams (25 g of soluble fiber and 25 g of insoluble fiber). Both diets had the same calorie level and percentages of fat, carbohydrate, and protein. After 6 weeks, the average daily blood sugar levels were 13 mg/dL lower in the group on the higher-fiber diet. Furthermore, the high-fiber diet also lowered the total area under the curve for 24-hour blood sugar levels, as well as insulin concentrations, and reduced total cholesterol concentrations by 6.7 percent, triglyceride concentrations by 10.2 percent, and very-low-density lipoprotein cholesterol concentrations by 12.5 percent. This study shows quite clearly that a high intake of dietary fiber, particularly of the soluble type, above the level recommended by the ADA, improves glycemic control, decreases hyperinsulinemia, and lowers plasma lipid concentrations in patients with type 2 diabetes. Similar studies looking at a low-GI diet versus a high-GI diet have shown quite clearly the advantages of a low-GI diet.[9,10]

Foundational Supplements for Individuals with Diabetes

Three key dietary supplements are critical to promote health and prevent disease:

1. A multiple vitamin and mineral supplement
2. A green drink
3. A pharmaceutical-grade fish oil supplement

In addition to these items, we recommend 500 to 1,500 mg of vitamin C and 400 to 800 IU of vitamin E daily as part of a foundation for nutritional supplementation for people with diabetes. In Chapter 9, we provide additional recommendations to greatly reduce appetite and improve glucose control with natural products, while in Chapter 11 we give recommendations for supplements to deal with the major complications of diabetes.

From Our Patient Files

Rick was a "meat and potatoes" kind of guy. He loved to fly-fish, watch football, and drink beer with his buddies. He had also smoked since he was 14 and enjoyed a good cigar two or three times per week. The problem was that Rick was now so heavy that he couldn't walk to his favorite fly-fishing holes without ending up exhausted. That was compounded by the fact that his fly-fishing shoulder was now so stiff and painful that he couldn't cast a line. "Can't you just give me something for this shoulder so I can cast a fishing line, doc?"

I wanted to look into things a bit deeper first. An X-ray showed that he had calcific tendonitis of the shoulder (a common accompaniment of diabetes). His fasting blood sugar was 220 mg/dL (12 mmol/L), confirming the diagnosis of diabetes. His cholesterol and triglycerides were elevated and his blood pressure was 140/95. His C-peptide level was elevated, confirming that he had elevated insulin levels and that he was in the early stages of type 2 diabetes. His hemoglobin A_1C level was 8.5, indicating that his average blood sugar was about 200 mg/dL (11 mmol/L) over the past 3 months.

What Rick needed, more than a strong painkiller, was a good heart-to-heart talk with his doctor. I leveled with him. He needed to know that his diet and lifestyle were killing him and that he might be disabled or dead within ten years if he didn't take the fork in the road that I was directing him to take. Rick was only 36, with three young children and a great job. The prospect of being disabled from work or not living to see his kids grow up was the wake-up call he needed. I had Rick in several times over the next few months for nutritional and lifestyle counseling and to help him quit smoking. Since Rick's wife did all the cooking, I made sure that she was there each time.

Rather than putting him on a strict diet that deprived him of enjoyment of food, I taught Rick and his wife about the principles of the low-glycemic-index/low-glycemic-load diet. I also gave them recipes to try, knowing that the average family gets most of its calories from seven to ten favorite recipes. Therefore, by helping them discover ten new recipes that were low-glycemic-index, high-fiber alternatives, along with acceptable snacks, Rick was able to cut way down on his daily calories, saturated fat, and glycemic load with almost no discomfort. He also had to exercise discipline in his choices at restaurants and in the size of his portions with each meal, but with the appetite-reducing supplements I prescribed, this was far easier than he imagined it could be. After getting cleared to exercise by a treadmill test, Rick began to walk his dog every day, gradually increasing the time and pace, and on the weekends he cycled or hiked to his favorite fishing holes with his wife. She had never shown an interest in his hobby before, but now that their future was at stake she gladly went along for the exercise. Once his diabetes was under good control, I began to help him with his shoulder, knowing that chronic pain problems are much easier to work with when diabetes is in good control.

A year later, Rick looked and felt like a new man! He had lost 43 pounds and he was amazed that he had enjoyed the whole process. He had learned a new way to eat, used the appetite-reducing low-glycemic-load diet along with appetite-reducing supplements, and lost weight without even feeling like he was dieting. I taught Rick to think of diabetes as a coach standing over his shoulder and telling him to be wise in his food choices and his decision to exercise. His blood tests improved steadily over that year until, around the anniversary of our first visit, I was pleased to let him know that according to all of the tests, he was no longer a diabetic. I helped him understand that he was like an alcoholic in recovery who was now living in sobriety, and that the disease was always around the corner, waiting for an opportunity to take over his life again. Even though the diabetes was gone, he had to live this new and careful lifestyle for the rest of his life if he wanted to keep diabetes from raising its ugly head once again. The payoff in how he looked and felt made it all worthwhile.

Multiple Vitamin and Mineral Supplements

A high-potency multiple vitamin and mineral formula is an absolute must for people with diabetes. Follow the guidelines given in Appendix H on pages 325–327 on how to select a high-quality formula. Supplying the diabetic with additional key nutrients has been shown to improve blood sugar control as well as to help prevent or reduce the development of the major complications of diabetes. Taking a multiple vitamin and mineral supplement has also been shown to boost immune function and reduce infections in diabetics.[11] Specific examples of nutrients that the diabetic needs more of include chromium, vitamin C, vitamin E, certain B vitamins, magnesium, zinc, and manganese. These nutrients will be discussed shortly and many will also be discussed in Chapters 8 and 9 as well. As you will see, supplementation with many of these nutrients leads to significant improvements not only in blood sugar control, but also in preventing complications.

CHROMIUM | The first nutrient to discuss is chromium, a trace element whose importance to human nutrition was not discovered until 1957. Chromium is vital to proper blood sugar control, as it functions in the body as a key constituent in the *glucose tolerance factor*. Chromium works closely with insulin in facilitating the uptake of glucose into cells. Without chromium, insulin's action is blocked and glucose levels are elevated. There is evidence that marginal chromium status is quite common in the United States. A chromium deficiency may be an underlying contributing factor to the tremendous number of Americans that have diabetes and hypoglycemia and are obese.

There have been more than twenty clinical studies of chromium supplementation in diabetes. In some of these studies, supplementing the diet with chromium in type 2 diabetes has been shown to decrease fasting glucose levels, improve glucose tolerance, lower insulin levels, and decrease total cholesterol and triglyceride levels, while increasing HDL cholesterol levels. Although other studies have not shown chromium to exert much effect in improving glucose tolerance in diabetes, there is no argument that chromium is an important mineral in blood sugar metabolism. At this time, however, it appears that chromium supplementation is likely to produce meaningful improvements in glycemic control only in people who are deficient in this essential trace element.[12]

Although there is no RDA for chromium, it appears that we need at least 200 mcg each day in our diet. People with diabetes need to supplement between 200 and 400 mcg per day. Chromium polynicotinate, chromium picolinate, and chromium-enriched yeast are suitable forms for supplementing the diet.

VITAMIN C | Since the transport of vitamin C into cells is enhanced by insulin,[13] many people with diabetes suffer from a relative deficiency of vitamin C inside their cells even if they consume an adequate amount of vitamin C in their diet. As a result, people with diabetes need to take extra vitamin C.

In addition to its role as an antioxidant, vitamin C is required in immune functions and the manufacture of collagen, the main protein substance of the human body. Since collagen is such an important protein for the structures that hold our body together (connective tissue, cartilage, tendons, and so on), vitamin C is vital for wound repair, healthy gums, and the prevention of easy bruising. A chronic, latent vitamin C deficiency leads to a number of problems for the diabetic, including an increased tendency to bleed (increased capillary permeability), poor wound healing, elevations in cholesterol levels, and a depressed immune system. Vitamin C supplementation has shown to exert a mild effect in improving glucose control, as evident by a slightly lower A_1C in the vitamin C group (8.5 percent) compared to a placebo (9.3 percent) in one double-blind study.[14] Probably more important than any significant effect on improving blood sugar control is the fact that vitamin C supplementation has been shown to reduce the formation of compounds linked to the development of diabetic complications such as sorbitol (this aspect will be discussed on pages 235–237).

In one of the most recent studies of vitamin C supplementation in type 2 diabetes, 30 patients age 45 to 70 who had not only type 2 diabetes but also high blood pressure were randomly assigned in a double-blind manner to take either a 500-mg vitamin C tablet or a placebo daily for 4 weeks. Vitamin C supplementation decreased systolic blood pressure from 142.1 to 132.3 and diastolic pressure from 83.9 to 79.5. Additional analytical methods designed to measure vascular resistance also demonstrated significant improvements in arterial stiffness. These results indicate that vitamin C supplementation is effective in improving the elasticity and function of blood vessels in patients with type 2 diabetes.[15]

While vitamin C supplementation is necessary, do not rely exclusively on supplements to meet all of your vitamin C requirements. Vitamin C–rich foods are rich in compounds, such as flavonoids and carotenes, which work to enhance the effects of vitamin C as well as exert favorable effects of their own. While most people think of citrus fruits as the best source of vitamin C, vegetables also contain high levels, especially broccoli, bell peppers, potatoes, and Brussels sprouts.

VITAMIN E | Vitamin E functions primarily as an antioxidant in protecting against damage to the cell membranes. Without vitamin E, the cells of the body would be quite susceptible to damage. Nerve cells are particularly vulnerable. Vitamin E supplementation or a high-vitamin-E diet has been shown to protect against many common health conditions, including diabetes. Diabetics appear to have an increased requirement for vitamin E. Vitamin E not only improves insulin action, it has a number of beneficial effects, when taken at dosages ranging from 400 to 800 IU, that may aid in preventing the long-term complications of diabetes, including the following:

- Prevents free radical damage to LDL cholesterol and the vascular lining.[16–18]
- Improves the functioning of blood vessels and the cells that line the blood vessels.[19,20]
- Increases the concentration of magnesium within cells.[21,22]
- Decreases the level of C-reactive protein and other inflammatory compounds.[23,24]
- Increases the level of glutathione, an important intracellular antioxidant, within cells.[25]
- Improves the rate of conduction of electrical impulses through the nervous system.[26]
- Improves blood flow to the eye and improves diabetic retinopathy.
- Improves kidney function and normalizes creatinine clearance—an indicator of kidney function—in diabetics with mild elevations.[27]

Be sure that the vitamin E that you take is a natural form. Such forms are designated *d-*, as in d-alpha-tocopherol, while synthetic forms are *dl-*, as in dl-alpha-tocopherol. (The letters *d* and *l* indicate mirror images of the vitamin E molecule.) The human body recognizes and responds only to the *d-* form; the *dl-* form may actually prevent the *d-* form from entering cell membranes. Because of the way the body uses vitamin E, people with diabetes will require lifelong supplementation for maximum benefits.[28]

NIACIN AND NIACINAMIDE | Enzymes containing niacin (vitamin B₃) play an important role in energy production; fat, cholesterol, and carbohydrate metabolism; and the manufacture of many body compounds, including sex and adrenal hormones. Niacin, like chromium, is an essential component of the glucose tolerance factor, making it a key nutrient for hypoglycemia and diabetes.

Supplementing the diet with vitamin B₃ in the form of niacinamide has been shown to exert many favorable effects. Foremost is its possible application in reversing recently diagnosed type 1 diabetes. This effect is discussed in more detail in Chapter 8.

Effects of Tomato Juice, Vitamin E, and Vitamin C in Type 2 Diabetes

Inflammation is an underlying factor in the progression of atherosclerosis and other complications of diabetes. Markers of inflammation and the potential for free radical damage include the measurement of circulating levels of C-reactive protein (CRP) and the susceptibility of LDL cholesterol to oxidation. These measurements were determined in fifty-seven patients with type 2 diabetes after they were randomized to receive either tomato juice (500 mL/day), vitamin E (800 IU/day), vitamin C (500 mg/day), or a placebo for 4 weeks.[29] Both the vitamin E and tomato juice groups demonstrated considerable protection against free radical damage to LDL, but only vitamin E reduced CRP. These findings highlight the importance of fat soluble antioxidants such as carotenes and vitamin E in the prevention of heart disease in patients with diabetes.

VITAMIN B$_6$ | Pyridoxine or vitamin B$_6$ is an extremely important B vitamin involved in the formation of body proteins and structural compounds, chemical transmitters in the nervous system, red blood cells, and hormonelike compounds known as prostaglandins. Vitamin B$_6$ is also critical in maintaining hormonal balance and proper immune function.

Vitamin B$_6$ supplementation appears to offer significant protection against the development of diabetic nerve disease (neuropathy).[30] Diabetics with neuropathy have been shown to be deficient in vitamin B$_6$ and to benefit from supplementation.[31] The neuropathy of a vitamin B$_6$ deficiency is indistinguishable from diabetic neuropathy. Individuals with long-standing diabetes or who are developing signs of peripheral nerve abnormalities should definitely supplement their diets with vitamin B$_6$. Vitamin B$_6$ is also important in preventing other diabetic complications.

Vitamin B$_6$ supplementation can be a very a safe and effective treatment for gestational diabetes (diabetes caused by pregnancy). In one study, fourteen women with gestational diabetes were given 100 mg of vitamin B$_6$ each day for two weeks, which resulted in eliminating the diagnosis in twelve out of the fourteen women.[32]

MAGNESIUM | Like chromium, magnesium is also involved in glucose metabolism. There is considerable evidence that diabetics should take supplemental magnesium: More than half of all people with diabetes show evidence of magnesium deficiency, and magnesium may prevent some complications of diabetes such as retinopathy and heart disease. Magnesium levels are usually low in diabetics and lowest in those with diabetic complications such as retinopathy and neuropathy. Clinical studies have shown that magnesium supplementation (usually 400 to 500 mg per day) improves insulin response and action, glucose tolerance, and the fluidity of the red blood cell membrane in patients with diabetes.[33,34]

The RDA for magnesium is 350 mg per day for adult males and 300 mg per day for adult females. Diabetics may need twice this amount because they tend to lose excessive magnesium through their kidneys.[35] Most of the magnesium should be derived from the diet. The average intake of magnesium by healthy adults in the United States ranges between 143 and 266 mg per day, far below the RDA. Food choices are the main reason; while magnesium occurs abundantly in whole foods, food processing refines out a very large portion of magnesium. The best dietary sources of magnesium are tofu, legumes, seeds, nuts, whole grains, and green leafy vegetables. Fish, meat, milk, and most commonly eaten fruits are quite low in magnesium. Most Americans consume a low-magnesium diet because their diet is high in refined foods, meat, and dairy products.

In addition to eating a diet rich in magnesium, diabetics should supplement their diet with 300 to 500 mg of magnesium daily. For best results, use highly absorbable sources of magnesium, such as magnesium aspartate or citrate. Also, diabetics should be sure to get at least 25 mg of vitamin B_6 per day, as the level of vitamin B_6 in body cells appear to be intricately linked to magnesium content. In other words, without vitamin B_6 (as well as vitamin E), magnesium will not get inside the cell and will, therefore, be useless.

ZINC | Zinc functions in more enzymatic reactions than any other mineral, as it is a cofactor in more than 200 different enzymes. Although severe zinc deficiency is very rare in developed countries, many individuals in the United States have marginal zinc deficiency—particularly the elderly as well as people with diabetes. Low zinc levels are associated with an increased susceptibility to infection, poor wound healing, a decreased sense of taste or smell, and skin disorders. Zinc deficiency, like chromium deficiency, has also been suggested to play a role in the development of diabetes.[36]

Zinc is involved in virtually all aspects of insulin metabolism: synthesis, secretion, and utilization. Zinc also protects against beta cell destruction and has well-known antiviral effects. Diabetics typically excrete too much zinc in the urine and therefore require supplementation. Diabetics should take at least 30 mg of zinc per day. Zinc is also found in good amounts in whole grains, legumes, nuts, and seeds.

MANGANESE | Manganese functions in many enzyme systems, including enzymes involved in blood sugar control, energy metabolism, and thyroid hormone function. Manganese also functions in the antioxidant enzyme superoxide dismutase, or SOD. In guinea pigs, a deficiency of manganese results in diabetes and the frequent birth of offspring who develop pancreatic abnormalities or no pancreas at all.

Diabetics have been shown to have only half the manganese of normal individuals. A good daily dose of manganese for a diabetic is 3 to 5 mg.

Green Drinks

We introduced the term "green drinks" in Chapter 5 to refer to green tea and a number of commercially available products containing dehydrated barley grass, wheat grass, or algae sources such as chlorella or spirulina. Such formulas are rehydrated by mixing with water or juice. These products—packed full of phytochemicals, especially carotenes and chlorophyll—are more convenient than trying to sprout and grow your own source of greens. An added advantage is that they tend to taste better than, for example, straight wheatgrass juice. Some of the more popular brands are Enriching Greens, Green Magma, Greens +, Barlean's Greens, and ProGreens. Of these, we rate Enriching Greens the highest.

Green foods such as young barley grass, wheat grass, spirulina, and chlorella are exceptionally high in nutritional value. Given their rich source of antioxidants, they are very important supplements for the diabetic. In addition, they may also help improve blood sugar control, based upon the results of a study with spirulina.[37] In the study, 2 months of spirulina supplementation (2 g/day) produced an appreciable lowering of fasting blood glucose (27 percent decline) and a significant reduction in A_1C levels (34 percent decline), clearly indicating improvements in long-term blood sugar regulation. Triglycerides declined by 22 percent and total cholesterol dropped 11 percent.

In another study, thirty-six type 2 diabetic patients received one of the following supplements daily for 4 weeks: 15 grams barley leaf extract, 200 mg vitamin C and 200 mg vitamin E, or barley leaf plus vitamins C and E.[38] The results indicated that the ingestion of the barley leaf extract along with the vitamins produced the greatest antioxidant protection compared to either barley leaf extract or vitamins C and E alone. Antioxidant protection was measured by looking at the effect that the supplements had on protecting different fractions of LDL cholesterol from oxidative damage.

While these studies used spirulina and barley leaf, we believe that using any of the popular brands listed earlier will likely produce similar results. We recommend drinking one to two servings daily. Try to consume these drinks 20 minutes before or 2 hours after a meal.

Pharmaceutical-Grade Fish Oil Supplements

The benefits of the omega-3 oils from fish oils have been described previously. We use the term *pharmaceutical-grade* to signify a high-potency fish oil product that is also free of heavy metals, environmental contaminants, lipid peroxides, and other harmful compounds. The specific product that we recommend is RxOmega-3 Factors from Natural Factors because we know firsthand the quality control steps employed to ensure that the product is free of contaminants. Each capsule provides 600 mg of long-chain omega-3 fatty acids (400 mg EPA and 200 mg DHA). We recommend one capsule daily for general health and two capsules daily for people with diabetes.

Two intensive investigations, one conducted at Oxford University and the other at the Mayo Clinic, analyzed data from eighteen double-blind clinical trials involving 823 participants followed for an average of 12 weeks.[39,40] Doses of fish oil (18 percent EPA and 12 percent DHA) ranged from 3 to 18 g/day. Both evaluations came to the same conclusions: Although fish oil supplementation has no statistically significant effect on glycemic control, it does appear to offer the same protection against heart disease in people with diabetes that it does to people without diabetes.[41] It is important to point out that many studies in patients with diabetes were conducted with lower-quality fish oil products that contained significant amounts of cholesterol and lipid peroxides; as a result, in some of these studies researchers noted an elevation in LDL cholesterol. This occurrence highlights the importance of using a pharmaceutical-grade fish oil product, as we have not seen increases in LDL cholesterol with these higher-quality products.

Fish oil supplements are best taken at or near the beginning of a meal to avoid any fishy aftertaste—some people burp up a little of the oil if they take it at the end of the meal on a full stomach.

Chapter Eight

Natural Products for Type 1 Diabetes

Individuals with type 1 diabetes absolutely require conventional treatment with the hormone insulin. We consider this approach consistent with natural medicine—after all, the goal is simply to provide the body with a critical *natural* hormone.

All of us have had our lives touched in miraculous ways by advances in medicine. Sometimes we lose perspective on just how much our lives have been changed by these advances. The modern treatment of type 1 diabetes provides an excellent example of a life-changing development.

Up until the twentieth century it was nearly impossible to live with diabetes. Most often children with the disease died within days of onset. The name *diabetes* was given to the disease sometime around 250 B.C. The literal translation, "to go through" or "to siphon," was used because the disease drained victims of more fluid than they could consume. In the first century A.D., the Greeks described the disease as "a melting down of the flesh and limbs into urine." Gradually the Latin word for honey, *mellitus,* was appended to *diabetes* because of its link with sweet urine.

Understanding what diabetes was all about was a slow process. In 1798 John Rollo actually documented excess sugar in the blood as well as the urine. But it was not until 1889 that scientists learned that type 1 diabetes could be produced in dogs by removing the pancreas. As soon as the link between the pancreas and diabetes was recognized, research focused on treating the disease with pancreatic extracts.

The real breakthrough came when John Macleod at the University of Toronto hired Frederick Banting to work on experiments with pancreatic extracts in dogs. Banting then enlisted Charles Best, a student, to assist him. In the summer of 1921, Banting and Best were able to make a pancreatic extract that had antidiabetic characteristics. They were successful in testing their extract on diabetic dogs. Encouraged by this success, the entire research team under the direction of Dr. MacLeod and James Collip worked on the production and purification of insulin.

The first tests were conducted on Leonard Thompson, a 14-year-old boy near death, early in 1922. With further purification of the pancreatic extract, Leonard's blood sugar levels dropped from 520 to 120 mg/dL in about 24 hours, and he quickly began to gain weight and strength. With Leonard's recovery, word of the miracle of insulin spread quickly around the world. Macleod and Banting were awarded Nobel Prizes in 1923 for their development of insulin, but both men eventually split their prize with other deserving members of the team; Banting split his prize with Best, and Macleod split his with Collip.

Modern Insulin Therapy

The insulin of today is much different from the preparation purified by the University of Toronto researchers back in 1922. Not long after the discovery of insulin, Eli Lilly and Company of Indianapolis, Indiana, was awarded a temporary exclusive license to manufacture the new miracle substance. Over the next decades, advances in laboratory techniques led to the production of more highly purified insulin, and long-acting

The University of Toronto—
Leading the Battle Against Diabetes

It is quite remarkable that some of the most exciting new discoveries for the treatment of diabetes are coming once again from the University of Toronto. Through the work directed by Dr. Vladimir Vuksan at the University of Toronto's Risk Factor Modification Centre, natural health products are being developed that have the potential to exceed the benefits and safety of any diabetic drug. Just as insulin was a lifesaving breakthrough for millions with type 1 diabetes, discoveries such as special fiber blends and very specific extracts from American and Korean ginseng may prove to be of equal or greater magnitude in helping to fight the frightening epidemic of diabetes that is sweeping across the globe.

and intermediate types were developed to provide more flexibility. Initially, all insulins were derived by extraction from either beef or pork pancreas tissue.

The biggest recent change in insulin came with the development of recombinant DNA technology that allowed synthesis of a "human" type of insulin from bacteria and yeast rather than relying on animal pancreatic tissue for extraction. In 1982 the Food and Drug Administration approved the first recombinant DNA human insulin, Humulin, made by Eli Lilly. Other human insulins, such as Novolin, followed. Human insulins now dominate the marketplace, and new insulin forms and ways of delivering them are being developed, including oral and inhaled forms. Currently insulin still must be injected via syringe, pump, or insulin pen.

Although there is little evidence to show that recombinant human insulin is superior to animal-derived insulins in safety or efficacy, pharmaceutical companies have effectively stopped manufacturing beef and pork insulins in favor of human insulin. Anecdotally, some people seem to achieve better control with human insulin, and others have a great deal of trouble with hypoglycemic episodes on human insulin. Animal insulin is different enough from human insulin that antibodies can form toward it and some degree of immune-mediated insulin resistance can occur. All in all, it is probably best to allow for greater choice and it would be in the interest of diabetics to provide ongoing availability of animal-derived insulins.

Insulin types are classified not by their source, but rather by how fast they start to work and how long their effects last. The types of insulin include the following:

TYPE OF INSULIN	ONSET	PEAK	DURATION
Very Rapid/ Immediate-Acting			
Insulin lispro (Humalog)	0–15 min.	1–3 hours	2–4 hours
Insulin aspart (Novalog)	0–15 min.	1–3 hours	2–4 hours
Rapid-Acting			
Regular (e.g. Humulin R)	½–1 hour	2–4 hours	3–6 hours
Velosulin (pump use)	½–1 hour	2–3 hours	5–7 hours
Intermediate-Acting			
NPH (e.g. Humulin N)	2–4 hours	4–12 hours	10–16 hours
Lente (e.g. Humulin L)	3–4 hours	4–12 hours	16–22 hours
Long-Acting			
Ultralente (U) (e.g. Humulin U)	4–6 hours	8–24 hours	24–28 hours
Insulin glargine (Lantus)	3–4 hours	none	20–24 hours
Pre-Mixed			
Humulin 70/30	½ hour	2–12 hours	18–24 hours
Novolin 70/30	½ hour	2–12 hours	18–24 hours
Humalog mix 50/50	½ hour	2–12 hours	18–24 hours
Humalog mix 75/25	0–15 minutes	1–12 hours	18 hours

There is not a single "one size fits all" approach with insulin therapy. You will need to work hard with your doctor to find out what type of insulin therapy is best for you. It is critical that you keep a detailed diary of blood glucose measurements to allow an insulin treatment program that is as close to ideal as possible. Table 8.1 provides a summary, but for more information on self-monitoring of blood glucose levels, see pages 124–132.

Table 8.1. Goals for Blood Glucose Measurements and A₁C in People with Type 1 Diabetes

TIME OF CHECK	GOAL (WHOLE-BLOOD MEASUREMENTS)
Before breakfast (fasting)	90–130 mg/dL (5–7.2 mmol/L)
Before lunch, supper, and snack	90–130 mg/dL (5–7.2 mmol/L)
2 hours after meals	Less than 150 mg/dL (8.3 mmol/L)
Bedtime	110–150 mg/dL (6.1–8.3 mmol/L)
A₁C (glycosylated hemoglobin)	≤ 7 percent

Intensive Insulin Therapy

For many years, insulin therapy involved administering a mixture of rapid- and intermediate-acting insulin, once or twice daily. This method has been replaced by intensified insulin therapy, where the insulin is given in increasingly sophisticated and complex regimens. The reason? Increasing evidence demonstrates that intensified insulin therapy significantly reduces the development of the chronic complications of diabetes. Intensive insulin therapy is designed to mimic as closely as possible the continuous variations in plasma insulin levels produced by a healthy pancreas.

Intensive insulin therapy has been made possible largely through the development of breakthrough immediate-acting insulins (insulin lispro [Humalog] and insulin aspart [Novolog]) as well as a novel very-long-acting insulin (insulin glargine [Lantus]). In the most recent protocols a basal-bolus system is used. In this approach, a daily dose of insulin glargine (Lantus) is given once a day, usually at bedtime (occasionally it is given twice per day instead). Lantus provides a near-constant (basal) release of insulin for one full day. This is much like the pancreas, which releases a constant basal level of insulin around the clock, even in a fasting state. In addition, multiple injections of immediate-acting insulin (Humalog or Novolog) are given, usually just before meals and snacks. These insulins act immediately and are much more like the normal action of the pancreas, which releases insulin immediately upon eating.

These breakthrough insulins are able to replicate much more closely the normal action of a healthy pancreas. Because the pancreas works by a basal (constant) release of insulin along with boluses (sudden bursts of insulin), giving one or two injections with Lantus and multiple (three or more) injections with Humalog or Novolog nearly replicates the normal action of the pancreas. Some diabetics will be put on a pump to achieve the same goals. In such cases, the pump may be used to deliver a constant small basal dose of insulin (nowadays usually Humalog or Novolog immediate-acting insulins) and the diabetic will choose a dose and activate a bolus of insulin through the pump just before meals and snacks.

In addition to more closely replicating the natural function of the pancreas, the greatest advantage of intensive insulin therapy is the way that it can bring about greater freedom to the lifestyle of the diabetic. Diabetics using only one or two scheduled injections of conventional insulin per day have to live by a very rigid schedule of mealtimes, exercise, and sleep. They must also eat exacting amounts of calories and carbohydrates with each meal because the injections they give take quite a while to achieve peak activity and then the dosages of insulin will dictate the diabetic's meal and activity schedule. If diabetics on conventional insulin regimens are late for a meal, if they eat too much or too little, or if they miss exercise or have too much exercise, it is likely that they will have wide swings of blood sugar and they risk serious hypoglycemic episodes.

On the other hand, although intensive insulin therapy requires much more frequent testing of blood glucose and frequent injections, the timing and dose of insulin can be easily adjusted to accommodate daily variations in the diabetic's eating and exercise schedule and food intake. Although the idea of checking blood sugar six times or more daily and giving four or more injections may sound bothersome, once a diabetic learns the fine art of intensive insulin therapy, it brings freedom and a much more normal lifestyle than before. Insulin pumps still require frequent blood glucose monitoring, but basal and bolus injections are taken care of by the pump (which is under the complete command of the diabetic). In the very near future, glucose monitoring will likely be done through a device connected directly to the insulin pump and the whole process will likely be almost completely taken care of by computerized electronics.

Although serious hypoglycemia is less likely to occur with the new immediate- and very-long-acting insulins, one of the goals of this therapy is, of course, to keep blood sugars under tight control. Because of this, serious hypoglycemia is still a risk and diabetics must become very adept at recognizing hypoglycemia and acting to correct it as soon as possible. The risk of hypoglycemia must be reduced by frequent blood glucose monitoring; adjustment of insulin dosage; alteration of the timing, frequency, and content of meals; and change in exercise/activity patterns. Thus, comprehensive self-management training is essential. Because children and older patients are more susceptible to hypoglycemia with intensive insulin therapy, treatment goals can be more flexible.

We have already mentioned the landmark Diabetes Control and Complications Trial (DCCT). The study design was simple. Two groups of patients were followed long term, one treated conventionally with the standard mixture of rapid- and intermediate-acting insulin, once or twice daily, and another treated intensively with more complex insulin regimens. Although normalization of blood glucose values was not achieved in the intensively treated group (average blood sugar values were 40 percent above normal limits), glycosylated hemoglobin levels were significantly better. As a result, there was a 60 percent reduction in risk between the intensive treatment group and the standard treatment group in diabetic retinopathy, nephropathy, and neuropathy. The benefit of intensive therapy resulted in a delay in the onset and a major slowing of the progression of these three complications. With the advent of more sophisticated insulins and insulin pumps since the DCCT, it is likely that with a more contemporary intensive insulin therapy program, the benefits to health will be even greater.

Another downside with intensive insulin therapy in the DCCT was weight gain. Insulin is a growth-promoting hormone, so one of the key goals is to follow the diet, lifestyle, and supplement strategies that are part of our program to support a lower dosage of insulin being needed to maintain blood sugar levels. Insulin resistance is also a common feature of type 1 diabetes and is related to the same risk factors as in type 2 diabetes (increased body fat, lack of exercise, lack of important nutritional factors, high-glycemic-index/high-glycemic-load diet). This is why the modifications of lifestyle and diet recommended for type 2 diabetics are equally valid in type 1 diabetics. Positive diet and lifestyle changes in type 1 diabetes will help ensure that the lowest possible daily dose of insulin is required to achieve optimal blood glucose control.

The methods of applying intensified insulin therapy are multiple daily injections (3 to 5 or more injections daily) with a syringe or insulin pen, or use of an insulin pump to administer a continuous supply of insulin. The decision to use multiple injections of insulin versus an

Preventing, Recognizing, and Treating Insulin Reactions (Hypoglycemic Episodes)

An insulin reaction or hypoglycemic episode occurs when the blood sugar level falls too low (usually below 60 mg/dL [3.3 mmol/L]).

To Prevent Insulin Reactions
- Eat regular meals on schedule
- Avoid sudden changes in diet, exercise, or insulin
- Eat a snack before exercising
- Always carry with you one of the following:
  - A couple of packets of sugar or honey
  - Insta-Glucose (1 tube)
  - Glucose tablets (2–3)
  - Destrasols (4–6)

Symptoms of Mild Hypoglycemia
- Hunger
- Cold sweat and a clammy feeling
- Dizziness, weakness, or shakiness
- Pounding heart or increased heart rate

Symptoms of Moderate Hypoglycemia
- Nervousness or confusion
- Headache
- Blurred or double vision
- Numbness or tingling in lips or fingers

Symptoms of Severe Hypoglycemia (*Note:* When the following symptoms are present, immediate medical assistance is always required. Don't wait; call 911 immediately. If glucagon, a hormone that raises blood sugar levels quickly, is available, administer it via injection.)
- Paleness and slurred speech
- Bizarre behavior
- Convulsions

Strategies to Treat Mild to Moderate Hypoglycemia
- Use one of the quick sugar supplies on hand
- In a pinch, go to a store or restaurant and get:
  - Lifesavers candies (4–6)
  - Cola or other soda (6 oz.)
  - Orange juice (4 oz.)
  - Jelly beans (6)
  - Milk (small carton)

Don't overtreat a mild to moderate insulin reaction by consuming more than the recommended amount. Stop what you are doing and sit or lie down. Wait 10 to 15 minutes. If you do not feel better, take the food again. After you feel better, if you are between meals, eat a low-glycemic-index snack. If it is close to mealtime, have your next meal.

Sample Snacks for After a Hypoglycemic Event
½ cup nuts or seeds
1 or 2 carrots or celery ribs
Low-glycemic-index food bar
Piece of fruit

After a reaction, you may feel tired and have high blood sugar, but don't make a permanent change in your insulin dosage without consulting your physician.

Be sure to wear diabetes identification to inform others of your condition in case of an accident or loss of consciousness due to a reaction. Teach your family, friends, teachers, and co-workers how to spot a reaction and how to help if you have one. If you ignore reaction warning symptoms and do not take sugar, you could become unconscious. While this occurrence is quite rare, you can protect yourself by teaching family and friends how to give an injection of glucagon in an emergency.

Blood Glucose Awareness Training

Many diabetics become relatively insensitive to hypoglycemia. This loss of hypoglycemia awareness has to do with diabetic damage to the autonomic nervous system, the part of the nervous system responsible for the most obvious hypoglycemia symptoms (such as sweating, shakiness, rapid heart rate, nervousness). These symptoms arise when blood sugar begins to drop and adrenaline is released by the adrenal glands and the autonomic nerve endings. As well, when any diabetic strives to achieve tighter blood glucose control, serious hypoglycemic episodes are more likely to occur. The fear of hypoglycemia and the serious lingering effects it can have on the brain cause many diabetics to be unwilling to strive for better blood sugar control. The Blood Glucose Awareness Training program, version two (BGAT-2), is now widely available and has been studied and shown to provide valuable skills to help diabetics recognize and effectively avoid serious hypoglycemic episodes.[1] Rather than relying on autonomic (adrenaline-driven) symptoms to recognize impending hypoglycemia, BGAT-2 teaches diabetics a system for keeping track of the subtle effects of blood sugar on brain function. Unlike autonomic symptoms of hypoglycemia, which often diminish over time, cognitive symptoms of hypoglycemia do not diminish. If you are a diabetic on insulin, we highly recommend that you seek out training for both intensive insulin therapy and hypoglycemia awareness with BGAT-2. Together, these two programs require a commitment of several days of training, but they will provide you with invaluable skills in managing your diabetes.

insulin pump depends on the preference of the patient and the ability of the health care provider and diabetes teaching unit to provide the necessary resources and support. We feel that the newer methods, the pump or pen, are preferable (see Table 8.2).

Table 8.2. Advantages of Intensive Insulin Therapy with the Insulin Pump or Pen

Greater flexibility of meals, exercise, and daily schedule
Improved physical and psychological well-being
Tighter control of blood glucose level
Lower glycosylated hemoglobin (hemoglobin A$_1$C)

The Insulin Pump

The insulin pump method involves filling a syringe with soluble insulin. The syringe is placed in a pump device and connected via a hollow flexible hose to a needle which is inserted into a site on the abdomen. The unit must be worn 24 hours a day. The plunger of the syringe is pressed slowly and constantly by a small pump so that a constant trickle of soluble insulin is delivered (basal insulin dosage). Fifteen minutes prior to a meal, the diabetic can press the pump manually to release a burst of insulin (bolus insulin dosage) in an amount determined by the premeal blood glucose level and the anticipated meal composition.

The insulin pump approximates the natural levels of insulin in the best of currently available techniques, but it is not without drawbacks. The device must be worn constantly and can be an irritation; the patient must be highly motivated to monitor blood sugar levels quite closely; the risk for hypoglycemia is greater; and not all physicians are familiar enough with the method. In all cases, diabetics should receive formal training in the proper use of their pump through a diabetes teaching unit (usually by a certified diabetes educator, or CDE). It is also wise to obtain blood glucose awareness training (BGAT-2) if it is available in your area. This program is now widely available and if it is not, you should request that your diabetes teaching unit make it available.

The use of the insulin pump is a great responsibility. Pump wearers must be highly motivated, able to operate the pump, willing to test blood glucose frequently, and astute enough to know when a problem is developing. They must also have access to a health care team familiar with pump therapy.

The Insulin Pen

Just as its name implies, this delivery method uses what looks like an old-fashioned fountain pen or cartridge pen, with two major differences: Instead of a cartridge of ink, the pen holds a cartridge of insulin, and instead of a nib, a needle attaches to the end. Drug companies usually give the pens away free—they make their money by supplying the cartridges.

As with the pump, there is a great deal of responsibility as the diabetic usually sets the dosage by setting the pen. Most pens hold cartridges containing 150 to 300 units of insulin. The person turns a dial to the required dosage, attaches a needle, and injects the insulin.

One of the key advantages of the insulin pen, convenience, is usually a strong motivator to make the switch from the syringe-and-needle approach. It is inconspicuous, quick, and easy. It is also less painful because smaller-gauge needles are used—another big plus with users.

Insulin pens have become extremely popular throughout the world; in some countries, 70 to 90 percent of all insulin is delivered by pen. However, in the United States only about 2 percent of insulin is injected via pen. The reason is probably difficulties with reimbursement from insurance companies. Although the insulin used in the pen is slightly more expensive, because the needles for the pen are slightly less expensive than disposable syringes the price evens out. Eventually the insurance companies will figure it out and insulin pens will be as popular here as they are elsewhere in the world.

Use of an insulin pen or pump requires the user to recognize factors that may cause a change in their blood sugar levels (see Table 8.3).

Table 8.3. Common Reasons for Blood Sugar Fluctuations

Changes in exercise or activity level
Snacks added or omitted
Delayed meals or a change in the type of amount of food eaten
Illness or infection
Emotional stress
Alcohol consumption
Insulin injected into a lumpy area or an exercising arm or leg
Overtreatment of an insulin reaction
Skipped insulin injection

Natural Products for Type 1 Diabetes Support

Achieving the goals of therapy in individuals with type 1 diabetes with supportive natural products involves the following:

1. Preserving beta cell function and possibly reversing the autoimmune process
2. Enhancing the effectiveness of insulin therapy to allow for lower dosages
3. Reducing after-meal elevations in blood sugar levels

Preserving Beta Cell Function

Can type 1 diabetes be stopped? Yes, and believe it or not, in some cases it can even be reversed. We know that statement may raise some eyebrows, but it is certainly possible with the recommendations we are going to make. Consistent with our other guidelines, there is scientific evidence to back them up. The key is to start therapy as soon as possible after the diagnosis or within the first year at the latest. The two key supplements are the niacinamide form of vitamin B$_3$ and green tea extract or the herb *Pterocarpus marsupium*.

NIACINAMIDE | Niacinamide, also called nicotinamide, has been shown to prevent some of the immune-mediated destruction of the pancreatic beta cells and may actually help reverse the process.[2,3] Research into using niacinamide for type 1 diabetes began with the observation that niacinamide can prevent the development of diabetes in experimental animals. This led to several pilot clinical trials that suggested that niacinamide can prevent type 1 diabetes from occurring, or, if given soon enough at the onset of diabetes, help restore beta cells or at least slow down their destruction. In one of the first pilot studies of newly diagnosed type 1 diabetics, seven patients were given 3 g of niacinamide daily and nine were given a placebo. After six months, five patients in the niacinamide group and two in the placebo group were still not taking insulin and had normal blood glucose and hemoglobin A$_1$C. At 12 months, three patients in the niacinamide group but none in the placebo group were in clinical remission.[4]

The results of this pilot study and others suggested that niacinamide can prevent type 1 diabetes from progressing in some patients if given soon enough at the onset of diabetes by helping restore beta cells. At present (2003) there have been ten studies of niacinamide treatment in recent-onset type 1 diabetes or type 1 diabetes of less than 5 years' duration and residual beta cell mass. Eight of these studies were double-blind placebo-controlled studies. Out of these eight, four studies showed a positive effect compared to placebo in terms of prolonged non-insulin-requiring remission, lower insulin requirements, improved metabolic control, and increased beta cell function as determined by C-peptide secretion. Again, it is important to point out that some newly diagnosed type 1 diabetics have experienced complete resolution with niacinamide supplementation. The main difference between the positive and negative studies in recent-onset type 1 diabetes was older age and higher baseline fasting C-peptide in positive studies.[5,6]

Based on the positive results in the studies in newly diagnosed type 1 diabetes, a couple of very large studies were designed to evaluate the effectiveness of niacinamide in preventing the development of type 1 diabetes in high-risk individuals—such as siblings of children who developed type 1 diabetes or individuals who already show elevations in antibodies directed against the beta cells. The first of these studies—the Deutsche Nicotinamide Intervention Study—did not show much of an effect with 1.2 grams of niacinamide daily, while results from the larger study, the European Nicotinamide Diabetes Intervention Trial (ENDIT), are not yet available.[7]

While we don't believe that niacinamide will work for all recent-onset type 1 diabetes patients or offer an effective prevention strategy on its own in most cases, it may work for some. The fact that some children have had complete reversal of their disease makes its use certainly worth the effort, especially since there is no other reasonable alternative.

The dosage recommendation is based on body weight: 25 to 50 mg of niacinamide for every 2.2 pounds of body weight.[8] Niacinamide is generally well tolerated and without side effects. In fact, no side effects have been reported in the clinical trials for type 1 diabetes. It does not cause the flushing of the skin characterized by high dosages of niacin. However, since it may harm the liver, we recommend a blood test for liver enzymes every three months to rule out liver damage.

How Much Proof Is Required When Human Lives Are at Stake?

In our current medical system there appears to be a unnecessary time lag between the time a vitamin or mineral is proven to be effective in preventing or treating a certain health condition and the time when it becomes widely accepted and recommended by physicians.

There are countless examples where supplementing the diet with an inexpensive vitamin or mineral can provide significant preventive or therapeutic effects, yet many physicians place an unnecessary burden of proof before they feel inclined to make the recommendation. Our message to these physicians is to rethink their position.

Instead of waiting for absolute proof, physicians should ask whether there is enough "reasonable certainty" that a particular recommendation may be beneficial. What do we mean by reasonable certainty? Basically, does the recommendation make sense? Is there a good chance that the recommendation may be of value? Does it provide a favorable cost to benefit ratio? Is the recommendation safe?

The potential role of niacinamide in the treatment of recent-onset type 1 diabetes or as a preventive measure in high-risk children is a good example. The results indicate an excellent cost-benefit ratio and safety profile. Most orthodox medical doctors would look at the information and say something like, "This research is very interesting, but, of course, I cannot recommend niacinamide until there is more absolute proof that it may be of value."

Again, we ask, how much proof is required when human lives are at stake? The results from larger double-blind studies with niacinamide are not yet available. What if the results of these larger studies are extremely positive? It would mean that by "playing it safe" and not supplementing niacinamide, many individuals who may have benefited would not have the opportunity, just like the thousands of children born with neural tube defects that could have been prevented with folic acid supplementation.

PTEROCARPUS MARSUPIUM **AND EPICATECHIN-CONTAINING PLANTS** |
The plant pterocarpus has a long history of use in India as a treatment
for diabetes. There is some evidence to justify this use as the flavonoid
(–)-epicatechin extracted from the bark has been shown to prevent beta
cell damage and actually regenerate functional pancreatic beta cells in
diabetic animals.[9,10]

In addition to pterocarpus, the dry weight percentage of epicatechin
is very high in a number of other plants, most notably green tea—1 to
3 percent epicatechin content.

As commercial sources of pterocarpus are lacking in the United
States, green tea may be a suitable alternative. The recommended dosage
is at least two cups of green tea per day or roughly 240 to 300 mg of
green tea polyphenols.

Enhancing the Effectiveness of Insulin

Managing diet, lifestyle, and optimal nutritional status is the first step
in enhancing the effectiveness of insulin. Chromium, vitamin E, magnesium, vanadium, manganese, and biotin are just some of the important nutrients required. In addition to taking a high-potency multiple
vitamin and mineral formula, individuals with poorly controlled type 1
diabetes should consider taking biotin, *Gymnema sylvestre,* or Korean
ginseng extract (only the one developed through research at University
of Toronto) to try to improve insulin utilization.

BIOTIN | Biotin is a B vitamin that functions in the manufacture and
use of carbohydrates, fats, and amino acids. Without biotin, sugar metabolism is severely impaired. Biotin supplementation has been shown
to enhance insulin sensitivity and increase the activity of the enzyme
glucokinase, the enzyme responsible for the first step in the use of glucose by the liver. Glucokinase concentrations in diabetics are very low.
Evidently, supplementing the diet with high doses of biotin improves
glucokinase activity and glucose metabolism in diabetics. In one study,
16 mg of biotin per day resulted in significant lowering of fasting blood
sugar levels and improvements in blood glucose control in type 1 diabetics; in another study, similar effects were noted in type 2 diabetics

with 9 mg of biotin per day.[11] Biotin therapy has also been shown to be quite helpful in the treatment of diabetic neuropathy (nerve disease).[12]

GYMNEMA SYLVESTRE | Gymnema is another plant from India that has long been used as a treatment for diabetes. Recent scientific investigation has upheld its effectiveness in both type 1 and type 2 diabetes. Gymnema extracts have been shown to enhance glucose control in diabetic dogs and rabbits. Interestingly, in animals that have had their pancreas removed, gymnema possesses no apparent effects, suggesting that it enhances the production or activity of insulin. As with pterocarpus, there is evidence in animal studies that gymnema promotes regeneration of the insulin-producing beta cells in the pancreas. Studies in humans also seem to support the possibility of pancreas regeneration.[13]

An extract of the leaves of *Gymnema sylvestre* given to twenty-seven patients with type 1 diabetes on insulin therapy was shown to reduce insulin requirements and fasting blood sugar levels and to improve blood sugar control.[14] These results indicate that gymnema enhances the action of insulin, as these diabetics were not recently diagnosed.

The dosage for *Gymnema sylvestre* extract (standardized to contain 24 percent gymnemic acid) is 200 mg twice a day. No side effects have been reported from gymnema extract; however, diabetics on insulin should be careful to monitor blood sugar when beginning this product because insulin dosages may have to be decreased to avoid hypoglycemia.

Reducing After-Meal Elevations in Blood Sugar Levels

Obviously, a low-glycemic-index and low-glycemic-load diet is the first step in reducing after-meal spikes in blood sugar levels, but a number of natural products can blunt postprandial (after-meal) blood sugar levels even further. These products are discussed in the next chapter as they have more to do with treating type 2 diabetes.

Additional Practical Recommendations

In addition to controlling blood sugar levels, a number of natural products are quite important in dealing with the complications that most

Bitter Melon—a Source of Phyto-Insulin

Bitter melon (*Momordica charantia*) is a green cucumber-shaped fruit with gourdlike bumps all over it. It looks like an ugly cucumber. In addition to being eaten as a vegetable in Asia, unripe bitter melon has been used extensively in folk medicine as a remedy for diabetes. The blood-sugar-lowering action of the fresh juice or extract of the unripe fruit has been clearly established in modern scientific studies in both type 1 and type 2 diabetes.

Bitter melon is composed of several compounds with confirmed blood-sugar-lowering properties. Charantin, extracted by alcohol, is a hypoglycemic agent composed of mixed steroids that is more potent than the oral hypoglycemic drug tolbutamide. Momordica also contains an insulin-like polypeptide, polypeptide-P, which lowers blood sugar levels when injected like insulin into type 1 diabetics. Since it appears to have fewer side effects than insulin, it has been suggested as a replacement for some patients, although the likelihood of this application ever being developed is extremely remote. Fortunately, taking as little as 2 ounces of the juice has shown good results in clinical trials.[15,16]

Unripe bitter melon is available primarily at Asian grocery stores. Health food stores may have bitter melon extract, but the fresh juice is probably the best to use as this was what was used in the studies. Bitter melon juice is, in my opinion, very difficult to make palatable. As its name implies, it is quite bitter. It is best simply to plug your nose and take a 2-ounce shot of the juice. The dosage of other forms should approximate this dose.

people with type 1 diabetes develop. These natural medicines will be discussed in Part III. In Appendix B on pages 295–300, we prioritize which product to use, based upon some of the additional benefits that each provides.

Chapter Nine

Natural Products for
Type 2 Diabetes

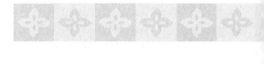

In this chapter we highlight key natural products to help improve blood sugar control in the treatment of type 2 diabetes. Before doing so, we want to remind you that diet and lifestyle are especially important in type 2 diabetes, as this condition is usually the result of many years of chronic metabolic insult. Even though the remedies discussed in this chapter possess significant effects, proper and effective treatment of type 2 diabetes requires careful integration of diet and lifestyle changes along with these natural medicines. Furthermore, some type 2 diabetics will also require conventional medical treatments (oral drugs or insulin) as well—depending on adequacy of pancreatic insulin production (which can be determined by C-peptide level) and the response of the diabetic to dietary and lifestyle measures. The most important determining factor as to whether the diabetic needs to be managed by drugs or insulin is the adequacy of blood sugar control. Even if insulin or oral drugs are used, diet and lifestyle factors still should be of primary importance in the management of type 2 diabetes. The use of insulin and oral antihyperglycemic drugs in the treatment of type 2 diabetes will be discussed later in this chapter.

Keep in mind that type 2 diabetes is usually a more complex condition to deal with than type 1 diabetes because it is most often associated with a multitude of other physiological stressors such as obesity and diminished insulin sensitivity. Achieving the goals of therapy in individuals with type 2 diabetes with natural medicine (or drugs) involves the following:

1. Reducing after-meal elevations in blood sugar levels.
2. Improving insulin function and sensitivity.

Remember that it is critical that blood glucose levels be monitored carefully, particularly if blood sugar levels have been relatively uncontrolled. Careful attention to symptoms, home glucose monitoring, and the hemoglobin A$_1$C test are critical in monitoring the effectiveness of treatment. Any change in your routine requires a closer eye on these measurements. Table 9.1 provides the blood sugar targets in people with type 2 diabetes.

We want to stress again that when diet and natural products are used to improve blood sugar control, insulin and/or drug dosages will have to be altered. A good working relationship with the prescribing doctor is extremely important.

Table 9.1. Goals for Blood Glucose Measurements and A$_1$C in People with Type 2 Diabetes

TIME OF CHECK	GOAL (WHOLE-BLOOD MEASUREMENTS)
Before breakfast (fasting)	80–110 mg/dL (4.4–6.1 mmol/L)
Before lunch, supper, and snack	80–130 mg/dL (4.4–7.2 mmol/L)
2 hours after meals	Less than 140 mg/dL (7.8 mmol/L)
Bedtime	110–140 mg/dL (6.1–7.8 mmol/L)
A$_1$C (glycosylated hemoglobin)	≤ 7%

Reducing After-Meal Elevations in Blood Sugar Levels

Elevations of blood glucose levels after a meal can wreak biochemical havoc in both type 1 and type 2 diabetics. In fact, an elevation in postprandial (after-meal) blood sugar levels is perhaps the major contributor to the development of diabetic complications, especially heart disease and diseases of the microvasculature (small blood vessels within the eyes, kidneys, and nerves). For example, patients who have normal fasting blood sugar measurement but have an average 2-hour-postprandial glucose level greater than 200 mg/dL (11 mmol/L) have a threefold increase in the incidence of diabetic eye disease (retinopathy).[1] Therefore, blunting the after-meal increase in blood sugar levels is a very important goal.

In addition to following dietary guidelines to reduce postprandial blood sugar levels (eating low-glycemic-index/low-glycemic-load meals), several natural products can be used. We will limit discussion to the most useful: fiber supplements, natural glucosidase inhibitors, and American ginseng extract (discussed later in this chapter).

Fiber Supplements

Fiber supplements have been shown to enhance blood sugar control, decrease insulin levels, and reduce the number of calories absorbed by the body. The best fiber sources for reducing postprandial (after-meal) blood sugar levels, lowering cholesterol levels, and promoting weight loss are those that are rich in water-soluble fibers such as glucomannan (from konjac root), psyllium, guar gum, defatted fenugreek seed powder or fiber, seaweed fibers (alginate and carrageenan), and pectin.

When taken with water before meals, these fiber sources bind to the water in the stomach and small intestine to form a gelatinous, viscous mass that not only slows down the absorption of glucose, but also induces a sense of satiety (fullness) and reduces the absorption of calories. In some of the clinical studies demonstrating weight loss, fiber supplements were shown to reduce the number of calories absorbed by 30 to 180 calories per day. While modest, this reduction in calories would,

Table 9.2. Examples of Clinical Studies with Dietary Fiber Supplements for Weight Loss

FIBER	NO. OF SUBJECTS	LENGTH OF STUDY	DOSAGE (G/DAY)
Guar	33	2.5 months	15
Glucomannan	20	2 months	3
Glucomannan	20	2 months	3
Mixture A	60	12 weeks	5
Mixture B	97	3 months	7
Mixture B	52	6 months	7

Mixture A = 80% fiber from grains, 20% fiber from citrus; mixture B = 90% insoluble and 10% soluble fiber from beet, barley, and citrus fibers

over the course of a year, result in a 3- to 18-pound weight loss (see Table 9.2).

We have two important recommendations for patients to help them choose fiber supplements:

- Avoid products that contain a lot of sugar or other sweeteners to camouflage the taste.
- Be sure to drink adequate amounts of water when taking any fiber supplement, especially if it is in a dry form (pill, cookie, capsule, or bar).

Because water-soluble fibers are fermented by intestinal bacteria, a great deal of gas can be produced, leading to increased flatulence and abdominal discomfort. Start with a dosage between 1 and 2 grams before meals and at bedtime, and gradually increase the dosage to 5 grams before meals and bedtime to reach the full daily dosage of 20 grams. Generally, the digestive system adapts to fiber over a few days and intestinal gas will become negligible.

PGX™ (POLYGLYCOPLEX) | Dietary fiber supplements appear to exert a dose-dependent effect in lowering cholesterol and blood glucose levels as well as body weight. Unfortunately, to achieve the greatest ben-

Table 9.2. Examples of Clinical Studies with Dietary Fiber Supplements for Weight Loss (continued)

CALORIE RESTRICTION	AVERAGE WEIGHT LOSS OF FIBER GROUP (LBS)	AVERAGE WEIGHT LOSS OF PLACEBO GROUP (LBS)
No	5.5	0.9
No	5.5	Gain, 1.5
No	8.14	0.44
Yes	18.7	14.7
Yes	10.8	7.3
Yes	12.1	6.1

efit, the dosage required (20 grams or more) is often difficult to achieve. That challenge has recently been overcome by the development of PGX™ (PolyGlycoPlex), a unique blend of selected, highly viscous soluble polysaccharide fibers that act synergistically to develop a higher level of viscosity and expansion with water than with the same quantity of any fiber alone. The synergistic effect of this unique blend means that PGX™ exerts an effect equal to three to five times that of other fibers alone. PGX™ is based on the intense scientific research at the University of Toronto led by Vladimir Vuksan, Ph.D., one of the most respected and recognized experts on the role of diet in the risk of diabetes, heart disease, and obesity. Dr. Vuksan and his colleagues have conducted extensive research with dietary fibers through his role as a director in the Risk Factor Modification Centre at St. Michael's Hospital at the University of Toronto. Hundreds of different fiber combinations were tested in laboratory, animal, and human studies before the PGX™ formulation was established.

Highly refined and uniquely processed PGX™ possesses the greatest viscosity (gelling property) of any single dietary fiber. It is three times as viscous as guar and approximately seven times as viscous as psyllium. By combining glucomannan with other soluble fibers, the viscosity of PGX™ is amplified further and has a viscosity three to five times that of any glucomannan alone (see Figure 9.1). The viscosity of soluble fiber is directly related to its physiological effects and ultimately its overall health benefits in humans.

Clinical studies conducted by Dr. Vuksan and his colleagues have repeatedly shown that after-meal blood sugar levels decrease as soluble

Figure 9.1. Viscosity of Soluble Fibers

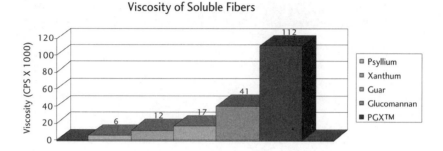

fiber viscosity increases.[2,3] This relationship has also been shown to hold true for the other physiological benefits produced by soluble fibers, including increased insulin sensitivity, diminished appetite, significant weight control, improved bowel movements, and decreased serum cholesterol. The impressive combination of effects produced by Dr. Vuksan's group led the American Dietetic Association to recognize his blend as one the first "evidence-based" dietary fibers in July 2002 and the U.S. Patent Office to grant a patent for its health applications (improvement of postprandial blood sugar levels, insulin sensitivity, and blood cholesterol levels).[4]

PGX™ lowers postprandial blood glucose by approximately 20 percent and also lowers insulin secretion by approximately 40 percent, producing a whole-body insulin sensitivity index improvement of nearly 50 percent—a phenomenal accomplishment that is unequaled by any drug or natural health product. Add to that its impressive effects on lowering blood cholesterol and triglyceride levels as well as its excellent safety profile and it is little wonder that we consider PGX™ a real superstar in the stable of natural products for diabetes. On top of that, University of Toronto researchers have recently found that higher doses of PGX™ can diminish appetite to such an extent that even the heaviest individuals have a dramatic and sustainable reduction in appetite. Table 9.3 provides a summary of the clinical effects of PGX™.

Because PGX™ can be given at much smaller quantities than other viscous dietary fibers to achieve comparable health benefits, it is a much more practical recommendation, especially when taken in capsule form. The typical dosage for PGX™ is 1,000 mg three times daily with

Table 9.3. Clinical Effects of PGX™

- Reduces postprandial (after-meal) blood glucose levels
- Reduces appetite and promotes effective weight loss
- Increases insulin sensitivity
- Improves diabetes control
- Lowers blood cholesterol
- Lowers blood pressure (an effect rarely seen with fiber)

meals. PGX™ also results in fewer gastrointestinal side effects than other viscous dietary fibers. Higher doses may be used for more significant appetite reduction.

Natural Glucosidase Inhibitors

Starches, complex carbohydrates, and even simple sugars (disaccharides) such as sucrose are broken down in the digestive tract into glucose by the action of certain enzymes. One of the most important enzymes

PGX™ Improves Syndrome X

Syndrome X refers to a collection of metabolic abnormalities including impaired glucose tolerance, high blood cholesterol and triglyceride levels, high blood pressure, and upper body (abdominal) obesity. The underlying metabolic factor in syndrome X is elevated insulin levels and insulin resistance. A complex similar to PGX™ was shown to significantly improve all aspects of syndrome X by increasing insulin sensitivity as evidenced by the reductions in total cholesterol (12.4 percent), LDL cholesterol (22.3 percent), the ratio of LDL to HDL cholesterol (15 percent), and serum fructosamine (5 percent).[5] In another study in similar patients, improvements were seen in postprandial blood glucose (27 percent), postprandial insulin levels (41 percent), and insulin resistance (48 percent).[6]

is the alpha-glucosidases that line the intestines. Because these enzymes are essential for the breakdown of starches, complex carbohydrates, maltose, and sucrose into absorbable glucose molecules, inhibiting them can diminish after-meal rises in both glucose and insulin.

Acarbose (Precose) and miglitol (Glyset) are approved drugs for treating diabetes in this application of inhibiting alpha-glucosidase. Although clinical studies have shown these drugs to be quite effective, their use is also characterized by a high frequency of mild-to-moderate gastrointestinal side effects, such as flatulence, diarrhea, and abdominal discomfort. While these side effects generally diminish in frequency and intensity with time, very few patients are willing to put in the necessary time to get over these troubling side effects.

Instead of the drug acarbose we recommend trying either touchi extract or mulberry extract, which are natural and superior to their drug counterparts.

TOUCHI EXTRACT | Touchi is a fermented soybean product that has been used in China and Japan for more than 3,000 years. Touchi extract is concentrated to possess high levels of naturally occurring alpha-glucosidase inhibitors. Several clinical studies have documented its effectiveness in reducing after-meal elevations in blood sugar levels. For example, let's look at the results from a study in which people with borderline diabetes were given 300 mg of Touchi extract and 75 grams of sucrose.[7] As you can see in Figure 9.2, the Touchi extract suppressed the rise in blood glucose compared to those taking only sucrose.

Longer-term studies have also shown benefit.[8,9] For example, when type 2 diabetes patients took 300 mg of Touchi extract before each meal for six months, there were moderate changes in fasting blood glucose and hemoglobin A_1C levels. The effects were apparent after only 1 month of use. As shown in Figure 9.3, after six months the fasting blood glucose level dropped more than 10 mg/dL in nearly 80 percent of the patients, and hemoglobin A_1C levels fell by more than 0.5 percent in 60 percent of patients. Surprisingly, Touchi extract also had a mild effect in lowering triglyceride and cholesterol levels, probably through a decrease in insulin resistance.

Unlike the drug alpha-glucosidase inhibitors, no side effects have ever been seen with Touchi extract and not a single subject in any of the clinical trials has ever complained of the gastrointestinal side effects,

Figure 9.2. Effects of Touchi Extract on Absorption of Sucrose

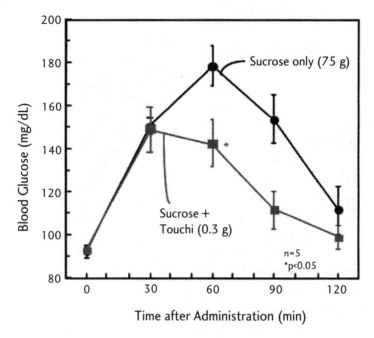

Figure 9.3. Effect of Touchi Extract on Blood Sugar Levels

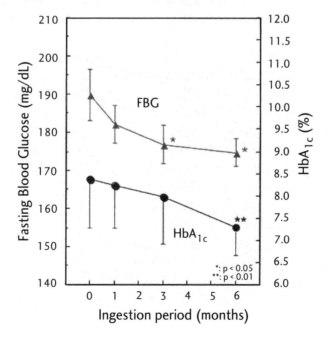

such as abdominal distension, abdominal pain, and flatulence that are so characteristic of acarbose.

MULBERRY EXTRACT | The mulberry plant (*Morus indica*) is probably best known as food for silkworms, but it has also been highly regarded in traditional Chinese and Japanese medicine. It has been shown to possess significant hypoglycemic effects in animal studies and it contains a very effective alpha-glucosidase inhibitor along with other compounds that appear to improve blood sugar control.[10,11] In fact, Coca-Cola is so convinced of the benefits of mulberry extract that the company includes it in a Coke product in Japan called Pocket Dr. Because mulberry extract has proven benefits, Pocket Dr. is actually a registered natural health product in Japan.

Mulberry extract has been studied in type 2 diabetes and the results are excellent. In one study, researchers decided to investigate its effect on blood and red blood cell lipids as well as compare its blood sugar–lowering actions to the oral antihyperglycemic drug glyburide.[12] Patients were given either mulberry dried leaves (3 g/day) or one tablet of glyburide (5 mg/day) for 4 weeks. Mulberry therapy significantly improved diabetic control in type 2 diabetic patients (Table 9.4). The results clearly show that the fasting blood glucose concentrations were significantly lowered with mulberry therapy, suggesting that mulberry therapy is effective in controlling diabetes. Compared to glyburide treatment, mulberry therapy reduced fasting blood glucose concentrations of diabetic patients by 27 percent. However, no significant differences were observed in blood glucose concentrations between pre- and posttreatments with glyburide. Mulberry extract was also superior to the approved drug in its ability to decrease hemoglobin A_1C, cholesterol, LDL, and triglycerides. It also resulted in an increase in HDL ("good cholesterol"). Although these changes were not statistically significant, there are strong suggestions that this natural product is clearly superior to an established pharmaceutical agent.

In addition to the benefits for blood sugar levels and blood lipids, mulberry therapy was also shown to reduce the amount of damage (lipid peroxidation) to the cell membranes of red blood cells, indicating a significant antioxidant effect. Additionally, mulberry therapy significantly decreased membrane cholesterol of type 2 diabetic patients.

**Table 9.4. Influence of Mulberry and Glyburide Treatments
on Blood Glucose, Glycosylated Hemoglobin, and Serum Lipids
of the Patients with Type 2 Diabetes**

	Glyburide			Mulberry		
PARAMETER	BEFORE	AFTER	CHANGE (%)	BEFORE	AFTER	CHANGE (%)
Fasting blood glucose (mg/dL)	154.4	141.8	−8	152.7	110.5	−27
A_1C (%)	12.5	12.4	0	12.5	11.2	−10
Cholesterol (mg/dL)	190	182	−4	193.7	170.3	−12
LDL cholesterol (mg/dL)	102.5	95.5	−7	102.1	78.7	−23
HDL cholesterol (mg/dL)	49.8	51.3	+3	50.1	59.2	+18
Triglycerides (mg/dL)	199.5	180	−10	200.4	168.0	−16
Free fatty acids (pmol/dL)	589.8	580	−2	590.1	520	−12

Improving Insulin Function and Sensitivity

The first step in improving insulin function and sensitivity is achieving ideal body weight and following the dietary and lifestyle recommendations given in Chapter 7, including taking a high-potency multiple - vitamin and mineral formula to ensure that the body has all of the necessary essential vitamins and minerals that proper insulin sensitivity requires. Using PGX or higher dosages of other sources of soluble fiber has been shown to increase insulin sensitivity. If additional support is needed to bring blood sugar levels under control, we recommend using one or more of the following, in isolation or in scientifically formulated combinations: *Gymnema sylvestre* extract, American ginseng, Korean ginseng, fenugreek seed extract, and increased intake of onions and garlic. Although we will provide general guidelines next, we also provide more specific single and combination product suggestions in Appendix C.

If even more support is necessary to further improve insulin utilization, prescription drugs must be used (discussed shortly).

Gymnema Sylvestre

Gymnema sylvestre, discussed in Chapter 8 on page 179, appeared on the U.S. market a few years ago. Originally it was hyped as a "sugar blocker." Manufacturers erroneously claimed that gymnema could block the absorption of sugar in the gastrointestinal tract and allow the sugar to pass through the intestinal tract unabsorbed. Ridiculous advertisement claims were made such as "how to cut down on sugar calories without cutting down on sugar." This claim was, in our opinion, blatant distortion of truth.

Gymnema components, like gymnemic acid, when applied to the tongue are able to block the sensation of sweetness. Clinically this has shown some significance. People who had gymnema extracts applied to the tongue have been shown to eat fewer calories at a meal compared to people who did not have the gymnema applied. It must be stressed that the gymnema extract was applied to their tongues. They did not swallow it in capsule or tablet form. Obviously this would not produce the same effect.

Gymnema extract appears to work in type 2 diabetes by enhancing the action of insulin. In one study, twenty-two type 2 diabetics were given gymnema extract along with their oral antihyperglycemic drugs.[13] All patients demonstrated improved blood sugar control; twenty-one out of the twenty-two were able to reduce their drug dosage considerably; and five were able to discontinue their medication and maintain blood sugar control with the gymnema extract alone.

The dosage for *Gymnema sylvestre* extract is 200 mg twice daily. Interestingly, gymnema extract given to healthy volunteers does not produce any blood-sugar–lowering effect.

American and Korean Ginseng

Research conducted at the University of Toronto's Risk Factor Modification Centre has uncovered important properties of some very ancient natural medicines. Along with the discovery of PGX™, the team of researchers led by Dr. Vladimir Vuksan has examined hundreds of different whole-herb preparations and unique extracts from dozens of different ginseng species from around the world for their effects on diabetes. In their first studies and published reports, Dr. Vuksan's group used whole powdered American ginseng root (*Panax quinquefolium*) and found that a dose of about 3 grams before each meal reduced postprandial (after-meal) blood sugar significantly in type 2 diabetics.[14–18] Later research has proven that a specific type of extract from American ginseng, containing a certain profile of ginsenosides, has a similar effect to the whole root with greater batch-to-batch consistency and with required intake far less than 3 grams per dose. Authorities now consider American ginseng the most evidence-based herbal therapy for type 2 diabetes.[19] Dr. Vuksan's team has determined that American ginseng works by the stimulation of pancreatic beta cells with a subsequent increase in insulin secretion. It also has significant antioxidant properties and improves cognitive function. American ginseng has also been shown to possess nerve protection and regeneration properties. This could prove to be valuable in diabetes where peripheral and autonomic nerve damage so often occurs. American ginseng has been used for centuries by Native Americans and it is likely to soon become one of the most sought after of all natural medicines.

As mentioned, Dr. Vuksan's research team has examined hundreds of different ginseng extracts prepared from dozens of different ginseng species from around the world in order to identify other possible treatments for diabetes. Their most important finding, apart from their discoveries with American ginseng, has been in a specific extract from a certain type of Korean ginseng (*Panax ginseng*). This extract is unique because it appears to lower blood sugar in diabetics by increasing insulin sensitivity rather than by increasing insulin release. Also, this specific extract from Korean ginseng exerts some effects that are similar to, yet more powerful than the drug Viagra. Although formal double-blind studies have not been done, it appears that Dr. Vuksan's Korean ginseng extract has the potential to improve blood sugar, sexual function, and hypertension. This would be a bonus for many diabetics who have erectile dysfunction and high blood pressure. So far, no side effects have been reported from this unique extract.

We are working with the University of Toronto to help make their unique, pharmaceutical-grade ginseng extracts commercially available soon. We are also working with the University of Toronto to conduct further clinical research on PGX™, American ginseng, and Korean ginseng at our clinic and research center, the Canadian Center for Functional

Medicine in Vancouver, Canada. In this research, we will examine the effects of various combinations of PGX™, American ginseng, and Korean ginseng extracts.

Fenugreek

Fenugreek seeds have demonstrated significant antidiabetic effects in experimental and clinical studies. The active ingredient is the special soluble fiber of fenugreek along with the alkaloid trigonelline. Fenugreek appears to be helpful in both type 1 and type 2 diabetes. Defatted fenugreek seed powder given twice daily in a 50-gram dose to type 1 diabetics resulted in significant reduction in fasting blood sugar and improved glucose tolerance test results.[20] There was also a 54 percent reduction in 24-hour urinary glucose excretion and significant reductions in LDL and VLDL cholesterol and triglyceride values. In type 2 diabetics, the addition of 15 grams of powdered fenugreek seeds soaked in water significantly reduced postprandial glucose levels during the meal tolerance test.[21]

In the most recent study, twenty-five patients with type 2 diabetes randomly received 1 gram per day of fenugreek seed extract or placebo capsules for two months.[22] Complex analysis of all of the data produced an interesting finding. The fenugreek group had improved blood sugar measurements (fasting blood sugar levels dropped from 148.3 to 119.9 mg/dL), but there was a significant decrease in insulin output. That finding indicates that a significant improvement in insulin sensitivity. Through our work at the Canadian Center for Functional Medicine, we are cooperating with Dr. Tappan Basu, professor of nutrition and agriculture at the University of Alberta, in a large project designed to further examine the potential of various extracts and fenugreek-derived products in type 2 diabetes.

Onions (Allium cepa) and Garlic (Allium sativum)

Onions and garlic appear to have significant blood-sugar-lowering action. The active ingredients are believed to be the sulfur-containing compounds allyl propyl disulphide (APDS) and diallyl disulphide oxide (allicin), respectively, although other constituents such as flavonoids may play a role as well.

Although garlic generally has more potent effects, onions can be given at higher dosages and the active compounds appear to be more stable than allicin. Graded doses of onion extracts (1 ml extract = 1 g whole onion) at levels sometimes found in the diet (1 to 7 ounces of onion) reduced blood sugar levels during an oral glucose tolerance test in a dose-dependent manner; that is, the higher the dose the greater the effect. The effects are similar in both raw and boiled onion extracts, indicating that the active components are probably very stable.[23]

The cardiovascular effects of garlic and onions—namely, reducing cholesterol and blood pressure—further substantiate the liberal intake of garlic and onions by the diabetic patient (see Chapter 11, pages 245–246, for dosage recommendations).

Supplementation Program for the Treatment of Type 2 Diabetes

The recommended supplementation program depends on the degree of blood sugar control as evident by self-monitored blood glucose and A_1C levels.

Initial Supplementation Programs

Level 1—Achievement of targeted blood sugar levels; A_1C below 7 percent, no lipid abnormalities, no signs of complications
- Foundation supplements:
  - High-potency multiple vitamin and mineral supplement— follow dosage recommendations on page 327.
  - Green drink—one serving daily
  - Fish oils—600 mg EPA and DHA daily

- Vitamin C—500 to 1,500 mg daily
- Vitamin E—400 to 800 IU daily

Level 2—Failure to achieve targeted blood sugar levels; A_1C between 7 and 8 percent
- Foundation supplements
- PGX™ (or other soluble source at equivalent dosage)—1,000 mg before meals

Level 3—Failure to achieve targeted blood sugar levels, A_1C between 8 percent and 9 percent.
- Foundation supplements.
- PGX™ (or other soluble source at equivalent dosage)—1,000 mg before meals.
- Insulin enhancer—use one of the following:
  - *Gymnema sylvestre* extract: 200 mg twice daily
  - Fenugreek extract: 1,000 mg daily
- Garlic—minimum 4,000 mcg of allicin per day

Level 4—Failure to achieve targeted blood sugar levels; A_1C above 9 percent
- Foundation supplements
- PGX™ (or other soluble source at equivalent dosage)—1,000 mg before meals.
- Insulin enhancer—use one of the following:
  - *Gymnema sylvestre* extract: 200 mg twice daily
  - Fenugreek extract: 1,000 mg daily
- Garlic: minimum 4,000 mcg of allicin per day.
- Glucosidase inhibitor—use one of the following:
  - Touchi extract: 300 mg before each meal
  - Mulberry extract: 100–200 mg before each meal

If self-monitored blood sugar levels do not improve after 4 weeks of following the recommendations for the current level, move to the next highest level. For example, if you start out with an A_1C

level of 8.2 percent and a fasting blood sugar level of 130 mg/dL, start on Level 2. After 4 weeks, if the average reading has not dropped to less than 110 mg/dL, then move to Level 3. If blood sugar levels and A_1C levels do not reach the targeted levels with Level 4, then a prescription medication (either an oral antihyperglycemic drug or insulin) is required.

Oral Antihyperglycemic Drugs

When type 2 diabetes cannot be controlled satisfactorily with weight loss, exercise, and diet therapy, oral antihyperglycemic agents or, when necessary, insulin are used for additional support. Remember, the importance of achieving optimal blood glucose control should outweigh any bias you may have against oral drugs and insulin. You need to do everything you can to improve your diabetes through lifestyle, diet, and supplements. However, if you do not achieve optimal blood glucose control, you must be willing to accept sound medical advice regarding medications or insulin. Above all, diabetics cannot be complacent and passively wait for the habits of a lifetime to change. Those who cannot or will not make the significant changes necessary to weight, lifestyle, exercise, and diet should still do whatever it takes to get their blood sugar under good control. Habits and weight can take quite a while to change for some people. On several occasions, we have failed to achieve adequate diabetic control through natural means initially, and have had to use medications or insulin. In some cases, given a good deal more time, patience, coaching and supplements, we were able to eventually reduce or stop medications.

Since most type 2 diabetics are obese and secrete large amounts of insulin each day to try to overcome insulin resistance, additional insulin is usually of only limited value. Unless C-peptide levels are normal or low, indicating partial pancreatic beta cell failure, improving insulin sensitivity should be the primary focus of treatment in type 2 diabetes. While healthy individuals secrete approximately 31 units of insulin daily, the obese type 2 diabetic secretes an average of 114 units daily. This amount is nearly four times the normal amount. In contrast to obese type 2 individuals, lean type 2 individuals produce about 14 units daily and individuals with type 1 diabetes secrete, on average, only 4 units of insulin daily. If a diabetic is overproducing insulin, it makes more sense to work on increasing insulin sensitivity by following the recommendations given previously or, when necessary, using appropriate oral hypoglycemic therapy. The major categories of these drugs are the following:

- Alpha-glucosidase inhibitors: acarbose (Precose), miglitol (Glyset)
- Sulfonylureas: acetohexamide (Dymelor), chlorpropamide (Diabinese, Insulase), glimepiride (Amaryl), glipizide (Glipizide, Glucotrol), glyburide (Diabeta, Micronase), repaglinide (Prandin), tolazamide (Tolinase), tolbutamide (Orinase)
- Biguanide type (nonsulfonylureas): metformin (Glucophage)
- Sulfonylurea/metformin combination: glyburide + metformin (Glucovance)
- Insulin-response enhancers: pioglitazone (Actos), rosiglitazone maleate (Avandia), troglitazone (Rezulin)
- Insulin-production enhancers: repaglinide (Prandin), nateglinide (Starlix)

Alpha-Glucosidase Inhibitors

We don't see much use for prescription alpha-glucosidase inhibitors, as there are natural compounds that can do the job just as well, without the gastrointestinal side effects. This is probably because the prescription forms inhibit both the starch-digesting enzyme pancreatic alpha amylase as well as the disaccharide-sugar-digesting intestinal alpha-glucosidase enzymes, so the result is a more profound maldigestion of carbohydrate. We recommend using natural alpha-glucosidase inhibitors (either Touchi extract or mulberry extract). These, especially if combined with PGX™, will control and slow the absorption of carbohydrates without creating the more severe carbohydrate malabsorption that results from alpha-glucosidase-inhibiting drugs.

Sulfonylureas

The sulfonylureas appear to stimulate the pancreas to secrete additional insulin by making beta cells more sensitive to glucose. Thus, as glucose levels rise, more insulin is released by beta cells than otherwise would occur. These drugs may also help enhance the action of insulin on the liver and peripheral tissues. As a group, when used alone these drugs are not very effective. After 3 months of continual treatment at an adequate dosage, only about 60 percent of users are able to control blood sugar levels using these drugs. Furthermore, these agents often lose their effectiveness over time. After an initial period of success, these drugs will fail to produce a positive effect in about 25 percent of cases. Overall, the improvements seen with this class of drug tend to be modest at best, with improvements in hemoglobin A_1C of usually no more than 1 to 2 percent.

In addition to being of limited value, some evidence indicates that sulfonylureas actually produce harmful long-term side-effects. For example, in a famous study conducted by the University Group Diabetes Program (UDGP) on the long-term effects of tolbutamide, it was shown that the rate of death due to a heart attack or stroke was 2.5 times greater than the group controlling their type 2 diabetes by diet alone. Since sulfonylureas enhance insulin secretion, they also promote fat deposition and weight gain. In obese diabetics, sulfonylureas actually fight against the diabetic's necessary efforts to lose weight. This can certainly be frustrating and can add to the chance of failure due to discouragement.

The major side effect of sulfonylureas is hypoglycemia. Other possible side effects include allergic skin reactions, headache, fatigue, indigestion, nausea and vomiting, and liver damage. Due to the high risk of side effects, these drugs must be used with caution. They should not be used in the following situations:

- Pregnancy
- Known allergy to sulfa drugs
- During infection, injury, or surgery
- During long-term corticosteroid use

In addition, sulfonylureas must be used with extreme caution in treating the elderly, alcoholics, those taking multiple drugs, and those with impaired liver or kidney function because serious, even lethal hypoglycemia can occur. In these groups, glicazide appears less likely to result in serious or prolonged hypoglycemia.

Sulfonylureas are of clearly of value in type 2 diabetics with some degree of pancreatic beta cell failure. Usually these diabetics are not overweight, but this is not always the case. We prefer to confirm a type 2 diabetic's ability to manufacture insulin by measuring C-peptide levels and use this as a determining factor. If C-peptide levels are normal or low in a type 2 diabetic, sulfonylureas are probably a reasonable choice.

As an alternative to sulfonylureas, we are inclined to recommend American ginseng. Although it also appears to enhance insulin secretion, it has other positive side benefits, such as its antioxidant effects and its positive effects upon cognition. We have not seen weight gain as a side effect of this agent, as commonly occurs with sulfonylureas.

Biguanide Types

Biguanide-type oral antihyperglycemics currently consist of only one approved medication—metformin (commercially known as Glucophage). Metformin is a drug with a profile that is generally more favorable than the sulfonylureas for most type 2 diabetics requiring medication. Metformin typically reduces blood glucose by 13 to 35 percent and hemoglobin A_1C by 1.5 to 2 percent. This medication also reduces triglycerides and LDL ("bad") cholesterol and increases HDL ("good") cholesterol. Unlike with sulfonylureas, which promote weight gain, diabetics taking metformin tend to lose weight (an average of 1 pound per week) without any other efforts to lose weight. This means that metformin complements positive lifestyle and dietary changes being undertaken by the diabetic. Importantly, the large-scale UKPDS study demonstrated that diabetics taking metformin had a decrease in heart attacks and all diabetes-related deaths.[24]

Metformin works by decreasing glucose production by the liver, increasing glucose uptake by muscles, and perhaps by mildly reducing appetite. Minor side effects (diarrhea, nausea, vomiting, abdominal bloating, and flatulence) are relatively common with metformin, but they usually lessen with time. Unlike sulfonylureas, metformin does not result in serious hypoglycemic episodes. A rare but very serious or potentially fatal side effect of metformin, referred to as lactic acidosis, can occur from metformin accumulation.[25] Lactic acidosis is most common in the elderly and in those with impaired kidney function, and so special caution needs to be taken in these groups.

Overall, metformin is the most proven and one of the safest oral drugs available.

Insulin-Response Enhancers—the Thiazolidinediones

The newest class of oral antihyperglycemic drugs are the thiazolidinediones, such as pioglitazone (Actose) and rosglitazone (Avandia). The first drug in this class, Rezulin (troglitazone), was removed from the market because widespread deaths occurred due to liver failure. Although the currently approved drugs have not been shown to cause the same effects, it is considered important to have liver enzymes checked every 2 months for the first year these drugs are taken. As well, serious fluid retention has been shown to occur with these drugs in animal studies, so they should be taken with caution by heart patients. Mild to moderate fluid retention is common with these drugs and, because they stimulate fat deposition, most people will gain weight on these agents. In addition, they also tend to raise triglycerides and LDL ("bad") cholesterol in most people.

Because these drugs promote weight gain, it would seem logical that they would worsen insulin resistance. However, they work by actually improving insulin sensitivity by inhibiting the fat cell factor known as resistin[26] described in Chapter 4, and thus may be one of the most effective ways to restore fertility in women with polycystic ovary syndrome, a condition related to insulin resistance. These drugs are also of value in the management of type 2 diabetes, although their side effects may outweigh their benefits in many cases.

Since there are proven natural products that improve insulin sensitivity (such as PGX™) and developments such as Korean ginseng extracts that also demonstrate insulin-sensitizing effects, we recommend giving these natural products a fair trial before considering a thiazolidinedione-class drug. Of course, we also recommend that everyone work on the important lifestyle, diet, and supplementation strategies we discuss in this book and that medications or insulin be used only when truly necessary to achieve optimal blood glucose control.

Niacinamide Improves Non-Insulin-Dependent Diabetes

In addition to offering possible benefits in type 1 diabetes, niacinamide may also help in type 2 diabetes. Eighteen patients with type 2 diabetes of normal body weight who failed to respond to oral antihyperglycemic drugs were randomly assigned to one of three treatments for six months: (1) insulin plus nicotinamide (500 mg three times daily); (2) insulin plus placebo; (3) oral antihyperglycemic drug plus niacinamide (500 mg three times daily). The parameters assessed included C-peptide (an indicator of insulin production, see Chapter 6, page 129, for more information), A_1C, and fasting and mean daily blood glucose levels. With detailed analysis, niacinamide administration was the only significant factor accountable for the improvement of C-peptide release. The data indicated that niacinamide improved C-peptide release and blood sugar control in type 2 diabetic patients who had previously failed to respond to oral antihyperglycemic drugs alone.[27]

Insulin Therapy in Type 2 Diabetes

Type 2 diabetics are not a uniform group. Although many type 2 diabetics go for years without any symptoms, and with relatively mild blood glucose elevations, some have a more severe presentation and may end up in the emergency department with dangerously elevated blood sugar. Although most type 2 diabetics have enough insulin production to prevent the potentially life-threatening complication ketoacidosis, it is not uncommon to see a type 2 diabetic with dangerously high blood glucose levels. These diabetics are usually placed appropriately on insulin. C-peptide levels in these people almost invariably are low, indicating serious pancreatic beta cell failure.

In other type 2 diabetics, who don't present in a crisis but still have very difficult-to-manage elevations in blood glucose, C-peptide levels can be checked for insulin deficiency. If C-peptide levels are normal or low in a poorly controlled type 2 diabetic, insulin therapy is probably the wisest choice in most cases. American ginseng extract (only the one from the University of Toronto, VV101, has been proven), *Gymnema sylvestre* extract, and fenugreek extract all enhance insulin secretion and may be tried in poorly controlled diabetics as long as blood sugar levels are only moderately elevated.

Insulin therapy in type 2 diabetes does not mean a death sentence. Since it has been shown that optimal blood sugar control is as important in type 2 diabetes as it is in type 1, insulin therapy has become increasingly used, but in selected cases where pancreatic beta cell failure has become significant (that is, where the person has a normal to low C-peptide level and, usually, is not obese). Type 2 diabetics in this category who mostly have significantly elevated fasting blood glucose elevations might benefit from one injection of intermediate-acting insulin (Humulin N) at night before bed. Supplements and often oral medications are used during the day. Those who have elevated blood sugars throughout the day might benefit by one injection of the new long-acting insulin glargine (Lantus) because of its smooth action over 24 hours. Again, supplements and often oral medications are usually used during the day. Type 2 diabetics with significantly low C-peptide levels are suffering from serious pancreatic beta cell failure and, in most cases, need to be referred for training in intensive insulin therapy. They should be treated much the same as a type 1 diabetic because, in essence, they are much the same.

Chapter Ten

Lifestyle and Attitude in Managing Diabetes

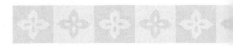

Perhaps no other condition has been as closely linked to our modern way of life as diabetes. The growing presence of both type 1 and type 2 diabetes has come about because of the influence of several dietary and lifestyle factors that are common to all developed societies. Diabetes was a rarity in cultures whose people ate diets composed entirely of wholesome, natural foods; who exercised vigorously; who lived and worked outdoors under natural sunlight; and who were exposed to a minimum of environmental pollutants. Unfortunately, economic and lifestyle factors have created thriving multitudes of consumers who congregate in polluted cities; who live sedentary, indoor lifestyles; who eat more calories than they expend; and who rely on all of the conveniences and pleasures offered to them through the powerful forces of marketing.

Addicted to the Consumer Lifestyle

For many people in our culture the comforts of inactivity and the temporary gratifications of an unnatural "junk food" diet eventually lead to the damaging and disabling effects of diabetes. Avoiding diabetes or reversing its harmful influence when it does occur is an achievable and very worthwhile goal. Many who succumb to diabetes may be addicted to the pleasures of a diet and lifestyle that will lead to pain, disability, and the degradation of good health.

Recapturing the enjoyment of vigorous health and avoiding catastrophic physical problems will require some discipline and willingness to change. Although some of these changes may be uncomfortable or difficult at first (any real change is), the payback is worth every effort. Being able to enjoy each day with the deep pleasure of true vitality is a far greater pleasure than any of the temporary pleasures that degrade our health. As well, by applying the sound principles outlined in this book, you will greatly reduce your chances of premature death and disability. If you knew that a cruel thief had made plans to break into your home, fully intending to beat and rob you, would you not take strong measures to keep this from happening? Of course you would! Diabetes can certainly be a cruel robber of health; however, this book gives you an effective strategy that you can use to thwart its merciless plan to degrade and eventually destroy the enjoyable and productive life that you were meant to live.

Choosing to Take a New Direction in Life

Frequently, throughout our years of practice, we have had the opportunity to detect diabetes for the first time in our patients. Any physician interested in preventive medicine should be on the lookout for the telltale signs of diabetes in all patients. When diabetes is first diagnosed, seriously leveling with the patient and letting the patient know that he or she must make some serious choices is usually the most successful approach.

Having diabetes is like being on a freeway that starts out smooth and without any speed limits. As time goes on, and health problems arise, the road begins to get rough (often years before diabetes is detected, when insulin resistance has begun to occur and a person starts to experience poor health). Later, as diabetes develops, potholes develop in the freeway that can damage the car (such as damage to organs that can begin to occur even before diabetes is diagnosed). If the diabetic continues down the freeway, major breaks in the road may be encountered along the way that can result in an unexpected and catastrophic end to the trip (such as heart attack, stroke, amputation, blindness, or kidney failure, all of which can result in profound disability or premature death).

As physicians, our primary goal is to help diabetic, prediabetic, or insulin-resistant patients take the first safe exit off that freeway and head in a completely new direction in their life. Of course there can still be rough spots along this new road, but we can greatly reduce their risk of harm and they can end up enjoying this new direction more than they ever did when they were on the bumpy freeway.

Developing a Winning Attitude

Helping an individual with diabetes or a prediabetic condition usually begins with strong wake-up call. Coming to grips with the fact that you are on the road to disaster is an important starting point, but it is equally important to realize that the power is in your hands to completely alter your future to achieve a much better outcome and enjoy a much better life. In dealing with diabetes it is important to realize that relying on conventional medicine alone sets in play a relentless worsening of the condition with little chance of successfully modifying the outcome.

Diabetics or those with a prediabetic condition such as impaired glucose tolerance or syndrome X need to make serious changes in their whole way of life. Rather than thinking about diabetes a great burden or dark disability, we have found it much more useful to have patients consider diabetes as a coach standing over their shoulder and helping them make the decisions they need to make to win. If the coach is standing there when you have to decide whether to eat that big piece of cheesecake with ice cream or skip your walk that day and watch TV instead, you will realize that you have to make the winner's choice and do what you need to do to achieve your positive goals.

A Personal Note from the Doctors

Both of us have a very strong genetic tendency toward obesity and diabetes, yet both of us are in great shape and fantastic health. The fact that we are both predisposed to obesity and diabetes has given us great motivation for the past 27 years to stay on a winning path. We exercise vigorously almost every day, we make wise food choices, we have a positive mental attitude, and we live with joy and passion. We are prime examples that people can overcome susceptible physiology by making the right health choices in their day-to-day lives, as we both enjoy a marvelous state of vitality and true health. For us, making the healthier lifestyle and dietary choices is a small price to pay to be able to enjoy the richness of life each day.

Breaking Down the Barriers to Change

If you have diabetes or a prediabetic condition, you will need to accept the need for change. Type 1 diabetics must accept the need for such things as intensive blood glucose monitoring and intensive insulin therapy. Type 2 diabetics or those with prediabetes or insulin resistance must be willing to look at a variety of factors that play a pivotal role in determining the outcome of their future. Research has shown that individuals with chronic illnesses who maintain an optimistic view of their life and circumstances tend to have better outcomes. Outcomes in chronic illness are also improved when individuals gain control over their illness by setting realistic goals for change.[1] Diabetes is then the perfect path to health because the diabetic has so much power in their own hands to change the direction of their condition.

Denial is a big barrier to change. As for those with addictive conditions, the first step in recovery is a willingness to see one's situation exactly as it is. Diabetics need to come to grips with the fact that their way of life is destroying their life. Most diabetics need to lose weight; if they smoke, they must stop; they cannot live a sedentary life and they must be careful about everything that goes in their mouth. These are facts and denial will not change them, so it is better face reality head on.

Depression, another common barrier to change, is a common occurrence in diabetes.[2] In fact, the diabetic brain is susceptible to clinical depression even years before diabetes is ever detected. Insulin resistance probably contributes to biochemical changes that render the brain more susceptible to depression. As well, obesity is commonly accompanied by diminished self-esteem, which can also render a person more likely to experience depression.[3] In any case, depression will erode a person's sense of self-worth and will make it very difficult for the diabetic to capture a positive winning attitude toward his or her circumstances. Diabetics suffering from even mild depression are more likely to maintain a fatalistic attitude and will find it very hard to remain motivated to make disciplined choices day after day. The catch-22 is this: If diabetes is brought under good control, depression will often diminish or disappear. On the other hand, if depression is not treated, it may be impossible to make the changes necessary for diabetes to be brought under control. Therefore, if clinical depression is evident, it is probably best to obtain adequate treatment through your physician at the same time that you embark upon the changes necessary to optimize control of blood glucose and other aspects of your diabetes.

So What Do I Need to Change?

Positive lifestyle changes hold the most important key to triumphing over diabetes. Five critical changes must occur and must be consistently maintained if you want to win good health and avoid catastrophic outcomes from diabetes. If you can achieve success with these five key areas, you will be making great strides toward achieving and maintaining good health:

1. Change your attitude
2. Learn to deal with stress
3. Don't smoke
4. Achieve ideal body weight
5. Exercise regularly

Could You Be Suffering from Depression?

Clinical depression may be present if several of these symptoms have been present consistently for at least 2 weeks:

- You're feeling down
- You find it hard not to focus on the negative
- You're feeling sad, with little energy or interest in things that used to be of interest to you
- You find it hard to concentrate
- You have a really hard time getting up in the morning, and you feel lethargic throughout the day
- You feel unable to sleep at all, or you wake up very early and can't get back to sleep
- Your appetite has gone away or you are eating just because of "nerves"

See your physician if you have noticed these or similar symptoms. Talk to him or her about opting to see a mental health expert who specializes in cognitive therapy (see page 211). If you need additional support, consider using safe and effective natural treatments for depression, such as St. John's wort extract or 5-HTP (for more information on these natural approaches to depression, see www. doctormurray.com).

The Importance of a Positive Mental Attitude

The first step in dealing with diabetes is developing a positive mental attitude. Researchers have shown that a person's attitude plays a major role in determining how well he or she deals with diabetes and blood sugar control. And since blood sugar control correlates with avoiding major complications such as heart attacks, blindness, and amputations, it is easy to conclude that attitude also determines the quality of life in diabetics as well.

As we have seen over and over in our patients' lives (and our own), it is not what happens in our lives that determines our direction; it is our *response* to those challenges that shapes the quality of our life and determines to a very large degree our level of health. Surprisingly, hardship, heartbreak, disappointment, and failure often serve as the spark for joy, ecstasy, compassion, and success. The determining factor is whether we view these challenges as stepping stones or stumbling blocks.

Fortunately, according to Martin Seligman, Ph.D., the world's leading authority on attitude and explanatory style (the manner in which we explain the events in our lives), humans are optimists by nature. Optimism is not only a necessary step toward achieving optimal health, it is critical to happiness and a higher quality of life.

Detailed evidence supports the contention that optimists live longer, suffer from fewer and less severe diseases, and are much healthier than pessimists. In a 30-year study conducted by researchers at the prestigious Mayo Clinic in Rochester, Minnesota, the survival rate among optimists was 19 percent greater than that of pessimists.[4]

To determine your level of optimism, we encourage you to take the self-assessment developed by Dr. Seligman; see Appendix E on page 308.

Our attitude is like our physical body; in order for it to be strong and positive it must be conditioned. Conditioning your attitude to be positive and optimistic means adopting specific healthy habits. Here are three key habits to help you develop a positive mental attitude:

- *Improve the way you talk to yourself.* We all conduct a constant running dialogue in our heads. In time the things we say to ourselves percolate down into our subconscious mind. Those inner thoughts, in turn, affect the way we think and feel. Naturally, if you feed yourself a steady stream of negative thoughts it will definitely have a negative impact on your mood, immune system, and quality of life. The cure is to become aware of your self-talk, and then consciously work to feed positive self-talk messages to your subconscious mind.
- *Ask better questions.* An expert in motivation, Anthony Robbins, believes that the quality of your life is equal to the quality of the questions you habitually ask yourself. For example, if you experience a setback, do you think, "Why am I so stupid? Why do bad

The Importance of Psychological Support in Diabetes

Helping people with diabetes deal with their diagnosis, develop a sense of empowerment, and make important lifestyle changes is an extremely important aspect of proper medical care. A type of psychological therapy known as cognitive therapy is emerging as the best approach, especially in people showing signs of depression. Cognitions are your whole system of thoughts, beliefs, mental images, and feelings. In the treatment of moderate depression, cognitive therapy can be as effective as the use of antidepressant drugs, and there is a lower risk of relapse—the return of depression—with cognitive therapy. One reason is that cognitive therapy teaches people practical skills they can use to combat depression any time, anywhere, every day for the rest of their lives. Cognitive therapy has proven especially effective in helping adolescents with type 1 diabetes deal with their disease, leading to improvements in both mood and blood sugar control.[5]

Mental health specialists trained in cognitive therapy seek to change the way the depressed person consciously thinks about failure, defeat, loss, and helplessness. To do so, they employ five basic tactics that help patients to do the following:

- Recognize the negative automatic thoughts that flit through consciousness at the times when they feel the worst
- Dispute the negative thoughts by focusing on contrary evidence
- Learn a different explanation to dispute the negative automatic thoughts
- Avoid rumination (the constant churning of a thought in one's mind) by helping the patient better control his or her thoughts
- Question depression-causing negative thoughts and beliefs, and replace them with empowering positive thoughts and beliefs

Cognitive therapy avoids the long, drawn-out (and expensive) process of psychoanalysis. It is a practical, solution-oriented psychotherapy that teaches skills a person can apply to improve the quality of life. If your thought processes are in need of a little rewiring, consider consulting a mental health professional who specializes in cognitive therapy.

things always happen to me?" Or do you think, "Okay, what I can learn from this situation so that it never happens again? What can I do to make the situation better?" Clearly, the latter response is healthier. Regardless of the situation, asking better questions is bound to improve your attitude. Here are some questions to start you off:

- What am I most happy about in my life right now?
- What am I most excited about in my life right now?
- What am I most grateful about in my life right now?
- What am I enjoying most in my life right now?
- What am I committed to in my life right now?
- Who do I love? Who loves me?
- What must I do today to achieve my long-term goal?

- *Set positive goals.* Learning to set achievable goals is a powerful method for building a positive attitude and raising self-esteem. Achieving goals creates a success cycle: You feel better about yourself, and the better you feel about yourself, the more likely you are to succeed. Here are some guidelines for setting health goals:
  - State the goal in positive terms and in the present tense; avoid negative words. It's better to say, "I enjoy eating healthy, low-calorie, nutritious foods" than to say, "I will not eat sugar, candy, ice cream, and other fattening foods."
  - Make your goal attainable and realistic. Start out with goals that are easily attainable, such as drinking six glasses of water a day and switching from white bread to whole wheat. By initially choosing easily attainable goals, you create a success cycle that helps build a positive self-image. Little things add up to make a major difference in the way you feel about yourself.
  - Be specific. The more clearly you define your goal, the more likely you are to reach it. For example, if you want to lose

weight, what is the weight you desire? What body fat percentage or measurements do you want to achieve?

Dealing with Stress

Stress adversely affects blood sugar control, as higher stress levels are associated with higher blood sugar levels in both type 1 and type 2 diabetes.[6] There is a very simple explanation for this phenomenon. Exposure to stress, whether it be physical, mental, or emotional, leads to activation of the "stress response" by the body and causes increases in the adrenal gland hormones adrenaline and cortisol. Among other things, these hormones cause blood sugar levels to rise and blunt the response to insulin. They also negatively affect the immune system by inhibiting white blood cells and causing the main organ of the immune system—the thymus gland—to shrink (involute). Since stress seems to be an inevitable part of modern living, it is critical to develop effective methods to deal with stress. Some studies have shown that methods such as relaxation training can improve blood sugar control, especially in individuals who are anxious or experiencing a lot of stress in their lives.[7,8]

Whether you are aware of it or not, you have developed a pattern for coping with stress. Unfortunately, most people have found patterns and methods that ultimately do not support good health. Negative coping patterns must be identified and replaced with positive strategies. Try to identify any negative or destructive coping patterns listed below that you may have developed and replace the pattern with more positive measures for dealing with stress, as shown in Table 10.1. Our experience is that in most individuals with type 2 diabetes, the most common coping pattern is overeating. Obviously, this coping pattern is not productive.

The most important coping mechanism to learn is how to calm the mind and body. In fact, it is an absolute essential in relieving stress and promoting a healthy mind, body, and attitude. Among the easiest methods to quiet the body and mind are relaxation exercises. The goal of relaxation techniques is to produce a physiological response known as *relaxation response*—a term coined by Harvard professor and cardiologist Herbert Benson, M.D., in the early 1970s to describe a physiological response. Although an individual may relax by simply sleeping, watching television, or reading a book, relaxation techniques are designed specifically to produce the relaxation response.

Table 10.1. Ways of Coping with Stress

NEGATIVE COPING PATTERNS	POSITIVE COPING STRATEGIES
Dependence on chemicals Drugs, legal and illicit Alcohol Smoking	Calming the mind Prayer Meditation Relaxation exercises
Escaping by distraction (e.g., watching television)	Physical exercise
Feelings of helplessness	Yoga or tai chi
Emotional outbursts	Constructive communication of feelings
Excessive behavior Overeating Overspending	Supporting the body's ability to deal with stress by eating healthfully

Producing the relaxation response requires breathing with the diaphragm, which dramatically changes a person's physiology by activating the relaxation centers in the brain. That translates to helping put the body and mind into proper balance. Relaxation exercises have been shown to not only help improve blood sugar control in diabetes, but also improve mood and relieve anxiety—critical goals for many diabetics. Here is a popular relaxation technique in which you breathe with your diaphragm.

1. Find a comfortable and quiet place to lie down or sit.
2. Place your feet slightly apart. Place one hand on your abdomen near your navel. Place the other hand on your chest.
3. You will be inhaling through your nose and exhaling through your mouth.
4. Concentrate on your breathing. Note which hand is rising and falling with each breath.
5. Gently exhale most of the air in your lungs.
6. Inhale while slowly counting to 4. As you inhale, slightly extend your abdomen, causing it to rise about 1 inch. Make sure that you are not moving your chest or shoulders.
7. As you breathe in, imagine the warmed air flowing in. Imagine this warmth flowing to all parts of your body.
8. Pause for 1 second, and then slowly exhale to a count of 4. As you exhale, your abdomen should move inward.

9. As the air flows out, imagine all your tension and stress leaving your body.
10. Focus on relaxing your toes and progressively move up the body as you imagine the stress melting away.
11. Repeat the process until a sense of deep relaxation is achieved.

Smoking and Diabetes—a Recipe for Disaster

Smoking and diabetes go together like nitro and glycerine! If you are diabetic and you smoke, you need to make smoking cessation the foremost goal of your life. You need to realize that the damaging effects of diabetes are multiplied over and over again if you smoke. Don't think that you escape this warning if you are only a "light" smoker. We consider a diabetic to be a heavy smoker if he or she smokes more than one cigarette per week. If you are exposed to secondhand smoke on a regular basis, it is absolutely essential to follow our dietary and supplemental strategies to protect yourself from the damaging compounds to which you are being exposed.

Quitting smoking is never easy, but it is always achievable—if 40 million Americans could do it over the last decade, you can do it too. A few simple principles can give you success over this horrible and degrading habit. First of all, let go of your denial and realize that smoking will virtually guarantee premature death and disability, especially if you are a diabetic. Smoking dramatically accelerates the progress of end organ disease (retinopathy, kidney disease, and neuropathy). It also greatly increases the likelihood that you will end up with blocked leg arteries with resulting amputation. It also greatly increases your risk of catastrophic cardiovascular events such as heart attack or stroke. Just because you don't have any chest pain now doesn't mean you are safe. At least 25 percent of the time, the first symptom of heart disease is sudden death. One minute you are here—the next minute you are gone!

Once you have come to grips with the fact that you must quit, the next step is to set a quit date. You should do this with the help and support of your physician. The quit date should be carefully decided, placed in your calendar, and made known to your physician, friends, and family members. The more accountability and leverage that you create, the more likely that you will be successful. It is best to provide at least 2 weeks between the time you decide to quit and your quit date. In that interim it probably doesn't help to cut down on your smoking. If you try to quit by gradually tapering, you will usually get to the point where you are only smoking cigarettes that you really crave. At that point, each cigarette will be especially pleasurable and will strongly reinforce your habit. It is probably better to continue smoking the same quantity as you have been right up to your quit date and then quit "cold turkey." Yes, it will be tough for a while, but the pain will pass and within a few weeks you will be free from your smoke-filled prison.

While you are counting down the days to your quit date, make a written inventory of your smoking habit. Smoking is both an addiction (to the drug nicotine and probably hundreds of other toxic chemicals in cigarette smoke) and a collection of habits that have been strongly integrated into your lifestyle. It is important that you carefully look at the various habits that make up your smoking lifestyle and develop strategies to cope with the loss of each of these small habits. For instance, if you light up a cigarette when you speak on the phone, think of a strategy to use when you quit smoking and you have to speak on the phone. For instance, instead of lighting up a smoke when you talk on the phone, get yourself a glass of water and slowly sip on the water while you're listening. The key is to purposefully enjoy the sensation of sipping water instead of smoking and tricking your brain into thinking that this is quite satisfactory.

In other situations you might have to avoid settings that trigger the desire to smoke. For instance, many smokers immediately want to light up as soon as they begin drinking a cup of coffee. The best thing to do is stop drinking coffee altogether and drink green tea instead, which is better for you anyway. You will be surprised how easy it is to quit drinking coffee if you start drinking green tea. Essentially, you must identify every subhabit embedded within your smoking habit and try to find a way to avoid the triggering behavior or replace the habit with something else. For example, if you feel that you need something in your hand, purchase one of those squishy stress balls that you typically see at checkout stands at office supply or computer supply stores. These balls are not called stress balls for nothing, as squishing them over and over during times of stress has a remarkable soothing effect. If you feel that you need something in your mouth, chew on toothpicks or chew gum.

As you approach your quit date, it is wise to purchase a supply of nicotine patches. Properly using the nicotine patch can make a huge difference in terms of the suffering that you will go through from nicotine withdrawal. The first patch goes on the morning of your quit date; generally one patch is used every day for up to 12 weeks. It is important to know that you never continue to smoke while you are using the patch. If you smoke one pack per day, start with a 21-mg patch and use one patch per day for 4 weeks; then go down to the 14-mg patch for 4 weeks; then begin the 7-mg patch for 4 weeks. If you smoke half a pack per day, you should start with the 14-mg patch. If you smoke a quarter pack per day, then start with the 7-mg patch. In all cases, it is generally wise to continue for 12 weeks; just be sure to drop down in the strength of the patch every 4 weeks until you are using a 7-mg patch, and then continue this patch until you have continued for 12 weeks in total. In general, it takes 12 weeks for the majority of addictive cravings to disappear and for major habits to be broken.

The benefit in using the nicotine patch is that it separates the nicotine addiction from the complex habit of smoking. When you quit "cold turkey" and begin using the patch, you will not have any significant nicotine withdrawal symptoms during the weeks that you are on the patch; during this time you can work on breaking the complex habits that have integrated smoking into your lifestyle. Once you have been on the 7-mg patch for 4 weeks you can usually stop with few or no nicotine withdrawal symptoms. The profound benefits achieved by quitting smoking far outweigh any minor concerns or dangers from using the nicotine patch. Even if you have heart disease, it is probably better to use a nicotine patch when you have quit smoking than to inhale one more filthy breath of smoke from the end of a cigarette.

Achieving Ideal Body Weight—the Key to Metabolic Control over Diabetes

Without a doubt, being overweight or obese is at the very heart of our diabetes epidemic. In particular, most people with type 2 diabetes are overweight or obese, which has profound implications in their management.[9] Determining the need for weight loss is one of the most important first steps in determining the treatment priorities in the diabetic. A simple measure known as the body mass index (BMI) is now the accepted

Ten Tips to Stop Smoking

1. List all the reasons why you want to quit smoking and review them daily.
2. Set a specific day to quit, tell at least ten friends that you are going to quit smoking, and then DO IT!
3. Use substitutes. Instead of smoking, chew on raw vegetables, fruits, or gum. If your fingers seem empty, play with a pencil or use one of those squishy stress balls.
4. Avoid situations that you associate with smoking.
5. When you need to relax, perform deep breathing exercises rather than reaching for a cigarette.
6. Realize that 40 million Americans have quit. If they can do it, so can you!
7. Visualize yourself as a nonsmoker with more available money, pleasant breath, unstained teeth, and the satisfaction that comes from being in control of your life.
8. Join a support group. Call the local American Cancer Society and ask for referrals. You are not alone.
9. Each day, reward yourself in a positive way. Buy yourself something with the money you've saved, or plan a special reward as a celebration for quitting.
10. Take one day at a time.

standard for classifying individuals with regard to their body composition. BMI generally correlates quite well to a person's total body fat. Your BMI can be calculated as follows:

1. $BMI = kg/m^2$ (kg = kilograms; m = height in meters) or
2. $BMI = (lbs \times 703)/in^2$ (lbs = pounds; in = height in inches)

Now calculate your BMI and consult Table 10.2 to see how you are classified.

Table 10.2. Classification of Body Mass Index

Underweight	< 18.5
Normal	18.5–24.9
Overweight	24.9–29.9
Obesity	30.0–39.9
Extreme obesity	> 40.0

Elevated blood sugar levels in type 2 diabetes results from a combination of insulin resistance, excessive production of glucose by the liver, and some degree of impairment of insulin secretion (even in the face of excessive levels of insulin, beta cells secrete insufficient insulin relative to the amount of blood glucose).[10] Weight loss in overweight or obese patients with type 2 diabetes results in a partial reversal of nearly every physiological abnormality associated with diabetes. Overall, insulin resistance begins to improve almost immediately upon weight loss—sometimes to normal levels—and in many cases of type 2 diabetes, a complete reversal of all signs of diabetes can occur.[11] Even when weight loss alone does not achieve optimal blood glucose control, an individual with type 2 diabetes who loses weight becomes much more responsive to other interventions such as supplements or medications.

People with type 2 diabetes, as well as those with type 1 diabetes who are beginning to experience insulin resistance, should aim to achieve three primary objectives in terms of weight management: prevention of weight gain, achievement of ideal body weight, and maintenance of weight loss.[12]

PREVENTION OF WEIGHT GAIN | Overweight and obesity are progressive states, and an important achievement is the avoidance of further weight gain. Without any caloric deprivation, a person can begin to develop an awareness of where excessive weight is coming from, and then he or she can develop strategies to prevent further weight gain. One of the most important things an overweight or obese person can do is to begin to record everything he or she eats or drinks in a food diary. The act of recording all intake can make an immense difference in helping to overcome "unconscious overeating." Many people who are overweight eat quickly or impulsively and often consume significant calories without even noticing what they have eaten. Maintaining a food diary and reviewing it with your physician on a regular basis can also help bring in a level of accountability and provide motivation to learn new health habits.

ACHIEVEMENT OF IDEAL BODY WEIGHT | Although everyone wants to look like a movie star, overweight and obese patients need to set more achievable goals, particularly when they are just embarking upon the weight loss program. In actual fact, achieving a 10 percent weight loss over a period of approximately 6 months is a realistic goal for most diabetics and will result in profound improvements in health. Most people will successfully lose 10 percent of their body weight by consistently learning to make wise food choices, avoiding overeating at all costs, and consistently finishing each day with a modest calorie deficit by eating slightly less than they need to maintain their weight in addition to burning some extra calories with moderate exercise. Generally, successful and long-lasting weight loss results from losing ½ to 2 pounds per week, depending on the amount of total weight to be lost (more weight lost per week when total weight loss requirements are greater). If a person can maintain a 10 percent weight loss for several months, further weight loss can be achieved until he or she reaches an ideal BMI. However, if this is done too quickly, the chances of successfully keeping the weight off is quite low. Generally, aiming to achieve a 10 percent weight loss slowly over several months through wise and sustainable dietary adjustments and moderate, regular exercise is the approach most likely to result in long-term success.

MAINTENANCE OF WEIGHT LOSS | Perhaps the most difficult goal to achieve is to maintain weight loss over the long term. Again, the keys to success lie in developing good eating habits, following the dietary principles outlined in this book, and moderate, regular exercise. The diet outlined in Chapter 7 forms an excellent foundation for prevention of weight gain, for weight loss, and for maintenance of weight loss. The low-glycemic-index/low-glycemic-load diet will avoid large surges of insulin after meals. This will also help prevent rapid drops in blood sugar 2 or 3 hours after meals, which would typically result in a ravenous appetite followed by overeating. This diet is also a high-volume diet, meaning that the high-fiber foods in this diet will fill the stomach with high volume but low calories. As well, supplementing the diet with water-soluble fiber supplements such as those made from PGX™ (discussed on pages 154–187) will bring about a profound sense of satiety (fullness) with very little contribution to daily calories. In fact, research at the University of Toronto's Risk Factor Modification Centre has shown that PGX™ given at higher doses effectively removes all hunger to the point where very few calories can be eaten in a day with little or no hunger at all.

Exercise and Diabetes

Exercise is absolutely essential in the prevention and management of diabetes as well as in prediabetic conditions such as glucose intolerance and syndrome X. Importantly, exercise as been shown to sustain weight loss more effectively than any other treatment available.[13] Exercise not only burns calories during the exercise session, it also results in a rise in the resting metabolic rate. In essence, exercise results in a rise in your personal thermostat so that you burn more calories 24 hours a day, 7 days per week, as long as you exercise nearly every day.

As well, exercise directly improves insulin sensitivity and blood sugar, probably from a combination of increased lean muscle mass and an improvement in muscle cell metabolism.[14] Exercise also has profound benefits on the cardiovascular system directly as well as indirectly by improvements in blood lipids, especially an improvement in HDL ("good") cholesterol. Exercise also decreases symptoms of anxiety and depression and improves sexual functioning, confidence, and self-esteem.

We feel that there are three important types of exercises for people with diabetes: aerobic exercise, strength training, and stretching exercises.

Aerobic exercise such as walking, jogging, aerobic dance classes, cycling, and swimming produce a rise in heart and respiratory rates. These activities are foundational in both the prevention and treatment of diabetes. You absolutely must incorporate at least 20 to 40 minutes of aerobic exercise into your daily routine. If you are not on a regular exercise program, please see Appendix G for some important guidelines. Aerobic activities should take place for ½ to 1 hour on 4 or 5 days of the week. In its simplest form, an aerobic exercise program would consist of a schedule of regular walking combined with cycling, swimming, or low-impact indoor exercise equipment such as an elliptical trainer.

Strength training should take place two or three times per week and should consist of light to moderate weights. This can be done at home with dumbbells, a compact weight machine, or even surgical rubber tubing. Fitness stores are excellent resources to show you the range of possibilities for strength training. Loss of lean body mass is a big problem for diabetics that increases with age. Losing lean muscle mass means that you have less tissue that actively absorbs glucose. The more muscle you have, the easier it is to control your blood sugar. Also, diabetics are particularly prone to developing chronic musculoskeletal complaints. Most of these problems are related to increased susceptibility to injury of joints, ligaments, and muscles as a result of loss of muscle mass.

Stretching exercises should be done daily. If you are not familiar with stretching, we recommend that you take a beginner's yoga class. If a class is not available to you, you can pick up a yoga video or well-illustrated book. Stretching is extremely important, as most people with diabetes suffer from premature stiffening of the spine and joints. Stretching on a daily basis helps you maintain flexibility and avoid the chronic pain problems that occur frequently in diabetics as a result of stiff muscles and joints.

In Appendix G we offer some key advice on how to really stick to a regular exercise program. One of the biggest mistakes that people make is thinking that they can repeat exactly the same exercise routine day after day, month after month. Unfortunately, doing the same exercise every day will almost invariably result in intolerable boredom and loss of interest in exercising. As well, if your exercise routine is monotonously repetitive, overuse or repetitive-strain injuries are much more likely. We highly recommend that you bring as much variety into your exercise routine as possible. For example, you might go for a walk twice a week, swim once a week, use a stationary bicycle in front of the television once a week, lift weights at home twice per week and stretch every morning.

Life Is Full of Choices

The question of health or disease in modern life often comes down to the habitual day-to-day choices that you have made over the years. We take these small decisions for granted, but they add up over a lifetime. Unfortunately, many of our health practices and lifestyle factors are

From Our Patient Files

Janine was a 69-year-old woman who had been on insulin for 18 years. In taking a careful medical history the first thing that really struck me was that she was started on insulin immediately upon finding sugar in her urine 18 years before. She was only 5'2" but she weighed 160 pounds at the time of her diagnosis. She now weighed 172 pounds. She was fastidious about her daily routine. Her insulin dosages were always exactly the same and given twice per day. She had her diet down to a fine science, avoiding sugar at all cost and measuring portions of food carefully with a scale. Surprisingly, she had never had a hemoglobin A_1C measurement and no one had ever suggested that she lose weight or exercise. She also had no concept of glycemic index and didn't realize that white flour products were essentially just sugar without the sweetness.

Janine's hemoglobin A_1C was 9.8, indicating that her blood sugar control was very poor even though she was on insulin and a very "controlled" diet. I checked her C-peptide levels and they were slightly elevated. This confirmed my suspicion that Janine's pancreas was still putting out insulin quite adequately even after 18 years of insulin injections. Unfortunately, an overzealous physician had placed her on insulin without any regard to the underlying causes behind her high blood sugar. I counseled her about the importance of exercise and the need for weight loss, and I spent time helping her understand the principles of the low-glycemic-index/low-glycemic-load diet.

Equipped with this new knowledge, Janine made some remarkable changes in her lifestyle. She started going to "aquacise" classes four times per week and she went for a walk on most other days, weather permitting. I showed her how to do some basic resistance exercises using surgical tubing and I went over some simple stretching exercises. She also began to eat a low-glycemic-index/low-glycemic-load diet, and we aimed for a 250- to 300-calorie-per-day deficit in addition to the exercise. She had to carefully monitor her blood sugar, and over the next few weeks she had to decrease her insulin dosage several times. Within 3 months she was taking only 5 units of intermediate-acting insulin every morning, and I suggested at this time that she stop her insulin altogether. Her blood sugar occasionally rose moderately but never to the point where there was pressure to put her on oral medication or back on insulin. Within six months she had lost 25 pounds and she felt better than she had in years. By that time I had initiated a supplement program and her blood sugars consistently stayed within an optimal range. Her hemoglobin A_1C after 6 months was 6.9, clear evidence that her blood sugars were in good control.

Janine took on a winning attitude and she was able to change the course of her life in a profound way. I only wished that I had seen her 18 years earlier!!

based on habit and marketing hype. The health practices and lifestyles of our parents usually become intricately woven into the fabric of our own lifestyles. Meanwhile, a great deal of time, energy, and money is spent to market bad health practices. The mass media constantly bombard us with messages affecting health, diet, and lifestyle. We urge you to ignore these messages and instead make a commitment to achieving optimal health. Build a strong foundation by making healthy choices over less healthy ones. By choosing to be positive, choosing to eat for optimum health, choosing to lead a health-promoting lifestyle, and choosing to support your body chemistry through proper nutritional supplementation, you are building a strong foundation for achieving ideal health and a long life, and, if needed, setting the stage for a possible cure.

Final Comments

Overall, the trend today is moving toward a more aggressive approach to managing blood glucose in diabetes. Oral medications are often prescribed in combinations of two or three and insulin, which was seldom being used in type 2 diabetics a few years ago, has been making a comeback as studies clearly demonstrate the benefits of optimal blood glucose control. Overall, our suggestion is for you to do as much as you can with the recommendations we make for lifestyle, diet, and weight loss. We also recommend that you work with the supplement programs that we have described and carefully monitor your blood sugar. If your blood sugar is still poorly controlled, medications and/or insulin may be required. Our goal is to help you find ways to improve your diabetes with every possible means, as long as it leads to benefits to your long-term health. Natural medicine may not provide all of the answers for every diabetic, but no diabetic should just rely on conventional drugs or insulin to manage his or her diabetes. Diet, lifestyle, and wise supplementation should always play an important role.

Part Three

Prevention and Treatment

of Diabetic Complications

Chapter Eleven

Diabetic Complications:
An Overview

Diabetes is such a serious medical condition because it wreaks havoc on the body's attempt to maintain homeostasis. The literal definition of this term is "same standing." Basically, homeostasis refers to all of the built-in checks and balances within the body and its cells designed to maintain a consistent internal environment. Every organism on the planet, from the simplest single-celled amoeba to a human being, relies on homeostasis to sustain life.

In diabetes, elevated blood sugar levels and the loss of sensitivity to insulin make it difficult or nearly impossible for cells to maintain homeostasis. The result is disease and complications. The complications of diabetes are divided into two major categories—acute and chronic.

Acute and Long-Term Complications of Diabetes

Acute Complications

- Hypoglycemia
- Diabetic ketoacidosis
- Nonketotic hyperosmolar hyperglycemia

Long-Term (Chronic) Complications

- Atherosclerosis and other vascular lesions
- Retinopathy and cataracts
- Neuropathy
- Nephropathy
- Poor wound healing
- Foot ulcers

Acute Complications

The acute complications of diabetes represent a medical emergency and a possible life-or-death situation. Any diabetic experiencing any symptom even remotely suggestive of an acute complication of diabetes should seek medical care immediately. The major acute complications of diabetes are hypoglycemia, ketoacidosis, and nonketotic hyperosmolar hyperglycemia.

Hypoglycemia, usually seen in type 1 diabetes, results from taking too much insulin, missing a meal, or overexercising. Severe hypoglycemia can also occur unpredictably in patients with "brittle" type 1 diabetes or in any diabetic on insulin or sulfonylurea drugs who neglects the need for proper monitoring of blood glucose. Daytime hypoglycemic episodes are usually recognized by the following symptoms: sweating, nervousness, tremor, and hunger. Nighttime hypoglycemia may be without symptoms or may manifest as night sweats, unpleasant dreams, or early morning headache. For information on the prevention and treatment of hypoglycemia, see pages 170–171.

Diabetic ketoacidosis is also more likely to occur in poorly controlled or untreated type 1 diabetes. The lack of insulin leads to extremely high blood sugar and a buildup of acidic ketone molecules in the body. If progressive, ketoacidosis can result in numerous metabolic problems and even coma or death. Since ketoacidosis is a medical emergency, prompt recognition is imperative. The coma is usually preceded by a day or more of increased urination and thirst as well as marked fatigue, nausea, and vomiting. A simple urine dipstick can be used at home by diabetics to measure the level of ketones in the urine. This procedure should be done during illness or severe stress. Inexperienced medical personnel occasionally make the mistake of not giving insulin to a type 1 diabetic who is fasting before surgery. This mistake can also be made at home by a misinformed diabetic who is too sick too eat. Generally, the stress of illness or surgery is sufficient to drive blood sugar up even when no food is taken. This is because the stress hormones cortisol and epinephrine (adrenaline) result in a massive release of glucose from the liver and muscles, and usual insulin doses are generally required.

Nonketotic hyperosmolar hyperglycemia is a very serious condition that occurs when blood sugar rises to extreme levels, usually in type 2 diabetics with some insulin production or type 1 diabetics who are receiving inadequate levels of insulin for their acute situation. Usually this occurs in already debilitated diabetics and it often evolves over days or weeks, resulting in severe dehydration and disturbances of electrolytes such as sodium and potassium. If the patient presents in a comatose state, this condition carries with it a mortality rate of over 50 percent. It is usually the result of deficient fluid intake and inadequate insulin to compensate for precipitating events such as pneumonia, burns, stroke, a recent operation, or certain drugs such as phenytoin, diazoxide, glucocorticoids, and diuretics. Symptoms include weakness, increased urination and thirst, and progressively worse signs of dehydration (weight loss, loss of skin elasticity, dry mucous membranes, rapid heartbeat, and low blood pressure). This condition is completely preventable by regular blood glucose monitoring, especially during times of illness or stress.

Long-Term (Chronic) Complications

Much more common than the acute complications of diabetes are certain long-term complications.

Atherosclerosis and other vascular lesions are the underlying factors in the development of many of the chronic complications of diabetes. Individuals with diabetes have a risk of dying prematurely of heart disease or stroke that is two to three times that of a nondiabetic individual; 55 percent of deaths in diabetes patients are caused by cardiovascular disease. Lesions to the microvascular system (small blood vessels) lead to reduced delivery of oxygen and nutrients to important tissue such as nerves, the eyes, and the kidneys.

Retinopathy of diabetes is a serious eye disease involving the retina—the collection of light-sensitive cells lining the back half of each eye. Diabetic retinopathy is the leading cause of blindness in the United States for people between ages 20 and 64. In diabetic retinopathy, the retina is damaged by microhemorrhages, scarring, and the attachment of glucose molecules (glycosylation) to structural proteins in the retina. Studies have shown that 20 years after the diagnosis of diabetes, 80 percent of type 1 and 20 percent of type 2 diabetics have significant retinopathy. Diabetics are also prone to *cataracts*—opacities that occur in the lens of the eye as a result of damage to the delicate protein structures of the lens.

Neuropathy (nerve disease) usually refers to the loss of peripheral nerve function and is characterized by tingling sensations, numbness, loss of function, and a characteristic burning pain known as neuropathic pain. Diabetic neuropathy first involves a subtle loss of sensation in the hands and feet in a pattern known as "stoking-glove" neuropathy. If it progresses, the neuropathy can affect deeper nerves of the autonomic nervous system, resulting in disturbances in stomach emptying, and later on, impaired heart function, alternating bouts of diarrhea and constipation, and inability to empty the bladder. Impotence is a very common occurrence and is caused by a damage to the small blood vessels of the penis combined with neuropathy of autonomic nerves controlling blood flow into the penis. Approximately 60 percent of all people with diabetes will eventually develop neuropathy.

Nephropathy (kidney disease) due to diabetes accounts for 40 percent of the cases of severe kidney disease and is the most common reason for hemodialysis and kidney transplant. In addition to monitoring blood sugar levels, it is important to monitor kidney function through various laboratory measurements (microalbuminuria, 24-hour urine protein, BUN, uric acid, creatinine, and creatinine clearance); see pages 266–267 for more information.

Poor wound healing is common in diabetes for several reasons, such as microvascular changes leading to poor circulation and functional deficiency of vitamin C (see pages 268–269 for more information).

Foot ulcers are common in individuals with diabetes due to the microvascular changes leading to a lack of blood supply, peripheral neuropathy, poor wound healing, and immune system dysfunction leading to chronic infections in the feet. More than 50 percent of cases of lower-limb amputation in the United States (70,000 each year) are due to diabetic foot ulcers.

Immune system dysfunction often begins to occur long before a diagnosis of diabetes is made. In fact, a recurrent vaginal or skin yeast infection is the clue that leads to the detection of diabetes in many cases. Immune system problems are made worse by poor glucose control, which puts the diabetic at risk for serious infections or complications of simple infections. For example, diabetics are far more likely to develop secondary pneumonia while recovering from influenza. Susceptibility to chronic, hidden infections may be a primary reason for increased risk of heart disease in diabetics. C-reactive protein, a measurement of smoldering inflammation, is often elevated in diabetics; this may be due, at least in part, to chronic infections of the oral cavity, respiratory tract, or blood.

Depression and cognitive difficulties are very common in diabetics. In fact, depression may begin to occur decades before the onset of type 2 diabetes when the individual first develops insulin resistance. The brain is more sensitive than any organ to its need for glucose, and it appears that brain cells may suffer from some degree of glucose deprivation when insulin resistance occurs.[1] Depression is also much more common in overweight and obese individuals, probably due to a combined effect from insulin resistance and diminished self-esteem. Cognitive changes begin to occur after the first severe hypoglycemic episode in diabetics. Hypoglycemia is profoundly stressful to the brain and, if severe hypoglycemia occurs many times, significant cognitive impairment is inevitable. Blood glucose awareness training has successfully helped thousands of diabetics avoid serious hypoglycemia. Frequent blood glucose monitoring and the use of the new immediate-acting and long-duration insulins have allowed optimal blood glucose control to be maintained without increasing the risk for serious hypoglycemia.

Contributors to the Long-Term Complications of Diabetes

While achieving good blood glucose control is a primary goal in preventing complications, so too is ensuring optimal nutritional status and using natural products that address some of the key mechanisms that create the complications. Here are the major contributors to the long-term complications of diabetes, followed by a brief description of each factor along with measures to deal with it:

- Poor glucose control
- Glycosylation of proteins
- Intracellular accumulation of sorbitol
- Increased oxidative damage
- Nutrient deficiency
- Homocysteine
- High blood pressure

Poor Glucose Control

A large body of evidence indicates that good blood sugar control significantly reduces the development of complications. The largest and most extensive study to date in type 1 diabetes is the Diabetes Control and Complications Trial (DCCT), while the largest and longest study on patients with type 2 diabetes is the United Kingdom Prospective Diabetes Study (UKPDS). Both of these studies conclusively demonstrated that improved blood glucose control reduces the risk of developing the long-term complications of diabetes, especially retinopathy, nephropathy, and neuropathy. Maintaining your hemoglobin A_1C levels near to normal (7.0 percent or less) can dramatically help to reduce your risk of eye problems (up to 76 percent), nerve damage (up to 60 percent), and kidney disease (up to 56 percent).

Glycosylation of Proteins

As described previously, glycosylation refers to the binding of glucose to proteins. The poorer the glucose control, the greater the binding, which leads to changes in the structure and function of the protein. Excessive glycosylation has many adverse effects: inactivation of enzymes, inhibition of regulatory molecule binding, and the formation of abnormal protein structures, to name a few. For example, when glucose molecules bind to cholesterol-carrying low-density-lipoprotein (LDL) molecules, it blocks the LDL from binding to receptors on the liver that essentially tell the liver to quit manufacturing cholesterol. As a result, the liver thinks there is a shortage of cholesterol in the body so it keeps making more and dumping it into the blood. That is one reason why diabetes is almost always associated with high cholesterol levels.

In addition to keeping blood sugar levels as close to ideal as possible, high intakes of antioxidants—especially vitamins C and E, flavonoids, and alpha-lipoic acid (discussed on page 238)—help to reduce glycosylation.

Intracellular Accumulation of Sorbitol

Sorbitol is a sugar molecule that is formed from glucose within cells. In people without diabetes, once sorbitol is formed it is quickly broken down into fructose, another simple sugar. This conversion to fructose is critical because it allows any excess sorbitol to be excreted from the cell, and sorbitol cannot exit the cell once it is formed. Increased sorbitol levels within cells create an osmotic effect.

Osmosis refers to the movement of water molecules from an area of high concentration to an area of low concentration. The cell works hard to maintain the concentration of water within cells. When there is an increase in the concentration of soluble compounds (such as sorbitol) that the cell can't get rid of, the cell will leak out small molecules such as amino acids, inositol, glutathione, niacin, vitamin C, magnesium, and potassium to maintain osmotic balance. Since these compounds function to protect cells from damage, their loss results in increased susceptibility to damage.

Intracellular accumulation of sorbitol is a major factor in the develop-

Vitamin C—an Efficient Way
to Lower Sorbitol Levels

Attempts to prevent sorbitol accumulation with drugs have failed due to severe side effects. In contrast, vitamin C is able to accomplish what these drugs could not—safe and effective inhibition of sorbitol accumulation.

In one study in young adults with type 1 diabetes, baseline measurement of sorbitol in red blood cells were nearly double in these patients despite "adequate" dietary intakes of vitamin C. Vitamin C supplementation at a dosage of either 100 or 600 mg normalized sorbitol in red blood cells within 30 days. This correction of sorbitol accumulation was independent of changes in diabetic control as monitored by fasting glucose or hemoglobin A_1C. In fact, overall diabetic control during the study was moderate to poor, indicating that the effect of vitamin C was not dependent on glucose concentration.

These results indicate that vitamin C may inhibit aldose reductase, the enzyme that converts glucose to sorbitol. A test-tube study was conducted to determine the necessary concentration of vitamin C required to inhibit aldose reductase in red blood cells.[2] At concentrations above 100 micromoles, vitamin C reduced sorbitol production by about 30 percent. Levels between 600 and 900 micromoles reduced sorbitol production by about 50 percent. Are these concentrations of vitamin C attainable with supplementation with vitamin C? Absolutely; in fact, the normal level of vitamin C in the plasma and red blood cells is 40 to 120 micromoles. One of the reasons that we recommend 500 to 1,500 mg of vitamin C daily is to boost blood levels into the higher range to inhibit sorbitol production. Remember that the transport of vitamin C into cells is facilitated by insulin, and as a result many diabetics do not have enough intracellular vitamin C. Therefore, a relative vitamin C deficiency exists in many diabetics despite adequate dietary consumption. Supplementation is required.

Sorbitol—the Sweetener

You may recognize sorbitol as a sweetener found in numerous food products—especially sugar-free chewing gum, because it has a smooth feel in the mouth with a sweet, cool, and pleasant taste. It is also used in many sugar-free or "dietetic" candies, cake mixes, syrups, and other foods. Sorbitol is about 60 percent as sweet as sucrose with one-third fewer calories (2.6 calories per gram versus 4.0 for sugar). It does not cause cavities, and because it is absorbed quite slowly and has a low glycemic index, it is perfectly fine as a sweetener for diabetics as are other "polyol" sweeteners such as xylitol, mannitol, and maltitol.

Polyol sweeteners are extremely safe at moderate dosages. However, because they are poorly absorbed at higher dosages (more than 10 grams daily) they can cause gastrointestinal symptoms ranging from mild discomfort to severe diarrhea. Children, because of their smaller size, may be affected by even smaller amounts. Currently, the FDA requires a laxative notice only on the few products that may lead to the consumption of 50 grams or more of sorbitol daily, though some companies voluntarily label additional products.

ment of the majority of the complications of diabetes, as evidenced by the fact that elevated sorbitol levels are found in high concentrations in the tissues commonly involved in the major diabetic complications: the lens of the eye, nerve cells, kidney cells, and the cells that line blood vessels.

In addition to controlling blood sugar levels, vitamin C, flavonoids such as quercetin, grapeseed extract, and bilberry extract can help lower intracellular sorbitol levels.

Increased Oxidative Damage

Increased oxidative stress is a major factor in the risk of the chronic complications of diabetes. As previously stated, individuals with diabetes typically have elevated levels of free radicals and oxidative compounds.[3] These highly reactive compounds bind to and destroy cellular compounds. They also greatly increase the inflammatory process by adding fuel to their destructive fire via increased formation of inflammatory mediators such as C-reactive protein.[4] One of the critical goals in diabetes prevention and treatment is to flood the body with a high level of antioxidant compounds to counteract the negative effects of free radicals and pro-oxidants. The implementation of this goal is achieved by following the dietary and supplement strategies given. In addition to the

Alpha-Lipoic Acid—Nature's Perfect Antioxidant

Alpha-lipoic acid is a vitamin-like substance that is often described as "nature's perfect antioxidant." First of all, alpha-lipoic acid is a very small molecule that is efficiently absorbed and easily crosses cell membranes. Unlike vitamin E, which is primarily fat-soluble, and vitamin C, which is water-soluble, alpha-lipoic acid can quench either water- or fat-soluble free radicals both inside the cell and outside in the intracellular spaces. Furthermore, alpha-lipoic acid extends the biochemical life of vitamin C and E as well as other antioxidants.

Alpha-lipoic acid is an approved drug in Germany for the treatment of diabetic neuropathy. In fact, it has been successfully used in Germany for more than 30 years. The beneficial effects of alpha-lipoic acid in diabetic neuropathy have been confirmed in several double-blind studies at a dosage of 300 to 600 mg daily.[5,6] Although alpha-lipoic acid's primary effect in improving diabetic neuropathy is thought to be the result of its antioxidant effects, it has also been shown to lead to an improvement in blood sugar metabolism, improve blood flow to peripheral nerves, and actually stimulate the regeneration of nerve fibers. Its ability to improve blood sugar metabolism is a result of its effects on glucose metabolism and an ability to increase insulin sensitivity. Its importance in treating diabetic neuropathy cannot be overstated.

basic supplementation program, supplementing the diet with super antioxidants such as alpha-lipoic acid and flavonoid-rich extracts is often useful in boosting antioxidant protection even more.

Nutrient Deficiency

As detailed in Chapter 7, people with diabetes have an increased need for many nutrients. A deficiency of any one of several nutrients has been shown to contribute to several chronic complications of diabetes. In general, it is very safe to say that the risk of long-term complications of diabetes is inversely proportional to micronutrient status. In other words, the risk of diabetic complications increases in proportion to the degree of nutrient deficiency. For example, the lower the levels of magnesium, the greater the severity of diabetic retinopathy.

Sometimes the symptoms of a nutrient deficiency can mimic very closely a chronic complication of diabetes. For example, vitamin B_{12} deficiency is characterized by numbness, pins-and-needles sensations, or a burning feeling in the hands and/or feet—symptoms virtually identical to diabetic neuropathy. Although vitamin B_{12} supplementation has been used with some success in treating diabetic neuropathy, it is really not clear if this success is due to correction of a B_{12} deficiency or the normalization of the deranged vitamin B_{12} metabolism seen in diabetics.

Again, we strongly assert that high-potency multiple vitamin and mineral supplementation is an absolute must in the management of diabetes. Supplying the diabetic with additional key nutrients improves blood sugar control and reduces the development of the major long-term complications of diabetes. Follow the guidelines given in Appendix H, pages 325–327, to ensure optimal intake of micronutrients.

Homocysteine

Homocysteine is a potentially harmful compound formed in the conversion of the amino acid methionine to cysteine. If a person is relatively deficient in folic acid, vitamin B_6, or vitamin B_{12}, there will be an increase in the level of homocysteine. This compound has been implicated in a variety of conditions, including atherosclerosis. Homocysteine is thought to promote atherosclerosis by directly damaging the artery and by reducing the integrity of the vessel wall, as well as by interfering with the formation of collagen (the main protein in connective tissue and bone).

Elevated homocysteine levels are an independent risk factor for heart attack, stroke, and peripheral vascular disease. In addition, recent research has implicated elevations of homocysteine in the development of the long-term complications of diabetes, especially diabetic retinopathy.[7]

Although folic acid has received the most attention as a nutritional supplement to lower homocysteine levels, several studies have shown quite clearly that the best reductions are seen when vitamin B_6 and B_{12} are supplemented along with folic acid. A good high-potency multiple vitamin and mineral should provide sufficient levels to see significant reductions in homocysteine levels.

High Blood Pressure

Blood pressure control is essential in preventing the complications of diabetes, especially kidney disease, retinopathy, and stroke. Maintaining blood pressure in the normal range (120/80) can reduce the risk of heart disease and stroke by approximately 33 to 50 percent and can reduce microvascular disease (eye, kidney, and nerve disease) by approximately 33 percent in patients with diabetes. More than half of all diabetics have high blood pressure.

Ultimately, the health of the artery is critical to maintaining normal blood pressure. Endothelial cell (cells that line arteries) dysfunction can lead to stiffening of arteries because normally endothelial cells produce nitric oxide, which relaxes the blood vessel wall. Also, when arteries become hard due to the buildup of plaque containing cholesterol and calcium, blood pressure increases due to arterial stiffness and narrowing. Therefore, it is very important to promote healthy arteries. The development of high blood pressure is closely related to lifestyle and dietary factors. Some important lifestyle factors that may cause high blood pressure include stress, lack of exercise, and smoking. Some of the dietary factors include obesity; a high sodium-to-potassium ratio; a low-fiber, high-sugar diet; a high saturated fat and low omega-3 fatty acid intake; and a diet low in calcium, magnesium, and vitamin C.

A Little DASH Goes a Long Way

The Dietary Approaches to Stop Hypertension (DASH) clinical studies are landmark studies funded by the National Heart, Lung, and Blood Institute (NHLBI) to fully evaluate the efficacy of a system of dietary recommendations in the treatment of hypertension. The DASH diet is rich in fruits, vegetables, and low-fat dairy foods, and low in saturated and total fat. It also is low in cholesterol; high in dietary fiber, potassium, calcium, and magnesium; and moderately high in protein. It is quite similar to the dietary program that we describe in Chapter 7.

The first DASH study showed that a diet rich in fruits, vegetables, and low-fat dairy products can reduce blood pressure in the general population and in people with hypertension.[8] The original DASH diet did not require either sodium restriction or weight loss—the two traditional dietary tools to control blood pressure—to be effective. The second study from the DASH research group found that coupling the original DASH diet with sodium restriction is more effective than either dietary manipulation alone.[9] In the first trial, the DASH diet produced a net blood pressure reduction of 11.4 points systolic and 5.5 points diastolic in patients with hypertension. In the second trial, sodium intake was also quantified at a "higher" intake of 3,300 mg per day; an "intermediate" intake of 2,400 mg per day; and a "lower" intake of 1,500 mg per day.

Compared to the control diet, the DASH diet was associated with a significantly lower systolic blood pressure at each sodium level. The DASH diet with the lower sodium level led to an average systolic blood pressure that was 7.1 points lower in participants without hypertension, and 11.5 points lower in participants with hypertension. These results are clinically significant and indicate that a sodium intake below the recommended level of 2,400 mg daily can significantly and quickly lower blood pressure.

Special foods for people with high blood pressure include celery, garlic and onions, nuts and seeds or their oils for their essential fatty acid content, cold-water fish (salmon, mackerel, and so on) or fish oil products concentrated for EPA and DHA, green leafy vegetables for their rich source of calcium and magnesium, whole grains and legumes for their fiber, and foods rich in vitamin C such as broccoli and citrus fruits.

Celery is a particularly interesting recommendation for high blood pressure. Two researchers at the University of Chicago Medical Center have performed studies on a compound found in celery, 3-n-butylphthalide (3nB), and found that it can lower blood pressure. In animals, a very small amount of 3nB lowered blood pressure by 12 to 14 percent.[10] The research was prompted by the father of one of the researchers, who after eating a quarter pound of celery every day for one week observed that his blood pressure dropped from 158/96 to a normal reading of 118/82. If you do not want to eat that much celery, you can take celery seed extract standardized to contain 85 percent 3nB at a dosage of 150 mg daily. 3nB appears to help lower blood pressure by acting as both a diuretic and a vasodilator by acting in a similar manner to drugs known as calcium channel blockers. 3nB has also been shown to lower blood cholesterol levels and reduce the formation of arterial plaque in experimental studies (animal and test-tube studies).[11] This effect increases the elasticity of the blood vessels and leads to lower blood pressure readings.

Garlic and onions are also important foods for lowering blood pressure. Although most recent research has focused on the cholesterol-lowering properties of garlic and onions, both have also been shown to lower blood pressure. Both garlic and onion should be used liberally in the diet. In addition, taking a garlic supplement that delivers at least 4,000 mcg of allicin daily may also be of benefit.[12]

POTASSIUM | It is a well-established fact that excessive consumption of dietary sodium chloride, coupled with diminished dietary potassium, is a common cause of high blood pressure, especially in "salt-sensitive" individuals. However, numerous studies have shown that sodium restriction alone does not significantly improve blood pressure control in most people—it must be accompanied by a high potassium intake. In a typical Western diet, only 5 percent of sodium intake comes from the natural constituents in food. Prepared foods contribute 45 percent of the sodium intake, 45 percent is added during cooking, and another 5 percent is added as a condiment.

Many studies have now shown that increasing dietary potassium intake or taking a potassium supplement can lower blood pressure.[13] Results from thirty-three clinical trials with 2,609 participants in which potassium supplementation was the only difference between the intervention and control conditions were used in one analysis. Potassium supplementation was associated with significant reductions in average blood pressure (4.44 points systolic and 2.45 points diastolic). However, some of the studies showed that potassium supplementation can lower systolic and diastolic blood pressure an average of 12 to 16 points.

Potassium supplements are available by prescription as well as over the counter (OTC). However, the FDA restricts the amount of potassium available in OTC potassium supplements to a mere 99 mg per dose because of problems associated with high-dosage prescription potassium salts, yet so-called salt substitutes such as the popular brands NoSalt and Nu-Salt are in fact potassium chloride and provide 530 mg of potassium per ⅙ teaspoon. Potassium salts are commonly prescribed in the dosage range of 1.5 to 3.0 grams per day. That dosage would translate to ½ to 1 teaspoon of NoSalt or Nu-Salt. Potassium supplementation is relatively safe, except for patients with kidney disease. Their inability to maintain appropriate potassium homeostasis may result in heart arrhythmias and other consequences of potassium toxicity. Potassium supplementation is also contraindicated when using a number of prescription medications, including digitalis, potassium-sparing diuretics, and the angiotensin-converting enzyme inhibitor class of antihypertensive drugs (ACE inhibitors).

MAGNESIUM | Potassium interacts in many body systems with magnesium, and low intracellular potassium levels may be the result of low magnesium intake. It is therefore appropriate to supplement magnesium (400 to 1,200 mg per day in divided dosages) along with potassium in diabetics with high blood pressure. A detailed analysis of fourteen clinical trials that tested the effects of magnesium supplementation on hypertension demonstrated that magnesium can lower systolic and diastolic blood pressure by 4 to 10 points.[14] However, our experience and the results from individual studies indicate that the hypertensive patients who respond best are those that have type 2 diabetes or who are taking a diuretic, have low magnesium levels, and have a high sodium-to-potassium ratio.

ANTI-ACE FISH PEPTIDES | The most effective natural product for lowering blood pressure currently available is a mixture of nine small peptides (proteins) derived from bonito (a member of the tuna family). It works to lower blood pressure by inhibiting ACE (angiotensin-converting enzyme), thereby inhibiting the formation of angiotensin II, a substance that increases both the fluid volume and the degree of constriction of the blood vessels. If we use a garden hose model, angiotensin II would be similar to pinching off the hose while turning up the faucet full blast. By inhibiting the formation of this compound, anti-ACE peptides relax the arterial walls and reduce fluid volume. Anti-ACE fish peptides exert the strongest inhibition of ACE reported for any naturally occurring substance available.

Three major clinical studies have been conducted with anti-ACE fish peptides.[15,16] The material appears to be effective in about two-thirds of people with high blood pressure—about the same percentage as many prescription drugs. The degree of blood pressure reduction in these studies was quite significant, typically reducing the systolic by at least 10 points and the diastolic by 7 points in people with borderline and mild hypertension. The typical dosage is three 500-mg capsules daily. No side effects were reported in the clinical studies, and a safety study showed no side effects with no dosages as high as 30 grams daily.

Anti-ACE fish peptides do not affect blood pressure in people without hypertension, do not interact negatively with potassium, and have no adverse drug interactions, so they can be used in combination with conventional antihypertensive drugs.

IF ADDITIONAL SUPPORT IS NEEDED TO LOWER BLOOD PRESSURE | It is extremely important to get blood pressure below 135/85 to reduce the risk of diabetic complications. In attempting to achieve this goal, sometimes conventional blood-pressure-lowering drugs are required. Currently most patients with type 2 diabetes are on at least three drugs to try to control their blood pressure. That is not good because these drugs are not without side effects. The four major categories of blood-pressure-lowering drugs are diuretics, beta-blockers, calcium channel blockers, and ACE inhibitors.

Daily Supplementation Strategies
for Lowering Blood Pressure

For Borderline Hypertension (130–139/85–89)

Foundational supplements
Potassium chloride—1,500 to 3,000 mg
Magnesium—150 to 400 mg three times daily
PGX™—1,000 mg before meals three times daily
Garlic—4,000 mcg of allicin

(*Note:* If after 2 months there is no change, add anti-ACE fish peptides—1,500 mg daily. If after 2 months there is still no change, discontinue anti-ACE fish peptides and replace with celery seed extract—150 mg daily.)

For Mild (140–160/90–104) to Moderate (140–180/105–114) Hypertension

Foundational supplements
Potassium chloride—1,500 to 3,000 mg
Magnesium—150 to 400 mg three times daily
PGX™—1,000 mg before meals three times daily
Garlic—4,000 mcg of allicin
Anti-ACE fish peptides—1,500 mg daily

(*Note:* If after 2 months there is no change, add celery seed extract—150 mg daily. If there is still no change, add coenzyme Q10—100 mg daily. If blood pressure has not dropped below 140/105, you will need to work with a physician to select the most appropriate medication. If a prescription drug is necessary, calcium channel blockers or ACE inhibitors appear to be the safest for diabetics.)

For Severe Hypertension (160+/115+)

Consult a physician immediately.
Foundational supplements
Potassium chloride—1,500 to 3,000 mg
Magnesium—150 to 400 mg three times daily
PGX™—1,000 mg before meals three times daily
Garlic—4,000 mcg of allicin
Anti-ACE fish peptides—1,500 mg daily
Celery seed extract—150 mg daily
Coenzyme Q10—100 mg daily

(*Note:* A drug may be necessary to achieve initial control. When satisfactory control over the high blood pressure has been achieved, work with the physician to taper off the medication.)

Diuretics lower blood pressure by reducing the volume of fluid in the blood and body tissues by promoting the elimination of salt and water through increased urination. In addition, diuretics also work to relax the smaller arteries of the body, allowing them to expand and increase the total fluid capacity of the arterial system. The net result of diuretics is lower pressure due to reduced volume in an expanded space.

There are important side effects to look for with all diuretics. The typical side effects of these drugs are increased blood sugar levels, lightheadedness, increased uric acid levels and aggravation of gout, and muscle weakness and cramps caused by low potassium levels. Decreased libido and impotence are also reported. Less frequent side effects include allergic reactions, headache, blurred vision, nausea, vomiting, and diarrhea.

Beta-blockers are drugs that block the binding of adrenaline (catecholamines) on beta-receptors on the heart and blood vessels, resulting in a reduced rate and force of contraction of the heart as well as relaxing the arteries. Beta-blockers have fallen out of favor due to a lack of effectiveness in reducing cardiovascular mortality as well as an increased risk of developing diabetes by about 30 percent.[17]

Beta-blockers produce some significant side effects in many patients. Because the amount of blood being pumped by the heart is reduced in a more relaxed arterial system, it is often difficult to get enough blood and oxygen to the hands, feet, and brain. This results in some typical symptoms in users of beta-blockers such as cold hands and feet, nerve tingling, impaired mental function, fatigue, dizziness, depression, lethargy, reduced libido, and impotence. Beta-blockers may also reduce HDL ("good" cholesterol). This effect may explain some of the negative effects in the clinical studies that failed to demonstrate any significant benefit of beta-blockers in reducing mortality from cardiovascular disease.

The other concern with beta-blockers in diabetics is that they can block the early symptoms of hypoglycemia mediated by adrenaline (sweating, shakiness, increased heart rate, weakness). This occurrence means that hypoglycemia can occur and a diabetic on a beta-blocker may not perceive the hypoglycemia it until it is too late to do anything. Beta-blockers may also worsen insulin resistance.

It is extremely important that a beta-blocker not be discontinued suddenly. Stopping the medication suddenly can produce a withdrawal syndrome consisting of headache, increased heart rate, and dramatic increase in blood pressure.

Calcium channel blockers, along with the ACE inhibitors, have taken over the top spots in the drug treatment of high blood pressure because they are better tolerated than diuretics and beta-blockers. While calcium channel blockers have been shown to lower the risk for strokes, they carry the same increased risk for heart attacks as the older approach of diuretics and beta-blockers.

Calcium channel blockers work by blocking the normal passage of calcium through certain channels in cell walls. Since calcium is required in the function of nerve transmission and muscle contraction, the effect of blocking the calcium channel is to slow down nerve conduction and inhibit the contraction of the muscle. In the heart and vascular system, this action results in reducing the rate and force of contraction, relaxing the arteries, and slowing the nerve impulses in the heart.

Although much better tolerated than beta-blockers and diuretics, calcium channel blockers still produce some mild side effects, including constipation, allergic reactions, fluid retention, dizziness, headache, fatigue, and impotence (about 20 percent of users). More serious side effects include disturbances of heart rate or function, heart failure, and angina.

ACE inhibitors work to block ACE (angiotensin-converting enzyme) in the formation of angiotensin II, a substance that increases both the fluid volume and the degree of constriction of the blood vessels. ACE inhibitors relax the arterial walls and reduce fluid volume. Unlike the beta-blockers and calcium channel blockers, however, ACE inhibitors actually improve heart function and increase blood and oxygen flow to the heart, liver, and kidneys. This effect may explain why ACE inhibitors are the only antihypertensive drugs that appear to reduce the risk of having a heart attack.[18] Unfortunately, they do not have any effect on reducing the risk for strokes.

The newer ACE inhibitors are generally very well tolerated, but share many of the same side effects as the other antihypertensives, including dizziness, light-headedness, and headache. The most common side effect is the development of a dry nighttime cough. ACE inhibitors can also cause potassium buildup and kidney problems (only if the arteries

---

ACE Inhibitors Are Now Given Prophylactically

It is now very common for diabetics to be placed on a very low dose of an ACE inhibitor drug (such as 2.5 mg Vasotec per day) because of the effects that these agents have in protecting the diabetic kidney from nephropathy (diabetic kidney disease). Because the evidence in favor of this intervention is so strong, and because the dosages used are so small that side effects are very unlikely, it is probably wise to ask your doctor to consider prescribing a low-dose ACE inhibitor if you have diabetes even if you don't have high blood pressure. Anti-ACE fish peptides may very well provide the same kind of benefits, but until this is proven, an ACE inhibitor drug should probably be used for this purpose. Anti-ACE fish peptides and other natural health products such as celery seed extract can still be used in addition to this if further blood pressure control is required.

to the kidneys are narrowed with atherosclerosis), so potassium levels and kidney function should be monitored.

CURRENT DRUG THERAPY OF HYPERTENSION | For many years, the drug of first choice for high blood pressure was a thiazide diuretic alone or in combination with a beta-blocker. As mentioned previously due to lack of effectiveness in reducing the cardiovascular death rate and side effects noted in numerous studies, this approach has somewhat fallen out of favor. Most often nowadays a diuretic is used alone or in combination with newer medications designed to relax the arteries such as calcium channel blockers and ACE inhibitors or the newer angiotensin receptor blocker drugs.

When a diuretic or any of these other drugs is used alone, it is referred to as a "Step 1" drug. Thiazide diuretics are still the most popular Step 1 drug, but may soon be displaced by calcium channel blockers, ACE inhibitors, or angiotensin receptor blockers. Beta-blockers are not often used as Step 1 drugs due to their known side effects, except in patients who have had heart attacks because they reduce the risk of a second cardiac event. A Step 2 drug approach uses two medications, a Step 3 approach uses three, and a Step 4 approach uses four. Physicians are instructed to try single therapies before combining medicines.

The Importance of Flavonoids in Preventing Diabetic Complications

We want to end this chapter by pointing out that one of the most important natural compounds to fight the complications of diabetes are the flavonoids, a group of plant pigments responsible for many of the colors of fruits, flowers, and medicinal herbs. Flavonoids are sometimes called "nature's biological response modifiers" because of their anti-inflammatory, antiallergic, antiviral, and anticancer properties. Recent research suggests that flavonoids may be useful in treating diabetes as well as in preventing long-term complications. Flavonoids such as quercetin promote insulin secretion and are potent inhibitors of glycosylation and sorbitol accumulation, while flavonoid-rich extracts such as bilberry and hawthorn extracts have been shown to be helpful in diabetic retinopathy and microvascular abnormalities.[19]

The beneficial effects of flavonoids in battling the complications of diabetes are numerous, including the fact that as antioxidants, flavonoids are generally more potent and effective against a broader range of oxidants than the traditional antioxidant nutrients vitamins C and E, beta-carotene, selenium, and zinc. Other beneficial effects include increasing intracellular vitamin C levels, decreasing the leakiness

Table 11.1. Choose the Right Flavonoid-Rich Extract

FLAVONOID-RICH EXTRACT	DAILY DOSE	INDICATION
Bilberry extract (25% anthocyanidins)	160 to 320 mg	Best choice in diabetic retinopathy or cataracts.
Ginkgo biloba extract (24% ginkgo flavon-glycosides)	120 to 240 mg	Best choice for most people over age 50. Protects brain and vascular lining. Very important in improving blood flow to the extremities, neuropathy, and foot ulcers.
Grapeseed extract or pine bark extract (95% procyanidolic oligomers)	150 to 300 mg	Systemic antioxidant; best choice for most people under 50, especially for retinopathy, high blood pressure, easy bruising, and poor wound healing. Also specific for the lungs, varicose veins, and protection against heart disease.
Green tea extract (60–70% total polyphenols)	150 to 300 mg	Best choice in the early stage of type 1 diabetes or if there is a family history of cancer.
Hawthorn extract (10% procyanidins)	150 to 300 mg	Best choice in heart disease or high blood pressure.
Milk thistle extract (70% silymarin)	100 to 300 mg	Best choice if showing signs of impaired liver function.
Mixed citrus flavonoids	1,000 to 2,000 mg	Least expensive choice, but may not provide same level of benefit. OK if no complication is present.
Quercetin	150 to 300 mg	Good choice if allergies, symptoms of prostate enlargement or bladder irritation, or eczema are also present.

and breakage of small blood vessels, preventing easy bruising, promoting wound healing, and providing immune system support. Good dietary sources of flavonoids include citrus fruits, berries, onions, parsley, legumes, green tea, and red wine.

In individuals with diabetes who are already showing signs of a long-term complication, we feel that it is extremely important to take a flavonoid-rich extract. Because certain flavonoids concentrate in specific tissues, it is possible to take flavonoids that target specific body tissue. For example, because the flavonoids of bilberry (*Vaccinium myrtillus*) have an affinity for the eye, including the retina, bilbery is probably the best choice in a diabetic already exhibiting signs of diabetic retinopathy. Identify which flavonoid or flavonoid-rich extract is most appropriate for you and take it according to the recommended dosage. There is tremendous overlap among the mechanisms of action and benefits of flavonoid-rich extracts; the key point is to take the one that is most specific to your personal needs (see Table 11.1).

Chapter Twelve

Recommendations for Specific Chronic Complications

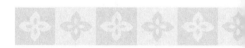

We have already introduced many of the natural tools useful in dealing with some of the specific complications of diabetes. Remember, the most important method for reducing the risk of these complications is achieving optimal blood sugar control.

One of the key goals in dealing with specific chronic complications is trying to improve blood flow and the delivery of vital nutrients and oxygen to all tissues. Diabetes is associated with significant damage to the vascular system of the body.[1] All of the mechanisms described in Chapter 11 play a role, especially glycosylation of proteins and increased oxidative damage, but another key disturbance greatly increases the development of vascular disease in diabetics—endothelial cell dysfunction. A single layer of endothelial cells lines all blood vessels to act as a metabolically active interface between the components of blood and the blood vessel. It is active in the sense that it regulates many important aspects of blood flow, coagulation, clot formation, and the formation of key regulating compounds, including those that control blood pressure. Endothelial cells are susceptible to damage by oxidized LDL cholesterol and other free radicals—hence the importance of high dietary antioxidant intake, flavonoids, and key supplemental antioxidants such as vitamin C and E, and alpha-lipoic acid. All of these factors have been shown to improve endothelial cell function and are critical in the battle against vascular disease in diabetes.[2–5]

In addition to the goal of improving endothelial cell function in diabetes, most diabetics will have to deal with high cholesterol.

Natural Products to Lower Cholesterol Levels

There are a number of specific natural medicines that we could recommend to lower cholesterol levels, but we are going to limit our recommendations to three: PGX™ (or other soluble fiber), garlic, and niacin.

Before taking a look at the effects of these compounds in lowering cholesterol levels, it is important that you understand exactly what all the different forms of cholesterol represent. First of all, cholesterol is a natural substance made by the liver to serve several important body functions including being the backbone for important hormones such as estrogen, testosterone, and cortisone.

Cholesterol travels from the liver and into your circulation by hitching a ride on protein molecules called low-density lipoprotein (LDL), often called "bad cholesterol." It is carried away from tissues and back to the liver aboard high-density lipoprotein (HDL) ("good" or "protective cholesterol"). Some people find it easier to remember the difference by labeling LDL "lousy" and HDL "healthy" or "happy."

The more LDL you have, the more cholesterol is in circulation and the greater your risk of heart disease. Currently, experts recommend that your total blood cholesterol level should be less than 200 mg/dL. The LDL level should be less than 130 mg/dL and the HDL level should be greater than 35 mg/dL. For every 1 percent drop in LDL levels, there's a 2 percent drop in the risk of heart attack. By the same token, for every 1 percent increase in HDL, the risk of heart attack drops 3 or 4 percent.

The ratio of your total cholesterol to HDL and the ratio of LDL to HDL are clues that indicate whether cholesterol is being deposited into tissues or is being broken down and excreted. The ratio of total cholesterol to HDL should be no higher than 4.2, and the LDL-to-HDL ratio should be no higher than 2.5.

Another important lipoprotein to be aware of is a form of LDL called lipoprotein (a), or Lp(a). This form of LDL has an additional molecule of an adhesive protein called apolipoprotein. That protein makes the molecule much more likely to stick to the artery walls and cause damage. New research suggests that high Lp(a) levels constitute a separate risk factor for heart attack. For example, it appears that high Lp(a) levels are ten times more likely to cause heart disease than high LDL levels. Lp(a) levels lower than 20 mg/dL are associated with low risk of heart disease; levels between 20 and 40 mg/dL pose a moderate risk, and levels higher than 40 mg/dL are considered extremely risky.

Soluble Fiber

In Chapter 9, we stressed the value of using soluble fiber supplements to reduce after-meal blood glucose levels. Supplemental dietary fiber, particularly soluble fiber, is also very effective in lowering cholesterol levels (see Table 12.1). One review article found a significant reduction in the level of serum total cholesterol in 68 of the 77 studies reviewed (88 percent). The effect of fiber, particularly soluble fiber, is clearly dose-dependent and, like its effect on reducing cholesterol levels, is related to the degree of viscosity.

Table 12.1. Impact of Various Sources of Fiber on Serum Cholesterol Levels

FIBER	DOSAGE (G)	TYPICAL REDUCTION IN TOTAL CHOLESTEROL
Oat bran (dry)	50–100	10–15%
Guar gum	9–15	10%
Pectin	6–10	5%
PGXTM	3	15–20%
Psyllium	10–20	10–15%
Vegetable fiber	25–30	10%

We feel that the most meaningful results are most easily obtained with PGX™, the special fiber complex based on the work by Dr. Vladimir Vuksan and his colleagues at the University of Toronto's world-renowned Risk Factor Modification Centre. Supplementation with a complex similar to PGX™ to individuals with syndrome X or diabetes reduced total and LDL cholesterol by up to 19 percent and 29 percent, respectively, even though these patients were kept on their regular cholesterol-lowering medication throughout the entire length of the study. In addition, the fiber complex was shown to lower systolic blood pressure by 8 points—an effect not seen with soluble fibers.[6]

Niacin

The cholesterol-lowering activity of niacin was first described in the 1950s. It is now known that niacin does much more than lower total cholesterol. Specifically, niacin has been shown to lower LDL cholesterol, Lp(a) lipoprotein, triglyceride, and fibrinogen levels while simultaneously raising HDL cholesterol levels. Despite the fact that niacin has demonstrated better overall results in reducing risk factors for coronary heart disease compared with other cholesterol-lowering agents, physicians are often reluctant to prescribe niacin. The reason is a widespread perception that niacin is difficult to work with because of the bothersome flushing of the skin. In addition, since niacin is a widely available "generic" agent, no pharmaceutical company stands to generate the huge profits that other lipid-lowering agents have enjoyed. As a result, niacin does not benefit from the intensive advertising that focuses on the "statin" drugs. Despite the advantages of niacin over other lipid-lowering drugs, it accounts for less than 10 percent of all cholesterol-lowering prescriptions.

Several studies have compared niacin to standard lipid-lowering drugs, including the statin drugs. These studies have shown significant advantages for niacin. For example, in one 26-week study, patients were randomly assigned to receive treatment with either lovastatin (Mevacor) or niacin.[7] The results are shown in Figure 12.1.

These results indicate that while lovastatin produced a greater LDL cholesterol reduction, niacin provided better overall results despite the fact that fewer patients could tolerate a full dosage of niacin because of

Figure 12.1. Lovastatin vs. Niacin in a 26-Week Study

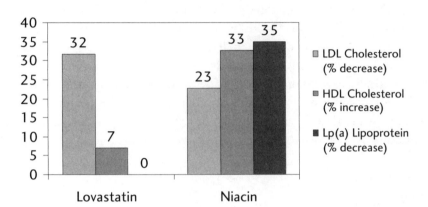

skin flushing. The percentage increase in HDL cholesterol, a more significant indicator for coronary heart disease, was dramatically in favor of niacin (33 percent versus 7 percent). Equally impressive was the percentage decrease in Lp(a) for niacin. While niacin produced a 35 percent reduction in Lp(a) lipoprotein levels, lovastatin did not produce any effect. Other studies have shown that niacin can lower Lp(a) levels by an average of 38 percent.[8,9]

The most recent comparative study involved niacin versus atorvastatin (Lipitor).[10] The average dosage was 3,000 mg per day for niacin and 80 mg per day for atorvastatin. The patients selected had abnormal LDL particle size in that the molecules were small and dense—these LDL molecules are considerably more atherogenic than larger, less dense LDL. The patients selected also had low levels (less than 40 percent) of a specific fraction of HDL associated with a greater protective effect than HDL alone. Although atorvastatin reduced total LDL cholesterol levels substantially more than niacin, niacin was more effective than atorvastatin in increasing LDL particle size and raising HDL and the even more protective HDL2 subfraction.

Because taking niacin at higher dosages (3,000 mg daily or more) can impair glucose tolerance, many physicians have avoided niacin therapy in diabetics, but newer studies with slightly lower dosages of niacin (1,000 to 2000 mg) have not shown it to adversely affect blood

Table 12.2. The Effect of Atorvastatin (Lipitor) and Niacin on Lipid Profiles

	Atorvastatin		Niacin		Atorvastatin + Niacin	
PARAMETER	BEFORE	AFTER	BEFORE	AFTER	BEFORE	AFTER
Total LDL (mg/dL)	110	56	111	89	123	55
LDL peak diameter	251	256	253	263	250	263
Lipoprotein (a) (mg/dL)	45	44	37	23	54	35
HDL (mg/dL)	42	43	38	54	38	54
HDL2 (%)	30	42	29	43	32	37
Triglycerides (mg/dL)	186	100	194	108	235	73

sugar regulation.[11] For example, during a 16-week, double-blind, placebo-controlled trial, 148 type 2 diabetes patients were randomized to placebo or 1,000 or 1,500 mg per day of niacin; in the niacin-treated groups there was no significant loss in glycemic control and the favorable effects on blood lipids were still apparent.[12] Other studies have actually shown hemoglobin A_1C to drop, indicating improvement in glycemic control.[13]

The most common blood lipid abnormality in type 2 diabetic patients is elevated triglyceride levels, decreased HDL cholesterol levels, and a preponderance of smaller, denser LDL particles. Niacin has been shown to address all of these areas much more significantly than the statin or other lipid-lowering drugs. However, one reason why niacin may not be as popular as it should be is the bothersome side effect of skin flushing—like a prickly, heat rash that typically occurs 20 to 30 minutes after the niacin is taken and disappears in about the same time frame. Other occasional side effects of niacin include gastric irritation, nausea, and liver damage.

To reduce the side effect of skin flushing you can use some of the newer time-released formulas, including the prescription version Niaspan, and take the niacin just before going to bed. Most people sleep right through the flushing reaction. Taking cholesterol-lowering agents at night is best because the liver manufactures most of its cholesterol at night. Another approach to reduce flushing is to use inositol hexaniacinate. This form of niacin has long been used in Europe to lower cholesterol levels and also to improve blood flow in intermittent claudication—a peripheral vascular disease that is quite common in diabetes. It yields slightly better clinical results than standard niacin, but is much better tolerated, in terms of both flushing and, more important, long-term side effects.[14] If you start out with inositol hexaniacinate and it does not work, try regular niacin. Our experience is that some people respond only to the regular niacin.

If regular niacin or inositol hexaniacinate is being used, start with a dose of 500 mg at night before going to bed for one week. Increase the dosage to 1,000 mg the next week and 1,500 mg the following week. Stay at the 1,500 mg dosage for 2 months before checking the response—dosage can be adjusted up or down depending on the response. If you are using a time-release niacin product such as Niaspan, start out at the full dosage of 1,500 mg at night.

Regardless of the form of niacin being used, we strongly recommend periodic checking (minimum every 3 months) of cholesterol, A_1C, and liver function.

Baby Aspirin Reduces Heart Attack Rates in Diabetes

Taking a baby aspirin just before each dose of niacin is another way to effectively block the flushing effects of niacin. Since many doctors now recommend low-dose aspirin to their diabetic patients as a way to lower heart attack and stroke risk, using aspirin along with niacin is a way to "kill two birds with one stone." Diabetes is associated with an increased risk of catastrophic events due to blood clotting (primarily stroke and heart attack). Taking a baby aspirin (80 mg) every day has been shown to lower the risk by about 10 percent without producing any significant side effects.[15]

Garlic

Garlic has a wide range of well-documented effects useful for the diabetic including helping to improve blood sugar control, lower cholesterol and blood pressure, and inhibit some of the factors associated with increased risk for vascular complications of diabetes such as increased fibrinogen levels.

The cardiovascular effects of garlic are attributed to its sulfur-containing compounds, especially allicin—the compound responsible for the pungent odor of garlic. It is formed by the action of the enzyme alliinase on the compound alliin. The enzyme is activated by heat, oxygen, or water. This fact accounts for the fact that cooked garlic as well as "aged garlic preparations" and garlic oil products produce neither as strong an odor as raw garlic nor nearly as powerful medicinal effects.

Since allicin is the component in garlic that is responsible for its easily identifiable odor, some manufacturers have developed highly sophisticated methods in an effort to provide the full benefits of garlic—they provide "odorless" garlic products concentrated for alliin because alliin is relatively "odorless" until it is converted to allicin in the body. Products concentrated for alliin and other sulfur components provide all of the benefits of fresh garlic if they are manufactured properly, but are more "socially acceptable."

Because alliin and alliinase are very stable when garlic is properly processed, manufacturers coat the specially prepared garlic in such a manner that the tablet does not break down until after it has passed through the stomach, to ensure that the allicin is not produced until the garlic powder mixes with the fluids of the intestinal tract. This method is referred to as "enteric coating."

If a nonenteric-coated garlic preparation is used, the stomach acid will destroy the majority of the formed allicin. So these preparations are not likely to produce results as good as a high-quality, enteric-coated product. The same can be said for aged garlic and garlic oil products, as these forms of garlic contain absolutely no allicin or allicin-degradation products.

There are a couple of vital considerations when choosing a garlic product. First of all, it is important to make sure that the product provides a sufficient level of allicin. Since allicin is not actually in the product at any significant levels, manufacturers often refer to the allicin potential or allicin yield. These terms signify the amount of allicin produced when alliinase is activated in the garlic tablet or powder.

The next issue, which is not so simple to tell from a label, involves the quality and character of the enteric coating of the tablet. In order for the allicin to be liberated within the intestinal tract, the tablet not only must be resistant to the stomach's acid, it must disintegrate rapidly when it reaches the small intestine. According to research conducted by the renowned garlic expert Dr. Larry D. Lawson, when twenty-four brands of enteric-coated garlic were analyzed for tablet dissolution using an approved method (USP dissolution method 724A), only one brand released the amount of allicin claimed on the label.[16] The second-best brand released only 44 percent of label claim, and 75 percent of the brands released less than 10 percent of label claim. Failure to deliver an effective dosage of allicin will most assuredly lead to failure to lower cholesterol or blood pressure.

Dr. Lawson discovered two major problems with garlic supplements. First of all, many of the garlic products contained little alliinase activity. There was plenty of alliin, but since the activity of alliinase was low, the level of alliicin formed was also low. Next, Dr. Lawson found that many of the tablets contained binders and fillers that actually inhibit alliinase activity. The alliinase activity in 63 percent of the brands was less than 10 percent of expected activity. The inability to release an effective dose of allicin would explain why so many studies with garlic supplements fail to show benefit in lowering cholesterol or blood pressure.[17]

The studies showing a positive effect of garlic and garlic preparations are those that deliver a sufficient dosage of allicin. The negative studies do not. In the positive double-blind studies in patients with initial cholesterol levels greater than 200 mg/dL, supplementation with garlic preparations providing a daily dose of at least a total allicin potential of 4,000 mcg, total serum cholesterol levels dropped by about 10 to 12 percent, LDL cholesterol decreased by about 15 percent, HDL cholesterol levels usually increased by about 10 percent, and triglyceride levels dropped by 15 percent. Blood pressure readings also dropped, with typical reductions of 11 points systolic and 5.0 points diastolic within a 1-to-3-month period.[18–20]

We currently know of only two brands that use the USP method 724A to ensure label claim for allicin potential—Garlicin (Nature's

Recommendations for the Complete
Cardiovascular Assessment

In Chapter 6 we highlighted tests that we feel are critical in assessing the risk for heart disease in people with diabetes. The general diet and lifestyle recommendations alone have been shown to improve all of these parameters, but we want to give you some additional specific recommendations when these values are abnormal:

- Total cholesterol above 200 mg/dL or LDL cholesterol above 135 mg (100 mg if history of heart attack):

  PGX™—1,000 mg three times daily before meals
  Niacin (or inositol hexaniacinate)—1,500 mg at night at bedtime
  Garlic—minimum of 4,000 mcg of allicin daily

Typically, this program will reduce total cholesterol by 50 to 75 mg/dL in patients with initial total cholesterol levels above 250 mg/dL within the first 2 months. In cases where the initial cholesterol level is above 300 mg/dL it may take 4 to 6 months before cholesterol levels begin to reach recommended levels. Once the cholesterol level is reduced below 200 mg/dL, reduce the dosage of niacin to 1,000 mg daily for 2 months. If the cholesterol levels creep up above 200 mg/dL, then raise the dosage of niacin back to 1,500 mg daily. If the cholesterol level remains below 200 mg/dL, then withdraw the niacin completely and check the cholesterol levels in 2 months. Reinstitute niacin therapy if levels creep up above 200 mg/dL. Garlic can be continued indefinitely, if desired.

- HDL cholesterol below 45 mg/dL: Niacin (or inositol hexaniacinate)—1,500 mg at night at bedtime
- Lipoprotein (a) above 40 mg/dL: Niacin (or inositol hexaniacinate)—1,500 mg at night at bedtime

- Triglycerides above 150 mg/dL: Niacin (or inositol hexaniacinate)—1,500 mg at night at bedtime
- C-reactive protein above 1.69 mg/L: Follow recommendations in Chapter 8, get more exercise, and add garlic and a flavonoid-rich extract
- Fibrinogen above 400 mg/L: Follow recommendations in Chapter 7, get more exercise, and add garlic.
- Homocysteine above 16 micromole/L: Be sure to take a high-potency multiple vitamin and mineral supplement.
- Ferritin (an iron-binding protein) above 200 mcg/L: Eliminate red meat from the diet, avoid iron supplements, and increase consumption of whole grains. Be sure to have an assessment for hemochromatosis (including transferrin saturation and genetic testing if indicated).
- Lipid peroxides elevated: Follow recommendations in Chapter 7 and add garlic and a flavonoid-rich extract

Way) and Garlic Factors (Natural Factors). So if you want to see results, we recommend using one of these two brands.

When Additional Support Is Needed

If the natural program described here does not bring cholesterol levels to where they should be, then additional support is required. That translates to being placed on one of the statin drugs. These drugs work by inhibiting a key enzyme in the liver, HMG-CoA reductase, required for the manufacture of cholesterol. Popular examples of statin drugs include atorvastatin (Lipitor); fluvastatin (Lescol); lovastatin (Mevacor); pravastatin (Pravachol); and simvastatin (Zocor). Lovastatin, the first drug in the statin family, was originally isolated from red yeast rice. Red yeast rice has shown benefit in clinical studies, but in an effort to protect the drug companies the FDA has restricted these products from having any active compounds.

The statins are very popular prescriptions for diabetics, but as shown earlier, niacin can be more effective. However, some people will be able to achieve target cholesterol levels only with the aid of a statin.

Statins are also gaining popularity as a prescription method to lower C-reactive protein (CRP), a marker of inflammation and a risk factor for heart disease. In one study, a group of 186 individuals with type 2 diabetes was selected to receive 10 mg daily of atorvastatin (Lipitor), 80 mg daily of atorvastatin, or a daily placebo for 30 weeks. In those given placebo, CRP levels increased 6.6 percent. CRP levels decreased by 15 percent in the 10-mg group and by 47 percent in the 80-mg group. In a study with pravastatin, 40 mg daily lowered CRP levels by 13 percent.[21] While many physicians appear to be aware of the effect of Lipitor and Pravachol on C-reactive protein, they do not seem to be aware that vitamin E (800 IU daily) lowered C-reactive protein by 49 percent and niacin (1,500 mg at night) lowered it by 20 percent.[22,23]

If You Use a Statin Drug, Take CoQ10

The statin drugs not only inhibit the manufacture of cholesterol, but also inhibit the making of coenzyme Q10 (CoQ10)—one of the most important nutrients for heart health. Its role in the heart is similar to the role of a spark plug in a car engine. Just as the car cannot function without that initial spark, the heart cannot function without CoQ10. More than twenty double-blind studies have shown that CoQ10 supplementation improves heart function by increasing energy production in the heart muscle and by acting as an antioxidant.[24]

Although the body makes some of its own CoQ10, considerable research shows significant benefits with supplementation. Also, people with any sort of heart disease, including high cholesterol levels and high blood pressure or those taking cholesterol-lowering drugs, are known to have low CoQ10 levels.

Supplementing CoQ10 (50 to 100 mg per day) is necessary to prevent the depletion of CoQ10 in body tissues while on these drugs.[25] Coenzyme Q10 is available primarily in tablets or capsules. Based on bioavailability studies, the best preparations appear to be soft gelatin capsules that contain CoQ10 in an oil base or in a soluble form. In order to further enhance absorption, CoQ10 should be taken with food.

Retinopathy and Cataracts

Diabetic retinopathy has two forms: "simple" retinopathy, consisting of bursting of blood vessels, hemorrhages, and swelling; and proliferative retinopathy, with newly formed vessels, scarring, more serious hemorrhage, and retinal detachment. The development of laser photocoagulation therapy is an important treatment for the more severe proliferative retinopathy, but is still not indicated in milder forms of retinopathy since the risk of visual loss due to the side effects usually outweighs the benefits.

As with other complications of diabetes, prevention is the best treatment, with the key factor being maintaining optimal blood sugar control. In particular, keep an eye on your hemoglobin A_1C. As shown in Figure 12.2, the higher the A_1C level, the greater the risk for retinopathy.

Extremely important in the battle against retinopathy are flavonoid-rich extracts, especially bilberry, pine bark, and grapeseed extracts. The flavonoids in these extracts exert many benefits in diabetes, including an ability to increase intracellular vitamin C levels, decrease the leakiness and breakage of small blood vessels, prevent easy bruising, and exert potent antioxidant effects. These effects are of particular value in dealing with the microvascular abnormalities of diabetes. Because the flavonoids

Figure 12.2. Risk of Retinopathy Progression by HbA$_{1c}$ Level and Years of Follow-Up

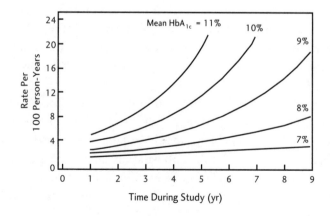

in bilberry, pine bark, and grapeseed extract have an affinity for the blood vessels of the eye and improve circulation to the retina, they are particularly helpful in slowing the progression of diabetic retinopathy as evidenced by positive results in more than a dozen clinical trials.[26,27] Follow the dosage recommendations given on page 250.

Neuropathy

In addition to alpha-lipoic acid and the basic supplementation program (magnesium is particularly important), we recommend some additional natural medicines for diabetic neuropathy.

Gamma-linolenic acid has been shown to improve and prevent diabetic neuropathy. Diabetes is associated with a substantial disturbance in essential fatty acid metabolism. One of the key disturbances is the impairment in the process of converting linoleic acid to gamma-linolenic acid (GLA). As a result, providing GLA in the form of borage, evening primrose, or black currant oils can bypass some of this disturbance. In the Gamma-Linolenic Acid Multicenter Trial, 111 patients with mild diabetic neuropathy were given either GLA at a dose of 480 mg per day or a placebo for one year. Sixteen different parameters were assessed, including conduction velocities, hot and cold thresholds, sensation, tendon reflexes, and muscle strength. After one year, all sixteen parameters improved, thirteen of them to a statistically significant degree. Treatment was more effective in relatively well-controlled than in poorly controlled diabetic patients. The latter finding highlights the need for a comprehensive approach in controlling blood sugar levels rather than expecting a single physiological aid (such as GLA) to compensate for poor control.

Capsaicin is the active component of cayenne pepper (*Capsicum frutescens*)—it is what makes chili peppers hot. When topically applied to the skin, capsaicin stimulates and then blocks the small nerve fibers that transmit the pain impulse. It works by depleting these fibers of a transmitting substance known as *substance P* (yes, the *P* stands for *pain*).[28] Topically applied capsaicin has been shown to be of considerable benefit in relieving the pain of diabetic neuropathy in numerous double-blind studies. Roughly 80 percent of people with diabetic neuropathy experience tremendous pain relief.[29] Commercial ointments containing 0.025 percent or 0.075 percent capsaicin are available over the counter without a prescription (Capzaicin and Zostrix are the most popular). We recommend that you apply the 0.75 percent cream twice daily to the affected area (cover your hand with plastic wrap to avoid the capsaicin coming in contact with your eyes or mucous membranes). It may take a few days for the cream to start working and it will only continue to work with regular application.

Alpha-lipoic acid, as mentioned in the previous chapter, is an approved drug in Germany for the treatment of diabetic neuropathy. In fact, it has been successfully used in Germany for more than 30 years. The beneficial effects of alpha-lipoic acid in diabetic neuropathy have been confirmed in several double-blind studies at a dosage of 300 to 600 mg daily.[30,31] Although alpha-lipoic acid's primary effect in improving diabetic neuropathy is thought to be the result of its antioxidant effects, it has also been shown to lead to an improvement in blood sugar metabolism, improve blood flow to peripheral nerves, and actually stimulate the regeneration of nerve fibers. Its ability to improve blood sugar metabolism is a result of its effects on glucose metabolism and an ability to increase insulin sensitivity. Its importance in treating diabetic neuropathy cannot be overstated.

If you are curious what conventional medicine has to offer for diabetic neuropathy, the answer is nothing but palliative care (pain relievers, antiepileptic drugs, and antidepressants).

Nephropathy

Be sure to undergo regular screening for the protein albumin in the urine, as its presence in a person with diabetes is a very strong predictor for progressing to end-stage kidney disease requiring dialysis or a kidney transplant.

Many of the previous recommendations also apply to preventing diabetic nephropathy. In fact, one more strong reason to adhere to the dietary principles laid out in this book is for the protection of the diabetic kidney. Diets that purport to control blood sugar by relying on very low carbohydrate and high protein (Atkins-style diets) work in the short term to keep blood sugar under control, but they put a strain on the kidneys, which are forced to dispose of a great deal more waste. The

Acupuncture for Diabetic Neuropathy

Acupuncture is a perhaps the most well-known treatment used in traditional Chinese medicine. It involves the use of extremely fine stainless steel needles inserted into points along what are traditionally believed to be energy channels known as meridians to direct the flow of energy. The scientific investigation of acupuncture in diabetes includes both experimental and clinical studies. For example, animal experiments have shown that acupuncture can act on the pancreas to enhance insulin synthesis, increase the number of receptors on target cells, and accelerate the use of glucose, resulting in lowering of blood sugar.[32] However, the best documentation for the clinical application of acupuncture is in treating chronic painful diabetic neuropathy. In one clinical study, 77 percent of patients treated with acupuncture noted significant improvement in their symptoms, with 21 percent noting that their symptoms were completely eliminated.[33] That success rate is excellent, considering the long-standing nature of the condition in most of the cases and the fact that no side effects were observed.

When done properly by trained personnel, acupuncture is extremely safe and side effects are rare. Make sure that any acupuncturist that you see has been accredited by the National Commission for Certification of Acupuncture and Oriental Medicine (NCCAOM), which ensures that he or she has had the proper training.

main waste materials disposed of by the kidneys are nitrogenous by-products of protein metabolism (such as ammonia and urea). When excessive protein is consumed, the amount of nitrogenous waste sent for disposal is greatly increased. Although a low-protein diet is not required except when nephropathy has progressed significantly, it is wise to adhere to a diet with a moderate amount of protein.[34] The low-glycemic-index/low-glycemic-load diet outlined in this book is the ideal diet to help preserve normal kidney function in diabetics.

Another feature of this diet that makes it excellent for the kidneys is that it is very high in dietary fiber. Dietary fibers (especially water-soluble fibers) are fermented in the colon to produce short-chain fatty acids. These by-products are the primary fuel for colonic cells and, if present in high amounts, they greatly increase the waste-removal capabilities of the colon. It has been shown that in the presence of a high-fermentable-fiber diet, the colon turns into the "second kidney" as it collects nitrogenous wastes out of the blood and disposes of them via the feces. This has been shown to greatly reduce the workload of and stress on the kidneys.[35] Therefore, in addition to keeping blood sugars well regulated, keeping with the high-fiber diet we have outlined and taking supplements such as PGX™ will provide benefits to the kidneys as well.

To highlight just how important some basic supplement recommendations are in halting the progression of diabetic nephropathy, let's look at the results of a study of thirty type 2 diabetes patients with elevated albumin in their urine who received vitamin C (1,250 mg) and vitamin E (680 IU) per day or a matching placebo for 4 weeks, followed by a 3-week washout period before being switched to the other treatment.[36] The results were that the vitamins reduced urinary albumin levels by an average of nearly 20 percent, indicating that antioxidant therapy may halt or slow the progression of kidney disease in diabetics.

Finally, achieving normal blood pressure is critically important in preventing diabetic nephropathy. If drugs are necessary, the ACE inhibitors (see page 248) offer the greatest benefits in helping deal with diabetic nephropathy. As discussed in the previous chapter, they are often prescribed in very low doses to help prevent nephropathy even in the absence of high blood pressure.

Poor Wound Healing

A deficiency of virtually any essential nutrient can lead to impaired wound healing. Key nutrients include vitamin C and zinc, both of which are often deficient in the diabetic. Taking a high-potency multiple vitamin and mineral formula should improve nutritional status and promote proper wound healing. For topical application we recommend using pure (100 percent) aloe vera gel. The wound healing effects of aloe vera are well known. Aloe vera contains a number of compounds necessary for wound healing, including vitamin C, vitamin E, and zinc. Aloe vera has been shown to stimulate many factors important to wound repair. Apply it to affected areas (not open wounds) two to three times daily.

Foot Ulcers

Lack of blood supply, poor wound healing, and peripheral neuropathy are the key factors in the development of diabetic foot ulcers. Key strategies in prevention and treatment are proper foot care, including professional care of nails and calluses, preferably by a podiatrist; regular physician's examination of the feet; avoidance of injury; avoidance of tobacco in any form; and employing methods to improve local circulation. Proper foot care also includes keeping the feet clean, dry, and warm, and wearing well-fitted shoes. Tobacco use in any form constricts the peripheral blood vessels and can lead to more serious peripheral vascular disease with severe arterial blockages. Remember, diabetes and smoking is like nitro and glycerin—a sure recipe for catastrophe.

Circulation can be improved by regular exercise and by avoidance of sitting with the legs crossed or in other positions that compromise circulation, and by massaging the feet lightly upward. We would also recommend consulting your physician for proper wound care (even minor nicks or slivers need immediate attention) and using either ginkgo biloba or grapeseed extract to support optimal circulation.

Ginkgo biloba extract (GBE) is probably best known for its ability to improve blood flow to the brain, but it also improves blood flow to the hands and feet. The most common symptoms of peripheral arterial disease are numbness, tingling, and intermittent claudication—a painful cramp or tightness produced with exertion. Intermittent claudication usually affects the calf muscle. More than twenty double-blind clinical trials have shown GBE to be very effective in improving peripheral vascular disease and intermittent claudication. The recommended dosage is 120 to 240 mg per day.

Practical Guidelines

Remember, the key to making any program for diabetes effective is to monitor blood sugar and hemoglobin A$_1$C levels. Also, remember that diet and lifestyle are the real keys to preventing the complications of diabetes, and that supplements are just that—supplements—to the dietary and lifestyle recommendations. For a summary of our supplement and natural product recommendations, go to Appendix B or C.

Appendices

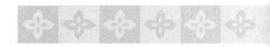

A Daily Plan for Preventing and Treating Diabetes

Constructing your own personal daily plan for preventing or treating diabetes involves strategies for strengthening the "four cornerstones of good health." You can liken these cornerstones to the four legs on a chair or table. If you want that chair or table to remain upright when stress is placed upon it, the four legs must be intact and strong. Likewise, if you want to have good or, better yet, ideal health it is essential that the following four areas be strong:

- A positive mental attitude
- A healthy lifestyle
- A health-promoting diet
- Supplementary measures

When your health is compromised by a disease such as diabetes, you need to be even more diligent in the area of supplementary measures. What do we mean by supplementary measures? Well, in this day and age we feel that everyone could use a little more support to supplement a health-promoting attitude, diet, and lifestyle. Examples of supplementary measures include medications, nutritional supplements, herbal medicines, and any other treatment measure designed to support or improve health. An example of an essential supplementary measure is the use of insulin in the treatment of people with insulin-dependent diabetes. At this time, insulin is absolutely essential to these individuals. Without it, they would either die or suffer greatly. There are numerous other examples where an appropriately used medication or surgery is absolutely essential to support good health. We also believe that several key nutritional supplements are absolutely essential to preventing and treating diabetes.

If you desire ideal health, it is a very good idea to develop a daily routine that is consistent with supporting and strengthening these four cornerstones of good health. Here is a sample daily routine based upon a nine-to-five workday.

6:30 A.M.—Wake up

6:40 A.M. to 7:30 A.M.—Exercise (including stretching, warmup, training in target heart range for 20 to 30 minutes, and a 5-minute cooldown)

7:30 A.M. to 9:00 A.M.—Personal time for shower, breakfast, catching up on the news, getting ready for the day, and commuting to work

10:30 A.M. to 10:45 A.M.—Healthy break

12:30 P.M. to 1:30 P.M.—Lunch break

3:00 P.M. to 3:15 P.M.—Healthy break

5:45 P.M. to 6:00 P.M.—Quiet time filled with deep breathing, prayer, or meditation

6:00 P.M. to 6:30 P.M.—Dinner preparation

6:30 P.M. to 7:15 P.M.—Dinner

7:15 P.M. to 10:30 P.M.—Engaging in social activities, development of relationships, and enjoyment of personal interests

10:30 P.M.—Bedtime

This sample routine most likely bears little resemblance to your daily routine; there are undoubtedly time obstacles in your life that will require you to modify it. The key point is that you absolutely must commit to engaging in a routine that supports optimal health and well-being. There are many variables in construction of your own personal routine; what is not variable is that in order to have a healthy and fulfilling life you will need to plug in positive social and personal relationships, regular exercise, time for enough sleep, a health-promoting diet, and nutritional supplementation.

Dietary Recommendations

Diet is a true cornerstone for good health. Our dietary program is based on scientific evidence on what constitutes the most health-promoting diet for anyone, but especially for people with diabetes (see Table A.1).

Table A.1. Daily Food Group Recommendations

FOODS	DAILY SERVINGS (2,000-CALORIE DIET)
Vegetables total servings	5 to 7
Green leafy and cruciferous vegetables	2 to 4
Low glycemic vegetables	2 to 3
Other vegetables	1 to 2
Good oils	
Total servings	4
Nuts and seeds	1
Olive, macadamia, flaxseed, or canola oil	2 to 3
Whole grains	3 to 5
Legumes	2 to 3 (4 to 5 if vegetarian)
High-quality protein	2 to 3
Fruit	2 to 3
Dairy	1 to 2 (optional)

Foods to Avoid Entirely
- Refined white-flour products: pastas, cakes, muffins, pretzels, and so on
- Refined sugar-loaded cereals, candies, baked goods, and so on
- Processed foods packed full of empty calories (sugar and fat) or salt (soups, theater-style popcorn, chips, and so on)
- Margarine, butter, and shortening
- Smoked or cured meats: bacon, hot dogs, smoked luncheon meats, sausages, ham, Spam, and so on
- Meats cooked at extremely high temperatures or cooked to well-done

- Heavily sweetened or artificially sweetened soft drinks, Kool-Aid, juice-flavored drinks, and so on
- Fried foods, including french fries, potato chips, corn chips, and doughnuts

Sample Menus and Recipes

To help you get started in planning out your own daily menus, we provide a 4-day program complete with menus and recipes. Since most people do not have the time to get to the grocery store every day, we want to show you how to shop for a 4-day period. That way you can get in the habit of planning out your meals well in advance and replenishing your perishables every 3 to 4 days.

We have chosen easy recipes that can be prepared and cooked within 30 minutes or less. We have also chosen recipes that have a short list of ingredients or readily available ingredients with no difficult steps to follow. In our own experiences we have been frustrated by vegetarian and other cookbooks designed for healthier eating whose recipes were

DAY 1	

BREAKFAST
Almond Butter Chocolate
  Truffle Smoothie
	DINNER
	Field Greens Salad with Bell
	  Peppers, Carrots, and
	  Radishes

MIDMORNING SNACK Green drink One cup of celery sticks	Minted Carrots with Pumpkin Seeds Steamed Broccoli

LUNCH
Field Greens Salad with
  Healthy Oil Dressing
Red Bean and Tomato Soup
Ry-Vita or WASA whole-grain
  rye crackers
	Asian Salmon
	Whole-grain bread or roll
	Fresh raspberries
	
	EVENING TEA
	One or two cups of herbal tea
	  (no caffeine)

MIDAFTERNOON SNACK One medium orange	

DAY 2

BREAKFAST
Whey-Enhanced Oatmeal
with Flaxseed or
Macadamia Nut Oil

MIDMORNING SNACK
Green drink
Three tablespoons of almonds

LUNCH
Tuna Salad Wrap

MIDAFTERNOON SNACK
Two medium plums

DINNER
Jicama Salad
Black Bean Chili
Whole-wheat tortillas
Sliced Pineapple

EVENING TEA
One or two cups of herbal tea
(no caffeine)

DAY 3

BREAKFAST
Tri-Berry Boost Smoothie

MIDMORNING SNACK
Green drink
Sliced pineapple

LUNCH
Italian White Bean Soup

MIDAFTERNOON SNACK
1 medium red pear

DINNER
Orange and Fennel Salad
Dr. Murray's Favorite Greens
Curried Chicken or Tofu over
Brown Rice
Blueberries

EVENING TEA
One or two cups of herbal tea
(no caffeine)

DAY 4

BREAKFAST
Whole-Grain Cereal with
Nuts and Seeds with Soy
milk or Nonfat Yogurt

MIDMORNING SNACK
Green drink
One cup of carrot sticks

LUNCH
Black Bean Salad

MIDAFTERNOON SNACK
One medium red apple

DINNER
Mediterranean Salad
Quick Acorn Squash
Polenta Puttanesca with Tofu
Fresh mango slices

EVENING TEA
One cup of herbal tea
(no caffeine)

packed full of difficult (or nearly impossible-to-get) ingredients, took too long to prepare, and required too many steps to prepare.

We have designed the menu selections to take advantage of foods such as oils, nuts, legumes, and high-fiber foods that slow gastric emptying, thereby significantly reducing the glycemic load as the carbohydrates in the meals are slowly absorbed.

Recipes

The recipes that we provide also allow for substitutions and modifications based on your own tastes. For example, if a recipe contains a vegetable that you do not like, substitute with one that you do like. The recipes are based on providing two servings; you can adjust the number of servings up or down as needed (for example, for four servings, simply double the recipe).

Shopping List

The following shopping list represents the items needed for the next 4 days.

HERBAL TEA

Most of the major brands of herbal tea (Celestial Seasonings, Bigelow, Republic of Tea, Traditional Medicinals, and so on) provide a sampler pack to help you identify teas that appeal to you. In general, avoid black teas. Try to choose decaffeinated varieties, especially for your nighttime cup of tea. If you feel you need a little caffeine in the morning, go with a cup of regular green tea.

PRODUCE

Try to buy organic, if possible, and be sure to wash all produce before consumption.

Acorn squash—1	Broccoli— 2 heads
Basil—1 bunch	Cabbage—½ head
Bell peppers—3 green, 2 red	Carrots—1 large bag
Blueberries—1 cup	Celery—2 bunches

Cilantro (fresh)—1 bunch
Cucumber—2
Fennel—1 small bulb
Garlic—2 bulbs
Green onions—1 bunch
Jicama—1
Kale—1 large bunch
Lemons—4
Mango—1
Mint (fresh)—½ cup
Mixed field greens—8 cups
Mushrooms—2 ounces
Onions—4
Oranges—4

Parsley (fresh)—1 bunch
Pear—1 red
Pineapple—1 medium
Plums—4 medium
Radishes—1 bunch
Raspberries—1 cup
Red or green grapes—1 cup
Romaine lettuce—1 head
Shiitake mushrooms—2 cups
Tomatoes, Roma or plum—
   2 medium
Tomatoes, cherry—6
Tomatoes, fresh—6 medium

FISH AND POULTRY

Salmon—½ lb fresh salmon
Tuna—1 can (or foil pouch)
   of low-sodium, chunk
   white tuna in spring water

Chicken breast—1 boneless,
skinless

MISCELLANEOUS GROCERY ITEMS

Balsamic vinegar—
   8 to 12 ounces
Dijon mustard—8 ounces
Honey (raw)—8 ounces
Kalamata olives—1 small jar
Soy milk, nonfat milk, or
   nonfat yogurt—32 ounces

Tofu—1 container (15 oz) of
   firm variety
Whey protein—chocolate
   and vanilla

NUTS, SEEDS, AND DRIED FRUIT

Almonds (raw)—1 cup
Almond butter—8 ounces
Flaxseeds (raw)—1 cup

Pumpkin seeds (raw)—1 cup
Sunflower seeds (raw)—1 cup
Walnuts (raw)—1 cup

OILS

Flaxseed oil—12 to 16 ounces
Olive oil (extra virgin) or macadamia nut oil—12 to 16 ounces

GRAINS AND PASTA

Brown rice (quick)—1 box
Rolled oats—1 small container
Polenta (quick)—1 box
Ry-Vita or WASA whole-grain
    rye crackers—1 packet

Whole-grain rolls—2
Whole-wheat tortillas—
    1 pack of eight

FROZEN FOODS

Corn (frozen)—2 cups

CANNED FOODS

Chicken or vegetable broth—
    6 11-ounce cans
Black beans—2 15-oz cans
Garbanzo beans—1 8-oz can
Red kidney beans—
    1 11-oz can
Refried black beans—
    1 15-oz can
Red kidney beans—
    1 8-oz can

Tomatoes, diced—
    1 7.5-oz can
Tomato sauce—1 4-oz can
    low-sodium; 1 12-oz can
    low sodium
Tomato soup (low-sodium)—
    1 11-oz can
White beans—1 15-oz can

SPICES AND SEASONINGS

Allspice or nutmeg
Capers
Curry powder
Chili powder
Cinnamon
Crushed red pepper
Cumin
Ginger (dried)

Ground black pepper
Italian herbs (seasoning)
No Salt or Nu-Salt—
    potassium chloride salts
    to use as a substitute for
    regular salt (sodium chloride)
Soy sauce (low-sodium)
Thyme

Recipes for Day 1

• BREAKFAST •

Almond Butter Chocolate Truffle Smoothie

Ingredients:

25 to 30 grams chocolate-flavored (sugar-free) whey protein powder
1 tbsp creamy almond butter
8 ounces nonfat milk or soy milk (chocolate)
4 ounces water
3 to 4 ice cubes
1 tbsp flaxseed or macadamia nut oil

Directions:

Place all ingredients in a blender and liquefy.

• LUNCH •

Field Greens Salad

Ingredients:

4 cups mixed field greens

Directions:

Most supermarkets and grocery stores now have mixed field greens in the produce section or in prepackaged plastic bags. This convenience makes a simple mixed field green salad a perfect quick and easy salad. Your serving size should be 2 cups along with 1 tablespoon olive (or flaxseed) oil salad dressing.

Healthy Oil Dressing

Ingredients:

4 ounces olive or macadamia nut oil
4 ounces organic flaxseed oil
2 tbsp lemon juice
2 tbsp balsamic vinegar
2 garlic cloves, finely minced
1 tbsp Italian herbs
1 tsp salt (use No Salt or Nu-Salt)
1 tsp black pepper

Directions:

Place all ingredients into a blender and blend for 2 to 3 minutes. Store in your refrigerator for a quick and easy health-promoting salad dressing.

Red Bean and Tomato Soup

Ingredients:

½ cup onion, chopped
1 clove of garlic, chopped
1 stalk celery, chopped in small chunks
1 tbsp olive oil
1 8-oz can red kidney beans, drained
1 11-oz can low-sodium tomato soup
2 tbsp Italian herbs
Salt (use No Salt or Nu-Salt) and pepper to taste

Directions:

Sauté onions, garlic, and celery in olive oil over medium-low heat for about 5 minutes in medium-sized soup pot, stirring often. Blend kidney beans, tomato soup, and spices in a blender for 2 to 3 minutes, and then add to soup pot and cook for 15 minutes. Add salt (use No Salt or Nu-Salt) and pepper to taste.

• DINNER •

Field Greens Salad with Bell Peppers, Carrots, and Radishes

Ingredients:

4 cups mixed field greens
1 green bell pepper, chopped
½ cup chopped carrots
½ cup chopped radishes

Directions:

Mix ingredients together. Your serving size should be 2 cups along with 1 tablespoon olive (or flaxseed) oil salad dressing.

Minted Carrots with Pumpkin Seeds

Ingredients:

3 medium carrots, peeled and cut into round slices
1 tbsp fresh chopped parsley
1 tbsp fresh chopped mint
2 tbsp coarsely chopped pumpkin seeds
1 tbsp lemon juice
1 tbsp olive oil
Salt (use No Salt or Nu-Salt) and pepper to taste

Directions:

Steam carrots until still slightly crunchy. Toss rest of ingredients with carrots when done.

Steamed Broccoli

Ingredients:

½ head broccoli

Directions:

Slice broccoli head lengthwise to separate out the florets of the head. Steam until tender.

Asian Salmon

Ingredients:

2 tsp low-sodium soy sauce
1 tbsp Dijon mustard
½ lb salmon, cut into 2 pieces
½ cup onion slices
1 garlic clove, chopped
¼ tsp dried ginger (or ½ tbsp minced fresh ginger)
2 cups sliced fresh shiitake mushrooms

Directions:

Preheat oven to 375°F. Mix the soy sauce into the mustard and coat the salmon. Sauté onion, garlic, ginger, and mushrooms in a medium sauté pan for about 5 minutes. Bake the salmon in a baking dish, depending on how thick it is (about 7 minutes if less than an inch thick). When cooked, place on bed of mushroom mixture.

Fresh Raspberries

Ingredients:

1 cup fresh raspberries

Directions:

Served chilled for a ½-cup serving size. A little vanilla soy milk or non-fat yogurt can be used to soak the berries as well.

Recipes for Day 2

• BREAKFAST •

Whey-Enhanced Oatmeal with Flaxseed or Macadamia Nut Oil

Ingredients:

1 cup cooked oatmeal
25 to 30 grams whey protein (vanilla)
¼ cup water, soy milk, or nonfat yogurt
1 tbsp flaxseed or macadamia nut oil
1 tbsp nuts and a sprinkle of cinnamon (optional)

Directions:

Cook oatmeal per instructions on package. While the oatmeal is cooking, stir whey protein into the ¼ cup water, soy milk, or nonfat yogurt. Adding additional liquid will thin the oatmeal, if desired. Add nuts and cinnamon if desired. Makes 1 serving.

• LUNCH •

Tuna Salad Wrap

Ingredients:

1 can (or foil pouch) low-sodium, chunk white tuna in spring water
¼ cup minced onion
1 celery stalk, chopped
1 tsp lemon juice
1 tbsp olive oil
1 tbsp chopped fresh parsley
¼ cup Dijon mustard
½ tsp salt (use No Salt or Nu-Salt)

½ tsp pepper
2 whole-wheat tortillas

Directions:

Mix all the ingredients except the tortillas in a bowl. Spoon the mixture onto the tortilla and wrap. Whole-grain bread may be substituted for the tortilla to make a sandwich.

• DINNER •

Jicama Salad

Ingredients:

1 cup julienne-cut peeled jicama
1 orange, peeled, sectioned, and cut into chunks
1 cucumber, seeded and thinly sliced
¼ cup chopped green onion
¼ cup chopped fresh cilantro
1 tbsp chopped fresh mint
¼ cup fresh orange juice
¼ cup fresh lemon (or lime) juice
¼ tsp salt (use No Salt or Nu-Salt)
¼ tsp pepper
¼ tsp chili powder

Directions:

Combine the jicama, orange, cucumber, onion, cilantro, and mint in a large bowl. In another bowl, mix the orange juice, lemon juice, and spices. Pour juice mixture over jicama mixture and toss gently. Cover and chill for at least 20 minutes.

Black Bean Chili

Ingredients:

½ medium onion, chopped
2 cloves garlic, chopped
1 green pepper, diced
1 15-oz can black beans, drained
1 cup frozen corn kernels
1 cup chicken or light vegetable broth
1 4-oz can low-sodium tomato sauce
2 tbsp cumin
2 tbsp red chili powder
2 tbsp Italian herbs
1 tbsp olive oil
½ tsp salt (use No Salt or Nu-Salt)
½ tsp pepper
¼ cup chopped fresh cilantro

Directions:

Sauté onion, garlic, and green pepper in a medium soup pot over medium-low heat for about 5 minutes, stirring frequently. Add the beans, corn, broth, tomato sauce, spices, oil, salt, and pepper and simmer for 15 minutes. Add cilantro as garnish and season with additional salt and pepper if needed. Serve with heated whole-wheat tortillas.

Sliced Pineapple

Slice a whole pineapple into bite-sized pieces. Place half of the sliced pineapple in the refrigerator for breakfast the next morning and serve the other half as a dessert.

Recipes for Day 3

• **BREAKFAST** •

Tri-Berry Boost Smoothie

Ingredients:

25 to 30 grams whey protein
8 oz nonfat milk or soy milk (vanilla)
⅓ cup strawberries (fresh or frozen)
⅓ cup raspberries (fresh or frozen)
⅓ cup blueberries (fresh or frozen)
3 to 4 ice cubes (optional)
1 tbsp flaxseed or macadamia nut oil

Directions:

Place all ingredients in a blender and liquefy.

• **LUNCH** •

Italian White Bean Soup

Ingredients:

½ onion, cut in half and thinly sliced
4 cloves garlic, sliced
2 cups chicken or light vegetable stock
2 cups finely chopped collard greens or kale
  (cut out stem)
1 7.5-oz can diced tomatoes
2 tsp Italian herb mixture
1 15-oz can navy beans, drained
Salt (use No Salt or Nu-Salt) and pepper to taste

Directions:

Sauté onion in medium soup pot over medium-low heat for 5 minutes, stirring frequently. Add garlic and continue to sauté for another minute. Add stock, greens, tomatoes, and herbs. Simmer for 15 minutes over medium heat. Add beans, salt, and pepper. Cook for another 5 minutes. Salt (use No Salt or Nu-Salt) and pepper to taste.

• DINNER •

Orange and Fennel Salad

Ingredients:

1 orange
1 small bulb fennel
1 head romaine lettuce, cut up
¼ cup chopped parsley
1 tbsp olive or flaxseed oil dressing

Directions:

Slice orange and fennel, then toss with greens and dressing in a large bowl.

Dr. Murray's Favorite Greens

Ingredients:

1 tbsp olive oil
1 tsp balsamic vinegar
1 large bunch kale; washed, trimmed, and coarsely chopped
½ cup diced green onion
1 clove garlic, thinly sliced
½ cup coarsely chopped walnuts or almonds
Lemon wedges
¼ tsp salt (use No Salt or Nu-Salt)
½ tsp black pepper

Directions:

Heat the olive oil and balsamic vinegar in a large skillet or wok over medium-high heat. Add greens, onions, garlic, and walnuts, and sauté until softened. Salt and pepper to taste. Serve with lemon wedges.

Curried Chicken or Tofu over Brown Rice

Ingredients:

½ cup uncooked quick brown rice
7.5 ounces firm tofu, cut into small cubes, or 1 boneless, skinless chicken
    breast, cut into bite-sized pieces
Olive oil for sautéing
½ cup chopped onion
1 clove of garlic, minced
ginger
2 tsp curry powder
1 tsp chili powder
1 cup chicken or vegetable stock
1 medium red bell pepper, chopped
½ cup coconut milk (make sure it is mixed well before using)
Salt (use No Salt or Nu-Salt) and pepper to taste

Directions:

Follow the instructions on the package of quick brown rice. While the water for the rice is coming to a boil, cut up the tofu or chicken and other ingredients. Sauté onion with a little olive oil in a medium sauté pan over medium-low heat for about 5 minutes, stirring frequently; add garlic and ginger, and continue to sauté for another minute, then remove from heat and add the curry powder and chili powder. Mix well. Return to heat and add stock, chicken, bell pepper, and coconut milk. Simmer until chicken is done, about 10 minutes. Salt (use No Salt or Nu-Salt) and pepper to taste.

Place rice on plate and top with the curry mixture.

Blueberries

Ingredients:

One cup fresh blueberries

Directions:

Served chilled for a ½-cup serving size. A little vanilla soy milk or non-fat yogurt can be used to soak the berries as well.

Recipes for Day 4

• BREAKFAST •

Whole-Grain Cereal with Nuts and Seeds with Soy Milk or Nonfat Yogurt

Ingredients (for each serving):

1 cup whole-grain cereal
1 tsp flaxseeds
1 tsp sunflower seeds
1 tsp coarsely chopped walnuts or almonds
1 cup vanilla soy milk or nonfat yogurt

• LUNCH •

Black Bean Salad

Ingredients:

1 15-oz can black beans, rinsed
1 cup frozen corn, thawed
6 cherry tomatoes, quartered
½ cup minced green onion
1 clove garlic, crushed or minced

½ cup diced red bell pepper
½ cup chopped cilantro
2 cups mixed field greens
1 tbsp olive or flaxseed oil
2 tbsp fresh lemon juice
¼ cup chopped cilantro
Salt (use No Salt or Nu-Salt) and pepper to taste

Directions:

Mix all ingredients together in a large bowl and serve.

• **DINNER** •

Mediterranean Salad

Ingredients:

1 cup chopped fresh tomato (cut out excess flesh if pulpy)
1 cup peeled and chopped cucumber
½ cup finely minced green onion
1 clove garlic, finely minced
1 8-oz can garbanzo beans, drained and rinsed
1 tbsp fresh lemon juice
1 tbsp fresh parsley
1 tsp Italian herbs
1 tbsp olive oil

Directions:

Mix all ingredients together and chill for at least 15 minutes.

Quick Acorn Squash

Ingredients:

1 acorn squash, cut in half with seeds removed
1 tbsp honey
Dash cinnamon

Directions:

Place the squash in a microwave-safe dish with cut side up. Cover and cook in the microwave for 10 to 13 minutes on high or until fork tender. Top with the honey and cinnamon. Serves 2.

Polenta Puttanesca with Tofu

Ingredients:

POLENTA:
3 cups water
1 tsp salt (use No Salt or Nu-Salt)
1 cup instant polenta

SAUCE:
1 onion, diced
1 clove garlic, crushed or minced
1 green pepper, diced
1 12-oz can tomato sauce
7.5 oz firm tofu, cut into small cubes
1 tbsp Italian herbs
1 tbsp crushed red pepper
2 tbsp capers, rinsed and drained
8–10 pitted Kalamata olives
1 tbsp finely chopped fresh parsley
¼ tsp salt (use No Salt or Nu-Salt)
¼ tsp black pepper
1 bay leaf

Directions:

Polenta: Bring water to a boil in a 2-quart saucepan. Add salt and reduce heat until water is simmering. Add polenta very slowly. To avoid lumps, stir quickly with a long-handled spoon while adding polenta. Cook, stirring continuously, for 5 minutes or until mixture is solid but still soft. Pour onto oiled 10½ × 15½" baking sheet. With wet hands or wet spatula, pat polenta into a smooth, flat rectangle. Let cool about 10 minutes or until firm.

Sauce: Sauté onion and garlic in a large saucepan over medium heat for 3 to 4 minutes. Add green pepper and sauté for 3 to 4 more minutes. Add water and drop in bay leaf and bring to a boil. Cover pot and simmer for 15 minutes. Add the rest of the ingredients and simmer for another hour, stirring occasionally. Remove from heat, remove the bay leaf, and allow to cool. Serve reheated or cold over spaghetti.

Supplementation Program for the Treatment of Type 1 Diabetes

The recommended supplementation program depends on the degree of blood sugar control as evident by self-monitored blood glucose and A_1C levels.

Initial Supplementation Programs

Recently diagnosed type 1 diabetes
- Foundation supplements:
  - High-potency multiple vitamin and mineral supplement—follow dosage recommendations on page 325–327.
  - Green drink—one serving daily
  - Fish oils—600 mg EPA and DHA daily
  - Vitamin C—500 to 1,500 mg daily
  - Vitamin E—400 to 800 IU daily
- Niacinamide—25 to 50 mg per kg (2.2 pounds) body weight
- Green tea extract—240 to 300 mg polyphenols

Level 1—Achievement of targeted blood sugar levels; A_1C levels below 7 percent, no lipid abnormalities, no signs of complications
- Foundation supplements:
  - High-potency multiple vitamin and mineral supplement—follow dosage recommendations on pages 325–327
  - Green drink—one serving daily
  - Fish oils—600 mg EPA and DHA daily

- Vitamin C—500 to 1,500 mg daily
- Vitamin E—400 to 800 IU daily

Level 2—Failure to achieve targeted blood sugar levels; A_1C between 7 and 8 percent.
- Foundation supplements
- *Gymnema sylvestre* extract (24 percent gymnemic acid)—200 mg twice daily
- Biotin—8 mg twice daily
- Optional: bitter melon juice—2 to 4 ounces daily

Level 3—Failure to achieve targeted blood sugar levels; A_1C between 8 and 9 percent.
- Foundation supplements
- *Gymnema sylvestre* extract (24 percent gymnemic acid)—200 mg twice daily
- Biotin—8 mg twice daily
- PGX™ (or other soluble source at equivalent dosage)—1,000 mg before meals
- Optional: bitter melon juice—2 to 4 ounces daily

Level 4—Failure to achieve targeted blood sugar levels; A_1C above 9 percent.
- Foundation supplements
- *Gymnema sylvestre* extract (24 percent gymnemic acid)—200 mg twice daily
- Biotin—8 mg twice daily
- PGX™ (or other soluble source at equivalent dosage)—1,000 mg before meals
- Glucosidase inhibitor—use one of the following:
  - Touchi extract—300 mg three times daily with meals
  - Mulberry extract—equivalent to 1,000 mg dried leaf three times daily
- Optional: bitter melon juice—2 to 4 ounces daily

If self-monitored blood sugar levels do not improve after 4 weeks of following the recommendations for the current level, move to the next highest level. For example, if you start out with an A_1C level of 8.2 percent and a fasting blood sugar level of 130 mg/dL, start on Level 2. After 4 weeks, if the average reading has not dropped to less than 110 mg/dL, then move to Level 3. If blood sugar levels and A_1C levels do not reach the targeted levels with Level 4, then a prescription medication (either an oral hypoglycemic drug or insulin) is required.

Additional Supplements for the Prevention and Treatment of Diabetic Complications

With the presence of any complication, add the following to the foundation supplement program:

- Alpha-lipoic acid—300 to 600 mg daily
- Grapeseed extract (or other appropriate flavonoid-rich extract; see pages 249–251)—150 to 300 mg daily

For specific complications, follow the foundation supplement program with the addition of alpha-lipoic acid and an appropriate flavonoid-rich extract, and add the specified supplement(s) listed next.

High Blood Pressure

For Borderline Hypertension (130–139/85–89)

- Foundational supplements
- Potassium chloride—1,500 to 3,000 mg
- Magnesium—150 to 400 mg three times daily
- PGX™—1,000 mg before meals three times daily
- Garlic—4,000 mcg allicin

(*Note:* If after 2 months there is no change, add anti-ACE fish peptides—1,500 mg daily. If after 2 months there is still no change, discontinue anti-ACE fish peptides and replace with celery seed extract—150 mg daily.)

For Mild (140–160/90–104) to Moderate (140–180/105–114) Hypertension

- Foundational supplements
- Potassium chloride—1,500 to 3,000 mg
- Magnesium—150 to 400 mg three times daily
- PGX™—1,000 mg before meals three times daily
- Garlic—4,000 mcg allicin
- Anti-ACE fish peptides—1,500 mg daily

(*Note:* If after 2 months there is no change, add celery seed extract—150 mg daily. If there is still no change, add coenzyme Q10—100 mg daily. If blood pressure has not dropped below 140/105, you will need to work with a physician to select the most appropriate medication. If a prescription drug is necessary, calcium channel blockers or ACE inhibitors appear to be the safest for diabetics.)

For Severe Hypertension (160+/115+)

- Consult a physician immediately.
- Foundational supplements
- Potassium chloride—1,500 to 3,000 mg daily
- Magnesium—150 to 400 mg three times daily
- PGX™—1,000 mg before meals three times daily
- Garlic—4,000 mcg of allicin
- Anti-ACE fish peptides—1,500 mg daily
- Celery seed extract—150 mg daily
- Coenzyme Q10—100 mg daily

(*Note:* A drug may be necessary to achieve initial control. When satisfactory control over the high blood pressure has been achieved, work with the physician to taper off the medication.)

High Cholesterol Levels and Other Cardiovascular Risk Factors

- Total cholesterol above 200 mg/dL or LDL cholesterol above 135 mg (100 mg if history of heart attack):

PGX™—1,000 mg three times daily before meals
Niacin (or inositol hexaniacinate)—1,500 mg at night at bedtime
Garlic—minimum of 4,000 mcg allicin daily

- HDL cholesterol below 45 mg/dL: Niacin (or inositol hexaniacinate)—1,500 mg at night at bedtime
- Lipoprotein (a) above 40 mg/dL: Niacin (or inositol hexaniacinate)—1,500 mg at night at bedtime
- Triglycerides above 150 mg/dL: Niacin (or inositol hexaniacinate)—1,500 mg at night at bedtime
- C-reactive protein above 1.69 mg/L: Vitamin E—800 IU daily
- Fibrinogen above 400 mg/L: Garlic extract—4,000 mcg daily
- Homocysteine above 16 micromole/L: No specific recommendation; be sure to take a high-potency multiple vitamin and mineral supplement.
- Ferritin (an iron-binding protein) above 200 mcg/L: Eliminate red meat from the diet, avoid iron supplements, and increase consumption of whole grains
- Lipid peroxides elevated: No specific additional recommendations; be sure to follow the foundation supplement program for type 1 diabetes

Diabetic Retinopathy

- Bilberry extract—160 to 320 mg daily; or grapeseed extract—150 to 300 mg daily

Diabetic Neuropathy

- Gamma-linolenic acid from borage, evening primrose, or blackcurrant oil—480 mg daily
- Capsaicin (0.075 percent) cream—apply to affected area twice daily

Diabetic Nephropathy

- Follow recommendations for high blood pressure unless kidney function falls below 40 percent of normal. In that situation, do not supplement with magnesium and potassium unless recommended to do so by physician.

Poor Wound Healing

- Aloe vera gel—apply to affected areas twice daily

Diabetic Foot Ulcers

- Ginkgo biloba extract—120 to 240 mg daily; or grapeseed extract—150 to 300 mg daily

Supplementation Program for the Treatment of Type 2 Diabetes

The recommended supplementation program depends on the degree of blood sugar control as evident by self-monitored blood glucose and A$_1$C levels.

Initial Supplementation Programs

Level 1—Achievement of targeted blood sugar levels; A$_1$C levels below 7 percent, no lipid abnormalities, no signs of complications
- Foundation supplements:
  - High-potency multiple vitamin and mineral supplement— follow dosage recommendations on pages 325–327.
  - Green drink—one serving daily
  - Fish oils—600 mg EPA and DHA daily
  - Vitamin C—500 to 1,500 mg daily
  - Vitamin E—400 to 800 IU daily

Level 2—Failure to achieve targeted blood sugar levels; A$_1$C between 7 and 8 percent
- Foundation supplements
- PGX™ (or other soluble source at equivalent dosage)—1,000 mg before meals.

Level 3—Failure to achieve targeted blood sugar levels; A$_1$C between 8 and 9 percent
- Foundation supplements

- PGX™ (or other soluble source at equivalent dosage)—1,000 mg before meals
- Insulin enhancer—use one of the following:
  - *Gymnema sylvestre* extract (24 percent gymnemic acid)— 200 mg twice daily
  - Fenugreek extract:
- Garlic—minimum 4,000 mcg allicin per day

Level 4—Failure to achieve targeted blood sugar levels; A_1C above 9 percent
- Foundation supplements
- PGX™ (or other soluble source at equivalent dosage)—1,000 mg before meals
- Insulin enhancer—use one of the following:
  - *Gymnema sylvestre* extract (24 percent gymnemic acid)— 200 mg twice daily
  - Fenugreek extract:
- Garlic—minimum 4,000 mcg allicin per day
- Glucosidase inhibitor—use one of the following:
  - Touchi extract—300 mg three times daily with meals
  - Mulberry extract—equivalent to 1,000 mg dried leaf three times daily

If self-monitored blood sugar levels do not improve after 4 weeks of following the recommendations for the current level, move to the next highest level. For example, if you start out with an A_1C level of 8.2 percent and a fasting blood sugar level of 130 mg/dL, start on Level 2. After 4 weeks, if the average reading has not dropped to less than 110 mg/dL, then move to Level 3. If blood sugar levels and A_1C levels do not reach the targeted levels with Level 4, then a prescription medication (either an oral hypoglycemic drug or insulin) is required.

Additional Supplements for the Prevention and Treatment of Diabetic Complications

With the presence of any complication, add the following to the foundation supplement program:

- Alpha-lipoic acid—300 to 600 mg daily
- Grapeseed extract (or other appropriate flavonoid-rich extract, see pages 249–251)—150 to 300 mg daily

For specific complications, follow the foundation supplement program with the addition of alpha-lipoic acid and an appropriate flavonoid-rich extract, and add the specified supplement(s) listed next.

High Blood Pressure

For Borderline Hypertension (130–139/85–89)

- Foundational supplements
- Potassium chloride—1,500 to 3,000 mg
- Magnesium—150 to 400 mg three times daily
- PGX™—1,000 mg before meals three times daily
- Garlic—4,000 mcg allicin

(*Note:* If after 2 months there is no change, add anti-ACE fish peptides—1,500 mg daily. If after 2 months there is still no change, discontinue anti-ACE fish peptides and replace with celery seed extract—150 mg daily.)

For Mild (140–160/90–104) to Moderate (140–180/105–114) Hypertension

- Foundational supplements
- Potassium chloride—1,500 to 3,000 mg
- Magnesium—150 to 400 mg three times daily
- PGX™—1,000 mg before meals three times daily
- Garlic—4,000 mcg allicin
- Anti-ACE fish peptides—1,500 mg daily

(*Note:* If after 2 months there is no change, add celery seed extract—150 mg daily. If there is still no change, add coenzyme Q10—100 mg daily. If blood pressure has not dropped below 140/105, you will need to work with a physician to select the most appropriate medication. If a prescription drug is necessary, calcium channel blockers or ACE inhibitors appear to be the safest for diabetics.)

For Severe Hypertension (160+/115+)

- Consult a physician immediately.
- Foundational supplements
- Potassium chloride—1,500 to 3,000 mg daily
- Magnesium—150 to 400 mg three times daily
- PGX™—1,000 mg before meals three times daily
- Garlic—4,000 mcg allicin
- Anti-ACE fish peptides—1,500 mg daily
- Celery seed extract—150 mg daily
- Coenzyme Q10—100 mg daily

(*Note:* A drug may be necessary to achieve initial control. When satisfactory control over the high blood pressure has been achieved, work with the physician to taper off the medication.)

High Cholesterol Levels and Other Cardiovascular Risk Factors

- Total cholesterol above 200 mg/dL or LDL cholesterol above 135 mg (100 mg if history of heart attack):
  PGX™—1,000 mg three times daily before meals
  Niacin (or inositol hexaniacinate)—1,000 to 1,500 mg at night at bedtime
  Garlic—minimum of 4,000 mcg allicin daily
- HDL cholesterol below 45 mg/dL: Niacin (or inositol hexaniacinate)—1,000 to 1,500 mg at night at bedtime
- Lipoprotein (a) above 40 mg/dL: Niacin (or inositol hexaniacinate)—1,500 mg at night at bedtime
- Triglycerides above 150 mg/dL: Niacin (or inositol hexaniacinate)—1,500 mg at night at bedtime
- C-reactive protein above 1.69 mg/L: Vitamin E—800 IU daily
- Fibrinogen above 400 mg/L: Garlic extract—4,000 mcg daily

- Homocysteine above 16 micromole/L: No specific recommendation; be sure to take a high-potency multiple vitamin and mineral supplement.
- Ferritin (an iron-binding protein) above 200 mcg/L: Eliminate red meat from the diet, avoid iron supplements, and increase consumption of whole grains
- Lipid peroxides elevated: No specific additional recommendations; be sure to follow the foundation supplement program for type 2 diabetes

Diabetic Retinopathy

- Bilberry extract—160 to 320 mg daily; or grapeseed extract—150 to 300 mg daily

Diabetic Neuropathy

- Gamma-linolenic acid from borage, evening primrose, or black-currant oil—480 mg daily
- Capsaicin (0.075 percent) cream—apply to affected area twice daily

Diabetic Nephropathy

- Follow recommendations for high blood pressure unless kidney function falls below 40 percent of normal. In that situation, do not supplement with magnesium and potassium unless recommended to do so by physician.

Poor Wound Healing

- Aloe vera gel—apply to affected areas twice daily

Diabetic Foot Ulcers

- Ginkgo biloba extract—120 to 240 mg daily; or grapeseed extract—150 to 300 mg daily

Open Letter to Physicians

Consider taking a copy of this letter to your physician when you discuss the use of alternative and complementary strategies for diabetes.

Dear Doctor,

We have written the book *How to Prevent and Treat Diabetes with Natural Medicine* as a guide that includes valuable and sensible information on how to incorporate diet, nutritional supplements, herbal medicine, and other strategies such as acupuncture into their diabetes treatment. Our goals are simple but important:

- Improve the sensitivity of cells to the action of insulin, thereby improving glucose tolerance and normalizing blood sugar
- Promote weight loss and reduce postprandial blood sugar levels
- Effectively reduce the complications of diabetes, including heart disease and retinopathy
- Improve the actions of drugs and insulin while at the same time reducing their side effects

Having painstakingly reviewed the medical literature, we base our recommendations on current scientific evidence and reasoning as well as our clinical experience. Should you wish to review the research that helped us form our opinions, please consult the references listed in the back of this book.

We urge you to work cooperatively with your patient to achieve the goal we all seek: the best possible outcome of care.

Sincerely,

Michael T. Murray, N.D.
Michael R. Lyon, M.D.

Table D.1. Doctor Visit Checklist

	QUARTERLY	ANNUALLY
Review Management Plan		
Blood glucose self-monitoring results	X	
Medication/insulin regimen	X	
Nutritional plan	X	
Exercise program	X	
Psychosocial support	X	
Physical Examination		
Weight	X	
Height (for children/adolescents)	X	
Sexual maturation (for children/adolescents)	X	
Skin, including insulin injection sites	X	
Feet: pulses, capillary refill, color, sensation, nails, skin, ulcers	X	
Neurologic: reflexes, proprioception, vibratory sensation, touch (distal temperature sensation, distal pinprick or pressure sensation, standardized monofilament)		X
Regular retinal exam	X	
Dilated retinal exam		X
Electrocardiogram		X
Laboratory Tests		
Fasting or random plasma glucose Normal/target range: 80–120 mg/dL before meals	X	
Glycosylated hemoglobin (A_1C) Target range: < 7 percent in adults, < 7.5 percent in children	X	
Urinalysis: glucose, ketones, microalbumin, protein, sediment	X	
Complete cardiovascular profile Test/Target: Cholesterol < 200 mg/dL Triglycerides < 200 mg/dL LDL < 130 mg/dL HDL > 35 mg/dL Lipoprotein (a) < 40 mg/dL C-reactive protein < 1.69 mg/L Fibrinogen < 400 mg/L Homocysteine < 16 micromole/L Ferritin 60 to 200 mcg/L (if elevated, transferrin saturation) Lipid peroxides < normal Serum creatinine (in adults; in children, do only if protein is present in urine)		X
	X	

A p p e n d i x   E

Are You an Optimist?

What distinguishes an optimist from a pessimist is the way in which they explain both good and bad events. Dr. Martin Seligman has developed a simple test to determine your level of optimism (from *Learned Optimism*, Knopf, 1981). Take as much time as you need. There are no right or wrong answers. It is important that you take the test before you read the interpretation. Read the description of each situation and vividly imagine it happening to you. Choose the response that most applies to you by circling either A or B. Ignore the letter and number codes for now; they will be explained later.

1. The project you are in charge of is a great success.   PsG
   A. *I kept a close watch over everyone's work.*   1
   B. *Everyone devoted a lot of time and energy to it.*   0

2. You and your spouse (boyfriend/girlfriend) make up
   after a fight.   PmG
   A. *I forgave him/her.*   0
   B. *I'm usually forgiving.*   1

3. You get lost driving to a friend's house.   PsB
   A. *I missed a turn.*   1
   B. *My friend gave me bad directions.*   0

4. Your spouse (boyfriend/girlfriend) surprises you with a gift.   PsG
   A. *He/she just got a raise at work.*   0
   B. *I took him/her out to a special dinner the night before.*   1

5. You forget your spouse's (boyfriend's/girlfriend's)
   birthday.   PmB
   A. *I'm not good at remembering birthdays.*   1
   B. *I was preoccupied with other things.*   0

6. You get a flower from a secret admirer.   PvG
   A. *I am attractive to him/her.*   0
   B. *I am a popular person.*   1

7. You run for a community office position and you win. PvG
   A. *I devote a lot of time and energy to campaigning.*   0
   B. *I work very hard at everything I do.*   1

8. You miss an important engagement.   PvB
   A. *Sometimes my memory fails me.*   1
   B. *I sometimes forget to check my appointment book.*   0

9. You run for a community office position and you lose. PsB
   A. *I didn't campaign hard enough.*   1
   B. *The person who won knew more people.*   0

10. You host a successful dinner.   PmG
    A. *I was particularly charming that night.*   0
    B. *I am a good host.*   1

11. You stop a crime by calling the police.   PsG
    A. *A strange noise caught my attention.*   0
    B. *I was alert that day.*   1

12. You were extremely healthy all year.   PsG
    A. *Few people around me were sick, so I wasn't exposed.* 0
    B. *I made sure I ate well and got enough rest.*   1

13. You owe the library ten dollars for an overdue book. PmB
    A. *When I am really involved in what I am reading,
       I often forget when it's due.*   1
    B. *I was so involved in writing the report that I forgot
       to return the book.*   0

14. Your stocks make you a lot of money.   PmG
   - A. *My broker decided to take on something new.*   0
   - B. *My broker is a top-notch investor.*   1

15. You win an athletic contest.   PmG
   - A. *I was feeling unbeatable.*   0
   - B. *I train hard.*   1

16. You fail an important examination.   PsB
   - A. *I wasn't as smart as the other people taking the exam.*   1
   - B. *I didn't prepare for it well.*   0

17. You prepared a special meal for a friend and he/she barely touched the food.   PvB
   - A. *I wasn't a good cook.*   1
   - B. *I made the meal in a rush.*   0

18. You lose a sporting event for which you have been training for a long time.   PvB
   - A. *I'm not very athletic.*   1
   - B. *I'm not good at that sport.*   0

19. Your car runs out of gas on a dark street late at night.   PsB
   - A. *I didn't check to see how much gas was in the tank.*   1
   - B. *The gas gauge was broken.*   0

20. You lose your temper with a friend.   PmB
   - A. *He/she is always nagging me.*   1
   - B. *He/she was in a hostile mood.*   0

21. You are penalized for not returning your income tax forms on time.   PmB
   - A. *I always put off doing my taxes.*   1
   - B. *I was lazy about getting my taxes done this year.*   0

22. You ask a person out on a date and he/she says no.   PvB
   - A. *I was a wreck that day.*   1
   - B. *I got tongue-tied when I asked him/her on the date.*   0

23. A game show host picks you out of the audience to
   participate in the show.   PsG
   A. *I was sitting in the right seat.*   0
   B. *I looked the most enthusiastic.*   1

24. You are frequently asked to dance at a party.   PmG
   A. *I am outgoing at parties.*   1
   B. *I was in perfect form that night.*   0

25. You buy your spouse (boyfriend/girlfriend) a gift he/she
   doesn't like.   PsB
   A. *I don't put enough thought into things like that.*   1
   B. *He/she has very picky tastes.*   0

26. You do exceptionally well in a job interview.   PmG
   A. *I felt extremely confident during the interview.*   0
   B. *I interview well.*   1

27. You tell a joke and everyone laughs.   PsG
   A. *The joke was funny.*   0
   B. *My timing was perfect.*   1

28. Your boss gives you too little time in which to finish a
   project, but you get it finished anyway.   PvG
   A. *I am good at my job.*   0
   B. *I am an efficient person.*   1

29. You've been feeling run-down lately.   PmB
   A. *I never get a chance to relax.*   1
   B. *I was exceptionally busy this week.*   0

30. You ask someone to dance and he/she says no.   PsB
   A. *I am not a good enough dancer.*   1
   B. *He/she doesn't like to dance.*   0

31. You save a person from choking to death.   PvG
   A. *I know a technique to stop someone from choking.*   0
   B. *I know what to do in crisis situations.*   1

32. Your romantic partner wants to cool things off
    for a while.   PvB
    A. *I'm too self-centered.*   1
    B. *I don't spend enough time with him/her.*   0

33. A friend says something that hurts your feelings.   PmB
    A. *She always blurts things out without thinking of others.* 1
    B. *My friend was in a bad mood and took it out on me.* 0

34. Your employer comes to you for advice.   PvG
    A. *I am an expert in the area about which I was asked.* 0
    B. *I'm good at giving useful advice.*   1

35. A friend thanks you for helping him/her get through
    a bad time.   PvG
    A. *I enjoy helping him/her through tough times.*   0
    B. *I care about people.*   1

36. You have a wonderful time at a party.   PsG
    A. *Everyone was friendly.*   0
    B. *I was friendly.*   1

37. Your doctor tells you that you are in good physical shape. PvG
    A. *I make sure I exercise frequently.*   0
    B. *I am very health-conscious.*   1

38. Your spouse (boyfriend/girlfriend) takes you away
    for a romantic weekend.   PmG
    A. *He/she needed to get away for a few days.*   0
    B. *He/she likes to explore new areas.*   1

39. Your doctor tells you that you eat too much sugar.   PsB
    A. *I don't pay much attention to my diet.*   1
    B. *You can't avoid sugar, it's in everything.*   0

40. You are asked to head an important project.   PmG
    A. *I just successfully completed a similar project.* 0
    B. *I am a good supervisor.*   1

41. You and your spouse (boyfriend/girlfriend) have
    been fighting a great deal.   PsB
    A. *I have been feeling cranky and pressured lately.*   1
    B. *He/she has been hostile lately.*   0

42. You fall down a great deal while skiing.   PmB
    A. *Skiing is difficult.*   1
    B. *The trails were icy.*   0

43. You win a prestigious award.   PvG
    A. *I solved an important problem.*   0
    B. *I was the best employee.*   1

44. Your stocks are at an all-time low.   PvB
    A. *I didn't know much about the business climate at the time.* 1
    B. *I made a poor choice of stocks.*   0

45. You win the lottery.   PsG
    A. *It was pure chance.*   0
    B. *I picked the right numbers.*   1

46. You gain weight over the holidays and you can't lose it.   PmB
    A. *Diets don't work in the long run.*   1
    B. *The diet I tried didn't work.*   0

47. You are in the hospital and few people come to visit.   PsB
    A. *I'm irritable when I am sick.*   1
    B. *My friends are negligent about things like that.*   0

48. They won't honor your credit card at a store.   PvB
    A. *I sometimes overestimate how much money I have.*   1
    B. *I sometimes forget to pay my credit card bill.*   0

SCORING KEY

PmB _____	PmG _____
PvB _____	PvG _____
PsB _____	PsG _____

Total B _____	Total G _____
	G – B _____

Interpreting Your Test Results

The test results will give you a clue as to your explanatory style. In other words, the results will tell you about the way in which you explain things to yourself. It tells you your habit of thought. Again, remember that there are no right or wrong answers.

There are three crucial dimensions to your explanatory style: permanence, pervasiveness, and personalization. Each dimension, plus a couple of others, will be scored from your test.

Permanence

When pessimists are faced with challenges or bad events, they view these events as being permanent. In contrast, people who are optimists tend to view the challenges or bad events as temporary. Here are some statements that reflect the subtle differences:

PERMANENT (PESSIMISTIC)	TEMPORARY (OPTIMISTIC)
"My boss is always a jerk."	"My boss is in a bad mood today."
"You never listen."	"You are not listening."
"This bad luck will never stop."	"My luck has got to turn."

To determine how you view bad events, look at the eight items coded PmB (for Permanent Bad): 5, 13, 20, 21, 29, 33, 42, and 46. Each statement with a "0" after it is optimistic; each one followed by a "1" is pessimistic. Total the numbers in the rightmost column for the questions coded PmB, and write the total on the PmB line in the scoring key.

If you totaled 0 or 1, you are very optimistic on this dimension; 2 or 3 is a moderately optimistic score; 4 is average; 5 or 6 is quite pessimistic; and 7 or 8 is extremely pessimistic.

Now let's look at the difference in explanatory style between pessimists and optimists when there is a positive event in their lives. It's just the opposite of what happened with a bad event. Pessimists view positive events as temporary, while optimists view them as permanent. Here again are some subtle differences in how pessimists and optimists might communicate their good fortune:

TEMPORARY (PESSIMISTIC)	PERMANENT (OPTIMISTIC)
"It's my lucky day."	"I am always lucky."
"My opponent was off today."	"I am getting better every day."
"I tried hard today."	"I always give my best."

Now total your score for the questions coded PmG (for Permanent Good): 2, 10, 14, 15, 24, 26, 38, and 40. Write the total on the PmG line in the scoring key.

If you totaled 7 or 8, you are very optimistic on this dimension; 6 is a moderately optimistic score; 4 or 5 is average; 3 is pessimistic; and 0, 1, or 2 is extremely pessimistic.

Are you starting to see a pattern? If you are scoring as a pessimist, you may want to learn how to be more optimistic. Your anxiety may be due to your belief that bad things are always going to happen, while good things are only a fluke.

Pervasiveness

Pervasiveness refers to the tendency to describe things either in universals (everyone, always, never, and so on) versus specifics (a specific individual, a specific time, and so on). Pessimists tend to describe things in universals, while optimists describe things in specifics.

UNIVERSAL (PESSIMISTIC)	SPECIFIC (OPTIMISTIC)
"All lawyers are jerks."	"My attorney was a jerk."
"Instruction manuals are worthless."	"This instruction manual is worthless."
"He is repulsive."	"He is repulsive to me."

Total your score for the questions coded PvB (for Pervasive Bad): 8, 17, 18, 22, 32, 44, and 48. Write the total on the PvB line in the scoring key.

If you totaled 0 or 1, you are very optimistic on this dimension; 2 or 3 is a moderately optimistic score; 4 is average; 5 or 6 is quite pessimistic; and 7 is extremely pessimistic.

Now let's look at the level of pervasiveness of good events. Optimists tend to view good events as universal, while pessimists view them as specific. Again, it's just the opposite of how each views a bad event.

Total your score for the questions coded PvG (for Pervasive Good): 6, 7, 28, 31, 34, 35, 37, and 43. Write the total on the PvG line in the scoring key.

If you totaled 7 or 8, you are very optimistic on this dimension; 6 is a moderately optimistic score; 4 or 5 is average; 3 is pessimistic; and 0, 1, or 2 is extremely pessimistic.

Hope

Our level of hope or hopelessness is determined by our combined level of permanence and pervasiveness. Your level of hope may be the most significant score for this test. Take your PvB and add it to your PmB score. This is your hope score.

If it is 0, 1, or 2, you are extraordinarily hopeful; 3, 4, 5, or 6 is a moderately hopeful score; 7 or 8 is average; 9, 10, or 11 is moderately hopeless; and 12, 13, 14, or 15 is severely hopeless.

People who make permanent and universal explanations for their troubles tend to suffer from stress, anxiety, and depression; they tend to collapse when things go wrong. According to Dr. Seligman, no other score is as important as your hope score.

Personalization

The final aspect of explanatory style is personalization. When bad things happen, we can either blame ourselves (internalize) and lower our self-esteem as a consequence, or we can blame things beyond our control (externalize). Although it may not be right to deny personal responsibility, people who tend to externalize blame in relation to bad events have higher self-esteem and are more optimistic.

Total your score for the questions coded PsB (for Personalization Bad): 3, 9, 16, 19, 25, 30, 39, 41, and 47.

A score of 0 or 1 indicates very high self-esteem and optimism; 2 or 3 indicates moderate self-esteem; 4 is average; 5 or 6 indicates moderately low self-esteem; and 7, 8, or 9 indicates very low self-esteem.

Now let's take a look at personalization and good events. Again, just the exact opposite occurs compared to bad events. When good things happen, the person with high self-esteem internalizes while the person with low self-esteem externalizes.

Total your score for the questions coded PsG (for Personalization Good): 1, 4, 11, 12, 23, 27, 36, and 45. Write your score on the PsG line in the scoring key.

If you totaled 7 or 8, you are very optimistic on this dimension; 6 is a moderately optimistic score; 4 or 5 is average; 3 is pessimistic; and 0, 1, or 2 is extremely pessimistic.

Your Overall Scores

To compute your overall scores, first add the three B categories (PmB + PvB + PsB). This is your B (bad event) score. Do the same for all of the G categories (PmG + PvG + PsG). This is your G score. Subtract B from G; this is your overall score.

If your B score is from 3 to 6, you are marvelously optimistic when bad events occur; 10 or 11 is average; 12 to 14 is pessimistic; anything above 14 is extremely pessimistic.

If your G score is 19 or above, you think about good events extremely optimistically; 14 to 16 is average; 11 to 13 indicates pessimism; and a score of 10 or less indicates great pessimism.

If your overall score (G minus B) is above 8, you are very optimistic across the board; if it's from 6 to 8, you are moderately optimistic; 3 to 5 is average; 1 or 2 is pessimistic; and a score of 0 or below is very pessimistic.

Hypoglycemia Questionnaire

Circle the number that best describes the intensity of symptoms suggestive of low blood sugar on the following scale:

0 = I do not experience this symptom
1 = Mild
2 = Moderate
3 = Severe

1. Dizziness when standing suddenly	0	1	2	3
2. Loss of vision when standing suddenly	0	1	2	3
3. Crave sweets	0	1	2	3
4. Headaches relieved by eating sweets or alcohol	0	1	2	3
5. Feel shaky	0	1	2	3
6. Irritable if a meal is missed	0	1	2	3
7. Wake up in middle of night craving sweets	0	1	2	3
8. Feel tired or weak if a meal is missed	0	1	2	3
9. Heart palpitations after eating sweets	0	1	2	3
10. Need to drink coffee to get started	0	1	2	3
11. Impatient, moody, nervous	0	1	2	3
12. Feel tired 1 to 3 hours after eating	0	1	2	3
13. Poor memory	0	1	2	3
14. Poor concentration	0	1	2	3
15. Forgetful	0	1	2	3
16. Calmer after eating	0	1	2	3

TOTAL _____

Scoring

12 or more: High priority
6–11: Moderate priority
1–5: Low priority

Interpretation

A score of 12 or higher indicates that hypoglycemia is a major factor on your health. A score of 6 to 11 indicates that hypoglycemia is likely responsible for some of your symptoms and every effort should be made to maintain better blood sugar control. A score of less than 6 indicates that hypoglycemia is not likely a significant factor on your health. The dietary approach to hypoglycemia involves the same basic principles as those given for diabetes.

Seven Steps to Creating an Effective Exercise Routine

Step 1: Recognize the Importance of Physical Exercise

The first step is realizing just how important it is to get regular exercise. We cannot stress enough just how vital regular exercise is to your health. But as much as we stress this fact, it means nothing unless it really sinks in and you accept it, too. You must make regular exercise a top priority in your life.

Step 2: Consult Your Physician

If you are not currently on a regular exercise program, get medical clearance if you have health problems or if you are over age 40. The main concern is the functioning of your heart. Exercise can be quite harmful (and even fatal) if your heart is not able to meet the increased demands placed on it.

It is especially important to see a physician if any of the following applies to you:

- Heart disease
- Smoking
- High blood pressure
- Extreme breathlessness with physical exertion
- Pain or pressure in chest, arm, teeth, jaw, or neck with exercise

- Dizziness or fainting
- Abnormal heart action (palpitations or irregular beat)

Step 3: Select an Activity You Enjoy

If you are fit enough to begin, the next thing to do is select an activity that you will enjoy. Using the following list, choose one to five of the activities that you think you may enjoy—or fill in a choice or two of your own. Make a commitment to do one activity a day for at least 20 minutes, and preferably an hour. Make your goal to enjoy the activity. The important thing is to move your body enough to raise your pulse a bit above its resting rate.

Bicycling	Jogging
Bowling	Stair climbing
Cross-country skiing	Stationary bicycling
Dancing	Swimming
Gardening	Tennis
Golfing	Treadmill
Heavy housecleaning	Walking
Jazzercise	Weight lifting

In general, the best exercises are the ones that get your heart moving. Aerobic activities such as walking briskly, jogging, bicycling, cross-country skiing, swimming, aerobic dance, and racquet sports are good examples. Brisk walking (4 to 5 miles per hour) for approximately 30 minutes may be the very best form of exercise for most people. Walking can be done anywhere, and the risk of injury is extremely low. It doesn't require any expensive equipment—just comfortable clothing and well-fitting shoes. If you are going to walk on a regular basis, we strongly urge you to first purchase a pair of high-quality walking or jogging shoes. They will not only make walking more enjoyable and comfortable, but they can also reduce the risk of injury.

Step 4: Monitor Exercise Intensity

Exercise intensity is determined by measuring your heart rate (the number of times your heart beats per minute). This determination can quickly be made by placing the index and middle finger of one hand on your opposite wrist, or on the side of your neck just below the angle of your jaw. Beginning with zero, count the number of heartbeats for six seconds. Simply append a zero to this number, and you have your pulse rate. For example, if you counted fourteen beats, your heart rate would be 140. Would this be a good number? It depends on your "training zone." A quick and easy way to determine your maximum training heart rate is to simply subtract your age from 185. For example, if you are 40, your maximum heart rate would be 145. To determine the bottom of the training zone, simply subtract 20 from this number. In the case of a 40-year-old, this would be 125. So the training range for a 40-year-old would be between 125 and 145 beats per minute. For maximum health benefits, you must stay within your training zone or range and never exceed it.

Step 5: Do It Often

You don't get in good physical condition by exercising once; it must be done on a regular basis. A minimum of 15 to 20 minutes of exercising at your training heart rate at least three times a week is necessary to gain any significant cardiovascular benefits from exercise. It is better to exercise at the lower end of your training zone for longer periods of time than it is to exercise at a higher intensity for a shorter period of time. It is also better if you can make exercise a part of your daily routine.

Step 6: Make It Fun

The key to getting the maximum benefit from exercise is to make it enjoyable. Choose an activity that you enjoy and have fun with. If you can find enjoyment in exercise, you are much more likely to exercise regularly. One way to make it fun is to get a workout partner. For example, if you choose walking as your activity, here is a great way to make it fun:

Find one or two people in your neighborhood with whom you would enjoy walking. If you are meeting others, you will certainly be more regular than if you depend solely on your own intentions. Commit to walking three to five mornings or afternoons each week, and increase the exercise duration from an initial 10 minutes to at least 30 minutes.

Step 7: Stay Motivated

No matter how committed you are to regular exercise, at some point you are going to be faced with a loss of enthusiasm for working out. Here is a suggestion: Take a break. Not a long break; just skip one or two workouts. It gives your enthusiasm and motivation a chance to recoup so that you can come back with an even stronger commitment. Here are some other things to help you to stay motivated:

- Read or thumb through fitness magazines like *Shape, Men's Fitness, Muscle & Fitness,* and *Muscular Development.* Looking at pictures of people in fantastic shape really inspires me. In addition, these magazines typically feature articles on new exercise routines that interest me.
- Set exercise goals. Because I am a goal-oriented individual, goals really help keep me motivated. Success breeds success, so set a lot of small goals that can easily be achieved. Write down your daily exercise goal and check it off when you have it completed.
- Vary your routine. Variety is important to help you stay interested in exercise. Doing the same thing every day becomes monotonous and drains motivation. Continually find new ways to enjoy working out.
- Keep a record of your activities and progress. Sometimes it is hard to see the progress you are making, but if you write in a journal you'll have a permanent record of your progress. Keeping track of your progress will motivate you toward continued improvement.

A p p e n d i x   H

What to Look for in a Multiple
Vitamin and Mineral Supplement

While a health-promoting diet is an essential component of good health, so too is proper nutritional supplementation. While some experts say that you can theoretically meet all of your nutritional needs through diet alone, the reality is that most Americans do not come anywhere near the optimal levels. During recent years the U.S. government has sponsored a number of comprehensive studies (HANES I, II, and III, Ten State Nutrition Survey, USDA nationwide food consumption studies, and so on) to determine the nutritional status of the population. These studies have revealed that marginal nutrient deficiencies exist in a substantial portion of the U.S. population (approximately 50 percent) and that for some selected nutrients in certain age groups, more than 80 percent of the group consumed less than the RDA.[1]

These studies indicate the that chance of consuming a diet meeting the recommended dietary allowance (RDA) for all nutrients is extremely unlikely for most Americans. In other words, while it is theoretically possible that a healthy individual can get all the nutrition he or she needs from foods, most Americans do not even come close. In an effort to increase their intake of essential nutrients, many Americans look to vitamin and mineral supplements.

Current estimates are that more than 70 percent of Americans now regularly take vitamin or mineral supplements.[2,3] It seems that taking vitamin and mineral supplements has become a way of life for most Americans. Sixty-seven percent of supplement users take only one supplement, with most of them taking a multiple vitamin and mineral product (46 percent). Unfortunately, most people taking a multiple vitamin and mineral formula are still not getting what they really need because they are being misled into thinking that a "one-a-day" multiple is meeting all their needs for optimum nutrition.

Giving Your Body the Tools It Needs

For optimum health, a high-quality multiple vitamin and mineral supplement is an absolute necessity. A high-quality multiple provides optimal levels of both vitamins and minerals. Your body needs all of the important building blocks in order to build health. The following recommendations provide an optimum intake range to guide you in selecting a high-quality multiple. (Note that different vitamins and minerals are measured in different units (IU = International Units; mg = milligrams; mcg = micrograms).

To find a multiple vitamin and mineral formula that meet these criteria, read labels carefully. Be aware that you will not be able to find a formula that can provide all of these nutrients at these levels in one single pill—it would simply be too large. Usually it will require at least four to six tablets to meet these levels. While many "one-a-day" supplements provide good levels of vitamins, they are woefully insufficient in the levels of minerals.

Realistic Expectations

In addition to the enormous number of studies showing benefits from the individual nutrients in a high-potency multiple, studies have shown that people taking a multiple vitamin and mineral formula may experience higher energy levels, improved brain function, fewer colds or infections, improved ability to deal with stress, a greater sense of well-being, and other health benefits.[4–8] However, the reality is that many people taking a multiple may feel nothing. But just because you may not feel anything doesn't mean that the higher nutrient levels you are ingesting are not being used by the body. For example, there is evidence that people taking nutritional supplements may have a lowered risk for heart disease, cancer, cataracts, and other degenerative diseases.[9–11] In a recent finding, women taking a multiple vitamin and mineral formula for more than 14 years had a 75 percent reduced rate of colon cancer.[12] While it is extremely unlikely that these women felt the awesome protection they were being given by their supplement, nonetheless they definitely realized the benefits.

VITAMIN	RANGE FOR ADULTS
Vitamin A (retinol)[a]	2,500–5,000 IU
Vitamin A (from beta-carotene)	5,000–25,000 IU
Vitamin B_1 (thiamin)	10–100 mg
Vitamin B_2 (riboflavin)	10–50 mg
Vitamin B_3 (niacin)	10–100 mg
Vitamin B_5 (pantothenic acid)	25–100 mg
Vitamin B_6 (pyridoxine)	25–100 mg
Vitamin B_{12} (cobalamin)	400 mcg
Vitamin C (ascorbic acid)	250–500 mg
Vitamin D[b]	100–600 IU
Vitamin E (d-alpha tocopherol)	100–400 IU
Niacinamide	10–30 mg
Biotin	100–600 mcg
Folic acid	400–800 mcg
Choline	10–100 mg
Inositol	10–100 mg
MINERAL	RANGE FOR ADULTS
Calcium[c]	250–1,000 mg
Chromium	200–400 mcg
Copper	1–2 mg
Iodine	50–150 mcg
Iron[d]	15–30 mg
Magnesium	250–350 mg
Manganese	10–15 mg
Molybdenum	10–25 mcg
Selenium	100–200 mcg
Silica	1–25 mg
Vanadium	50–100 mcg
Zinc	15–20 mg

[a] Women of child-bearing age who might become pregnant should not take more than 2,500 IU of retinol daily, because of the possible risk of birth defects. (*Note:* Beta-carotene is safe during pregnancy and lactation.)

[b] People living in northern latitudes should supplement at the high range.

[c] Women should take 800 to 1,000 mg of calcium to reduce the risk of osteoporosis.

[d] Men and postmenopausal women rarely need supplemental iron.

Glycemic Index, Carbohydrate Content, Fiber Content, and Glycemic Load of Selected Foods

A complete list of the glycemic index and glycemic load of all tested foods is beyond the scope of this book—it would be a book in itself. So we have selected the most common foods. This listing will give you a general sense of what is a high-GL and low-GL food. We have listed the items by food groups, from low to high glycemic loads. You may notice that certain food groups are not listed. For example, you won't see nuts, seeds, fish, poultry, and meats listed; these foods have little impact on blood sugar levels because they are low in carbohydrates.

If you would like to see an even more complete listing, visit www. mendosa.com—a free Web site operated by medical writer Rick Mendosa. It is an excellent resource.

FOOD	GI	CARBS (G)	FIBER (G)	GL
Beans (Legumes)				
Soybeans, cooked, ½ cup, 100 g	14	12	7	1.6
Peas, green, fresh, frozen, boiled, ½ cup, 80 g	48	5	2	2
White navy beans, boiled, ½ cup, 90 g	38	11	6	4.2
Kidney beans, boiled, ½ cup, 90 g	27	18	7.3	4.8
Peas, split, yellow, boiled, ½ cup, 90 g	32	16	4.7	5.1
Lentils, ½ cup, 100g	28	19	3.7	5.3
Lima beans, baby, ½ cup cooked, 85 g	32	17	4.5	5.4
Black beans, canned, ½ cup, 95 g	45	15	7	5.7
Pinto beans, canned, ½ cup, 95 g	45	13	6.7	5.8
Chickpeas, canned, drained, ½ cup, 95 g	42	15	5	6.3
Kidney beans, canned and drained, ½ cup, 95 g	52	13	7.3	6.7
Broad beans, frozen, boiled, ½ cup, 80 g	79	9	6	7.1
Peas, dried, boiled, ½ cup, 70 g	22	4	4.7	8
Baked beans, canned in tomato sauce, ½ cup, 120 g	48	21	8.8	10
Blackeyed peas, soaked, boiled, ½ cup, 120 g	42	24	5	10
Bread				
Multigrain, unsweetened, 1 slice, 30 g	43	9	1.4	4
Oat Bran & Honey Loaf, 1 slice, 40 g	31	14	1.5	4.5
Sourdough, rye, 1 slice, 30 g	48	12	0.4	6
Stoneground whole-wheat, 1 slice, 30 g	53	11	1.4	6
Wonder enriched white, 1 slice, 20 g	73	10	0.4	7
Sourdough, wheat, 1 slice, 30 g	54	14	0.4	7.5
Pumpernickel, 1 slice, 60 g	41	21	0.5	8.6
Whole-wheat, 1 slice, 35 g	69	14	1.4	9.6
Healthy Choice, hearty 7-grain, 1 slice, 38 g	56	18	1.4	10
White (wheat flour), 1 slice, 30 g	70	15	0.4	10.5
Healthy Choice, 100% whole grain, 1 slice, 38 g	62	18	1.4	11
Gluten-free multigrain, 1 slice, 35 g	79	15	1.8	12
French baguette, 30 g	95	15	0.4	14

FOOD	GI	CARBS (G)	FIBER (G)	GL
Bread (cont.)				
Hamburger bun, 1 prepacked bun, 50 g	61	24	0.5	15
Rye, 1 slice, 50 g	65	23	0.4	15
Light rye, 1 slice, 50 g	68	23	0.4	16
Dark rye, black, 1 slice, 50 g	76	21	0.4	16
Croissant, 1, 50 g	67	27	0.2	18
Kaiser roll, 1, 50 g	73	25	0.4	18
Pita, 1 piece, 65 g	57	38	0.4	22
Bagel, 1, 70 g	72	35	0.4	25
Breakfast Cereals				
Oat bran, raw, 1 tablespoon, 10 g	55	7	1	4
Bran with psyllium, 1/3 cup, 30 g	47	12	12.5	5.6
Bran, 1/3 cup, 30 g	58	14	14	8
All-Bran Soy 'n Fiber, 1/2 cup, 45 g	33	26	7	8.5
All-Bran, 1/2 cup, 40 g	42	22	6.5	9.2
Oatmeal (cooked with water), 1 cup, 245 g	42	24	1.6	10
Shredded wheat, 1/3 cup, 25 g	67	18	1.2	12
Mini-Wheats (whole wheat), 1 cup, 30 g	58	21	4.4	12
All-Bran Fruit 'n Oats, 1/2 cup, 45 g	39	33	6	13
Weet-Bix, 2 biscuits, 30 g	69	19	2	13
Cheerios, 1/2 cup, 30 g	74	20	2	15
Frosties, 3/4 cup, 30 g	55	27	1	15
Corn Bran, 1/2 cup, 30 g	75	20	1	15
Honey Smacks, 3/4 cup, 30 g	56	27	1	15
Wheatbites, 30 g	72	22	2	16
Total, 30 g	76	22	2	16.7
Healthwise for Heart Health, 45 g	48	35	2	16.8
Mini-Wheats (black currant) 1 cup, 30 g	71	24	2	17
Puffed wheat, 1 cup, 30 g	80	22	2	17.6
Bran Flakes, 3/4 cup, 30 g	74	24	2	18
Crunchy Nut Cornflakes (Kellogg's), 30 g	72	25	2	18
Froot Loops, 1 cup, 30 g	69	27	1	18
Cocoa Puffs, 3/4 cup, 30 g	77	26	1	20

FOOD	GI	CARBS (G)	FIBER (G)	GL
Breakfast cereals (cont.)				
Team, 30 g	82	25	1	20.5
Corn Chex, 30 g	83	25	1	20.75
Just Right, ¾ cup, 30 g	60	36	2	21.6
Corn flakes, 1 cup, 30 g	84	26	0.3	21.8
Rice Krispies, 1 cup, 30 g	82	27	0.3	22
Rice Chex, 1 cup, 30 g	89	25	1	22
Crispix, 30 g	87	26	1	22.6
Just Right Just Grains, 1 cup, 45 g	62	38	2	23.5
Oat 'n Honey Bake, 45 g	77	31	2	24
Raisin Bran, 1 cup, 45 g	73	35	4	25.5
Grape-Nuts, ½ cup, 58 g	71	47	2	33.3
Cake				
Cake, angel food, 1 slice, 30 g	67	17	< 1	11.5
Cake, sponge, 1 slice, 60 g	46	32	< 1	14.7
Cupcake, with icing and cream filling, 1 Cake, 38 g	73	26	< 1	19
Cake, chocolate fudge (Betty Crocker), 73 g cake + 33 g frosting	38	54	< 1	20.5
Cake, banana, 1 slice, 80 g	47	46	< 1	21.6
Cake, pound, 1 slice, 80 g	54	42	< 1	22.6
Cake, French vanilla (Betty Crocker), 73 g cake + 33 g frosting	42	58	< 1	24.4
Cake, Lamington's, 1, 50 g	87	29	< 1	25
Flan, 1 slice, 80 g	65	55	< 1	35.75
Scones, made from packet mix, 1 scone, 40 g	92	90	< 1	83
Crackers				
Corn Thins, puffed corn cake, 2, 12 g	87	9	< 1	7.8
Crackers, Kavli, 4, 20 g	71	13	3	9.2
Breton wheat crackers, 6, 25 g	67	14	2	9.4
Ryvita or Wasa, 2, 20 g	69	16	3	11
Stoned Wheat Thins, 5, 25 g	67	17	1	11.4
Premium soda crackers, 3, 25 g	74	17	0	12.5
Water crackers, 5, 25 g	78	18	0	14
Crackers, graham 1, 30 g	74	22	1.4	16
Rice cakes, 2, 25 g	82	21	0.4	17

FOOD	GI	CARBS (G)	FIBER (G)	GL
Milk, Soy Milk, and Juices				
Milk, whole, 1 cup, 250 mL	27	12	0	3
Soy, 1 cup, 250 mL	31	12	0	3.7
Milk, skim, 1 cup, 250 mL	32	13	0	4
Grapefruit juice, unsweetened, 1 cup, 250 ml	48	16	1	7.7
Nesquik chocolate powder, 3 tsp in 250 mL milk	55	14	0	7.7
Milk, chocolate flavored, low-fat, 1 cup, 250 mL	34	23	0	7.8
Orange juice, 1 cup, 250 mL	46	21	1	9.7
Gatorade, 1 cup, 250 mL	78	15	0	11.7
Pineapple juice, unsweetened, canned, 250 mL	46	27	1	12.4
Apple juice, unsweetened, 1 cup, 250 mL	40	33	1	13.2
Cranberry juice cocktail (Ocean Spray USA), 240 mL	68	34	0	23
Coca-Cola, 375 mL	63	40	0	25.2
Soft drink, 375 mL	68	51	0	34.7
Milk, sweetened condensed, ½ cup, 160 g	61	90	0	55
Fruit				
Cherries, 20, 80 g	22	10	2.4	2.2
Plums, 3–4 small, 100 g	39	7	2.2	2.7
Peach, fresh, 1 large, 110 g	42	7	1.9	3
Apricots, fresh, 3 medium, 100 g	57	7	1.9	4
Apricots, dried, 5–6 pieces, 30 g	31	13	2.2	4
Kiwi, 1 raw, peeled, 80 g	52	8	2.4	4
Orange, 1 medium, 130 g	44	10	2.6	4.4
Peach, canned, in natural juice, ½ cup, 125 g	38	12	1.5	4.5
Pear, canned in pear juice, ½ cup, 125 g	43	13	1.5	5.5
Watermelon, 1 cup, 150 g	72	8	1	5.7
Pineapple, fresh, 2 slices, 125 g	66	10	2.8	6.6
Apple, 1 medium, 150 g	38	18	3.5	6.8
Grapes, green, 1 cup, 100 g	46	15	2.4	6.9
Apple, dried, 30g	29	24	3.0	6.9

FOOD	GI	CARBS (G)	FIBER (G)	GL
Fruit (cont.)				
Prunes, pitted (Sunsweet), 6 prunes, 40 g	29	25	3.0	7.25
Pear, fresh, 1 medium, 150 g	38	21	3.1	8
Fruit cocktail, canned in natural juice, ½ cup, 125 g	55	15	1.5	8.25
Apricots, canned, light syrup, ½ cup, 125 g	64	13	1.5	8.3
Peaches, canned, light syrup, ½ cup, 125 g	52	18	1.5	9.4
Mango, 1 small, 150 g	55	19	2.0	10.4
Figs, dried, tenderized (water added), 50 g	61	22	3.0	13.4
Sultanas, ¼ cup, 40 g	56	30	3.1	16.8
Banana, raw, 1 medium, 150 g	55	32	2.4	17.6
Raisins, ¼ cup, 40 g	64	28	3.1	18
Dates, dried, 5, 40 g	103	27	3.0	27.8
Grains				
Rice bran, extruded, 1 tablespoon, 10 g	19	3	1	0.57
Barley, pearled, boiled, ½ cup, 80 g	25	17	6	4.25
Millet, cooked, ½ cup, 120 g	71	12	1	8.52
Bulgur, cooked, ⅔ cup, 120 g	48	22	3.5	10.6
Brown rice, steamed, 1 cup 150 g	50	32	1	16
Couscous, cooked, ⅔ cup, 120 g	65	28	1	18
Rice, white, boiled, 1 cup 150 g	72	36	0.2	26
Arborio risotto rice, white, boiled, 100 g	69	35	0.2	29
Rice, basmati, white, boiled, 1 cup, 180 g	58	50	0.2	29
Buckwheat, cooked, ½ cup, 80 g	54	57	3.5	30
Rice, instant, cooked, 1 cup, 180 g	87	38	0.2	33
Tapioca (steamed 1 hour), 100 g	70	54	< 1	38
Tapioca (boiled with milk), 1 cup, 265 g	81	51	< 1	41
Rice, jasmine, white, long grain, steamed, 1 cup, 180 g	109	39	0.2	42.5

FOOD	GI	CARBS (G)	FIBER (G)	GL
Ice Cream				
Ice cream, low-fat French vanilla, 100 mL	38	15	0	5.7
Ice cream, full-fat, 2 scoops, 50 g	61	10	0	6.1
Jam				
Jam, no sugar, 1 tbsp, 25 g	55	11	< 1	6
Jam, sweetened, 1 tbsp	48	17	< 1	8
Muffins and Pancakes				
Muffins, chocolate butterscotch, from mix, 50 g	53	28	1	15
Muffins, apple, oat, and sultana, from mix, 50 g	54	28	1	15
Muffins, apricot, coconut, and honey, from mix, 50 g	60	27	1.5	16
Muffins, banana, oat, and honey, from mix, 50 g	65	28	1.5	18
Muffin, apple, 1, 80 g	44	44	1,5	19
Muffin, bran, 1, 80 g	60	34	2.5	20
Muffin, blueberry, 1, 80 g	59	41	1.5	24
Pancake, buckwheat, from dry mix, 40 g	102	30	2	30
Pancake, from dry mix, 1 large, 80 g	67	58	1	39
Pasta				
Tortellini, cheese, cooked, 180 g	50	21	2	10.5
Ravioli, meat-filled, cooked, 1 cup, 220 g	39	30	2	11.7
Vermicelli, cooked, 1 cup, 180 g	35	45	2	15.7
Rice noodles, fresh, boiled, 1 cup, 176 g	40	44	0.4	17.6
Spaghetti, whole-meal, cooked, 1 cup, 180 g	37	48	3.5	17.75
Fettucini, cooked, 1 cup, 180 g	32	57	2	18.2
Spaghetti, gluten-free in tomato sauce, 1 small can, 220 g	68	27	2	18.5
Macaroni and cheese, packaged, cooked, 220 g	64	30	2	19.2
Star pastina, cooked, 1 cup, 180 g	38	56	2	21
Spaghetti, white, cooked, 1 cup, 180 g	41	56	2	23
Rice pasta, brown, cooked, 1 cup, 180 g	92	57	2	52

FOOD	GI	CARBS (G)	FIBER (G)	GL
Sugars				
Fructose, 10 g	23	10	0	2.3
Honey, ½ tbsp, 10 g	58	16	0	4.6
Lactose, 10 g	46	10	0	4.6
Sucrose, 10 g	65	10	0	6.5
Glucose, 10 g	102	10	0	10.2
Maltose, 10 g	105	10	0	10.5
Snacks				
Corn chips, Doritos original, 50 g	42	33	< 1	13.9
Snickers, 59 g	41	35	0	14.3
Tofu Frozen Dessert (nondairy), 100 g	115	13	< 1	15
Real Fruit bars, strawberry, 20 g	90	17	< 1	15.3
Twix cookie bar (caramel), 59 g	44	37	< 1	16.2
Pretzels, 50 g	83	22	< 1	18.3
Mars Bar, 60 g	65	41	0	26.6
Skittles, 62 g	70	55	0	38.5
Soups				
Tomato, canned, 220 mL	38	15	1.5	6
Black bean, 220 mL	64	9	3.4	6
Lentil, canned, 220 mL	44	14	3	6
Split pea, canned, 220 mL	60	13	3	8
Vegetables				
Carrots, raw, ½ cup, 80 g	16	6	1.5	1

Low glycemic vegetables:
    Asparagus, 1 cup cooked or raw
    Bell peppers, 1 cup cooked or raw
    Broccoli, 1 cup cooked or raw
    Brussels sprouts, 1 cup cooked or raw
    Cabbage, 1 cup cooked or raw
    Cauliflower, 1 cup cooked or raw
    Cucumber, 1 cup
    Celery, 1 cup cooked or raw
    Eggplant, 1 cup
    Green beans, 1 cup cooked or raw
    Kale, 1 cup cooked, 2 cups raw
    Lettuce, 2 cups raw
    Mushrooms, 1 cup
    Spinach, 1 cup cooked, 2 cups raw
    Tomatoes, 1 cup
    Zucchini, 1 cup cooked or raw
	≈20	≈7	≈1.5	≈1.4

FOOD	GI	CARBS (G)	FIBER (G)	GL
Vegetables (cont.)				
Carrots, peeled, boiled, ½ cup, 70 g	49	3	1.5	1.5
Beets, canned, drained, 2–3 slices, 60 g	64	5	1	3
Pumpkin, peeled, boiled, ½ cup, 85 g	75	6	3.4	4.5
Parsnips, boiled, ½ cup, 75 g	97	8	3	8
Sweet corn on the cob, boiled 20 min, 80 g	48	14	2.9	8
Corn, canned and drained, ½ cup, 80 g	55	15	3	8.5
Sweet potato, peeled, boiled, 80 g	54	16	3.4	8.6
Sweet corn, ½ cup boiled, 80 g	55	18	3	10
Potato, peeled, boiled, 1 medium, 120 g	87	13	1.4	10
Potato, with skin, boiled, 1 medium, 120 g	79	15	2.4	11
Yam, boiled, 80 g	51	26	3.4	13
Potato, baked in oven (no fat), 1 medium, 120 g	93	15	2.4	14
Potatoes, mashed, ½ cup, 120 g	91	16	1	14
Potatoes, instant, prepared, ½ cup	83	18	1	15
Potatoes, new, unpeeled, boiled, 5 small (cocktail), 175 g	78	25	2	20
Cornmeal (polenta), ⅓ cup, 40 g	68	30	2	20
French fries, fine cut, 120g	75	49	1	36
Gnocchi, cooked, 1 cup, 145 g	68	71	1	48
Yogurt				
Yogurt, low-fat, artificial sweetener, 200 g	14	12	0	2
Yogurt, with fruit, 200 g	26	30	0	8
Yogurt, low-fat, 200 g	33	26	0	8.5

Resources

Acupuncture

Accreditation Commission for Acupuncture and Oriental
  Medicine (ACAOM)
7501 Greenway Center Drive, Suite 820
Greenbelt, MD 20770
(301) 313-0855
Fax (301) 313-0912
www.acaom.org

American Diabetes Association

American Diabetes Association
1701 North Beauregard Street
Alexandria, VA 22311
(800) 342-2383
www.diabetes.org

The American Diabetes Association (ADA) is the nation's leading
nonprofit health organization providing diabetes research, information, and advocacy.

Health Food Store Locator

The National Nutritional Foods Association (NNFA)
www.nnfa.org

The NNFA, founded in 1936, represents the manufacturers and retailers of the natural foods industry. To find a health food store retailer in your area, go to the NNFA Web site.

Naturopathic Medical Schools

Bastyr University
14500 Juanita Drive
Kenmore, WA 98028
(425) 602-3000
www.bastyr.edu

Canadian College of Naturopathic Medicine
1255 Sheppard Ave. East
North York, Ontario M2K 1E2
Canada
(416) 498-1255
www.ccnm.edu

National College of Naturopathic Medicine
049 S.W. Porter
Portland, OR 97201
(503) 499-4343
www.ncnm.edu

Southwest College of Naturopathic Medicine & Health Sciences
2140 E. Broadway Road
Tempe, AZ 85282
(480) 858-9100
www.scnm.edu

Naturopathic Physician Associations and Referrals

The American Association of Naturopathic Physicians
8201 Greensboro Drive, Suite 300
McLean, VA 22102
(877) 969-2267
www.naturopathic.org

Canadian Naturopathic Association
1255 Sheppard Ave. East
North York, Ontario M2K 1E2
Canada
(416) 496-8633
www.naturopathicassoc.ca

References

The primary resources for the materials presented in this book are the personal files of Dr. Murray. Over the past 25 to 30 years Dr. Murray has painstakingly collected thousands of scientific articles from medical journals on the healing power of foods and food components. The references provided are by no means designed to represent a complete reference list for all of the studies reviewed or mentioned in *How to Prevent and Treat Diabetes with Natural Medicine.* We have chosen to focus on key studies and comprehensive review articles. In general, these sorts of scientific references are usually of value only to health care professionals.

In addition to finding the articles listed here useful, we encourage interested parties to access the Web site for the National Library of Medicine (NLM), www.ncbi.nlm.nih.gov/entrez/query.fcgi, for additional studies.

The NLM Gateway is a Web-based system that lets users search simultaneously in multiple retrieval systems at the NLM. From this site you can access all of the NLM databases, including the PubMed database. This database was developed in conjunction with publishers of biomedical literature as a search tool for accessing literature citations and linking to full-text journal articles at Web sites of participating publishers. Publishers participating in PubMed electronically supply NLM with their citations before or at the time of publication. If the publisher has a Web site that offers the full text of its journals, PubMed provides links to that site, as well as links to other biological data, sequence centers, and so on. User registration, a subscription fee, or some other type of fee may be required to access the full text of articles in some journals.

PubMed provides access to bibliographic information, which includes Medline—the NLM's premier bibliographic database covering the fields of medicine, nursing, dentistry, veterinary medicine, the health care system, and the preclinical sciences. Medline contains bibliographic citations and author abstracts from more than 4,000 medical journals published in the United States and seventy other countries. The file contains more than 11 million citations dating back to the mid-1960s. Coverage is worldwide, but most records are from English-language sources or have English abstracts (summaries). Conducting a search is quite easy and the site has a link to a tutorial that fully explains the process.

Chapter 1. An Ounce of Prevention . . .

1. Cox D, Gonder-Frederick L, Kovatchev B, et al. Reduction of severe hypoglycemia (SH) with blood glucose awareness training (BGAT-2). Diabetes. 1995;4(suppl):27A.
2. Barr RG, Nathan DM, Meigs JB, Singer DE. Tests of glycemia for the diagnosis of type 2 diabetes mellitus. Ann Intern Med. 2002;137:263–272.
3. Ko GT, Chan JC, Woo J, et al. The reproducibility and usefulness of the oral glucose tolerance test in screening for diabetes and other cardiovascular risk factors. Ann Clin Biochem. 1998;35:62–67.
4. Vuguin P, Saenger P, Dimartino-Nardi J. Fasting glucose insulin ratio: a useful measure of insulin resistance in girls with premature adrenarche. J Clin Endocrinol Metab. 2001;86:4618–4621.
5. Kraft JR. Detection of diabetes mellitus in situ (occult diabetes). Laboratory Med. 1975;6:10–22.
6. Wiener K, Roberts NB. The relative merits of haemoglobin A1c and fasting plasma glucose as first-line diagnostic tests for diabetes mellitus in non-pregnant subjects. Diabet Med. 1998;15:558–563.
7. Perry RC, Shankar RR, Fineberg N, McGill J, Baron AD. HbA1c measurement improves the detection of type 2 diabetes in high-risk individuals with nondiagnostic levels of fasting plasma glucose: the Early Diabetes Intervention Program (EDIP). Diabetes Care. 2001;24:465–471.

Chapter 2. A Closer Look at Risk Factors for Type 1 Diabetes

1. Kelly MA, Mijovic CH, Barnett AH. Genetics of type 1 diabetes. Best Pract Res Clin Endocrinol Metab. 2001;15:279–291.
2. Akerblom HK, Vaarala O, Hyoty H, Ilonen J, Knip M. Environmental factors in the etiology of type 1 diabetes. Am J Med Genet. 2002;115: 18–29.
3. Knip M, Akerblom HK. Environmental factors in the pathogenesis of

type 1 diabetes mellitus. Exp Clin Endocrinol Diabetes. 1999;107(suppl 3):S93–S100.

4. Kaprio J, Tuomilehto J, Koskenvuo M, et al. Concordance for Type 1 (insulin-dependent) and Type 2 (non-insulin-dependent) diabetes mellitus in a population-based cohort of twins in Finland. Diabetologia. 1992;35:1060–1067.

5. Redondo MJ, Yu L, Hawa M, et al. Heterogeneity of Type I diabetes: analysis of monozygotic twins in Great Britain and the United States. Diabetologia. 2001;44:354–362.

6. Guo SW. Does higher concordance in monozygotic twins than in dizygotic twins suggest a genetic component? Hum Hered. 2001;51:121–132.

7. Guo SW. The behaviour of some heritability estimators in the complete absence of genetic factors. Hum Hered. 1999;49:215–228.

8. Pociot F, McDermott MF. Genetics of type 1 diabetes mellitus. Genes Immun. 2002;3:235–249.

9. Metcalfe KA, Hitman GA, Rowe RE, et al. Concordance for type 1 diabetes in identical twins is affected by insulin genotype. Diabetes Care. 2001;24:838–842.

10. Onkamo P, Vaananen S, Karvonen M, Tuomilehto J. Worldwide increase in incidence of type 1 diabetes—analysis of the data on published incidence trials. Diabetologia. 1999;42:1395–1403.

11. Willis J, Scott R, Brown L, Zimmet P, MacKay I, Rowley M. Type 1 diabetes in insulin-treated adult-onset diabetic subjects. Diabetes Res Clin Pract. 1998;42:49–53.

12. Feltbower RG, Bodansky HJ, McKinney PA, et al. Trends in the incidence of childhood diabetes in south Asians and other children in Bradford, UK. Diabet Med. 2002;19(2):162–166.

13. Bodansky HJ, Staines A, Stephenson C, Haigh D, Cartwright R. Evidence for an environmental effect in the aetiology of insulin dependent diabetes in a transmigratory population. BMJ. 1992;304:1020–1022.

14. Elliott RB. Epidemiology of diabetes in Polynesia and New Zealand. Pediatr Adolesc Endocrinol. 1992;21:66–71.

15. Vaarla O. The gut immune system and type 1 diabetes. NY Acad Sci. 2002;958:39–46.

16. Hypponen E, Kenward MG, Virtanen SM, et al. Infant feeding, early weight gain, and risk of type 1 diabetes. Childhood Diabetes in Finland (DiMe) Study Group. Diabetes Care. 1999;22:1961–1965.

17. Kohno T, Kobashiri Y, Sugie Y, et al. Antibodies to food antigens in Japanese patients with type 1 diabetes mellitus. Diabetes Res Clin Pract. 2002;55:1–9.

18. Monetini L, Cavallo MG, Manfrini S, et al. Antibodies to bovine beta-

casein in diabetes and other autoimmune diseases. Horm Metab Res. 2002;34:455–459.

19. Zunt S. Recurrent aphthous stomatitis. Dermatol Clin. 2003;21(1): 33–39.

20. Hyoty H. Enterovirus infections and type 1 diabetes. Ann Med. 2002;34:138–147.

21. The EURODIAB Substudy 2 Study Group. Vitamin D supplement in early childhood and risk for Type I (insulin-dependent) diabetes mellitus. Diabetologia. 1999;42:51–54.

22. Hypponen E, Laara E, Reunanen A, Jarvelin MR, Virtanen SM. Intake of vitamin D and risk of type 1 diabetes: a birth-cohort study. Lancet. 2001;358:1500–1503.

23. Stene LC, Ulriksen J, Magnus P, Joner G. Use of cod liver oil during pregnancy associated with lower risk of Type 1 diabetes in the offspring. Diabetologia. 2000;43:1093–1098.

24. Krishna Mohan I, Das UN. Prevention of chemically induced diabetes mellitus in experimental animals by polyunsaturated fatty acids. Nutrition. 2001;17:126–151.

25. Zhao HX, Mold MD, Stenhouse EA, et al. Drinking water composition and childhood-onset Type 1 diabetes mellitus in Devon and Cornwall, England. Diabet Med. 2001;18:709–717.

26. Parslow RC, McKinney PA, Law GR, et al. Incidence of childhood diabetes mellitus in Yorkshire, northern England, is associated with nitrate in drinking water: an ecological analysis. Diabetologia. 1997;40:550–556.

Chapter 3. Preventing Type 1 Diabetes

1. Vickerstaff-Joneja J. *Dietary Management of Food Allergies and Intolerances.* 2nd ed. Vancouver, BC: J. A. Hall Publications; 1998:263.

2. Blot WJ, Henderson BE, Boice JD Jr. Childhood cancer in relation to cured meat intake: review of the epidemiological evidence. Nutr Cancer. 1999;34:111–118.

3. Nijveldt RJ, van Nood E, van Hoorn DE, et al. Flavonoids: a review of probable mechanisms of action and potential applications. Am J Clin Nutr. 2001;74:418–25.

4. Nihal A, Hasan M. Green tea polyphenols and cancer: biological mechanisms and practical implications. Nutr Rev. 1999;57:78–83.

5. Chakravarthy BK, Gupta S, Gode KD. Functional beta cell regeneration in the islets of pancreas in alloxan induced diabetic rats by (–)-epicatechin. Life Sci. 1982;31:2693–2697.

6. Mukoyama A, Ushijima H, Nishimura S, et al. Inhibition of rotavirus and enterovirus infections by tea extracts. Jpn J Med Sci Biol. 1991;44:181–186.

7. Phuapradit P, Varavithya W, Vathanophas K, et al. Reduction of rotavirus infection in children receiving bifidobacteria-supplemented formula. J Med Assoc Thai. 1999;82(suppl 1):S43–S48.
8. Qiao H, Duffy LC, Griffiths E, et al. Immune responses in rhesus rotavirus-challenged BALB/c mice treated with bifidobacteria and prebiotic supplements. Pediatr Res. June 2002;51(6):750–755.
9. Bouglé D, Roland D, Lebeurrier N, Arhan F. Effect of propionibacteria supplementation on fecal bifidobacteria and segmental colonic transic time in healthy human subjects. Scand J Gastroenterol. 1999;34:144–148.

Chapter 4. A Closer Look at Risk Factors for Type 2 Diabetes

1. Guerre-Millo M. Adipose tissue hormones. J Endocrinol Invest. 2002;25: 855–861.
2. Trayhurn P, Beattie JH. Physiological role of adipose tissue: white adipose tissue as an endocrine and secretory organ. Proc Nutr Soc. 2001;60:329–339.
3. Tschritter O, Fritsche A, Thamer C, et al. Plasma adiponectin concentrations predict insulin sensitivity of both glucose and lipid metabolism. Diabetes 2003;52(2):239–243.
4. Spranger J, Kroke A, Mohlig M, et al. Adiponectin and protection against type 2 diabetes mellitus. Lancet 2003;361(9353):226–228.
5. Gloyn AL, McCarthy MI. The genetics of type 2 diabetes. Best Pract Res Clin Endocrinol Metab. 2001;15:293–308.
6. Bennett PH. Type 2 diabetes among the Pima Indians of Arizona: an epidemic attributable to environmental change? Nutr Rev. 1999;57:S51–S54.
7. Nelson KM, Reiber G, Boyko EJ. Diet and exercise among adults with type 2 diabetes: findings from the third national health and nutrition examination survey (NHANES III). Diabetes Care. 2002;25:1722–1728.
8. van Dam RM, Rimm EB, Willett WC, Stampfer MJ, Hu FB. Dietary patterns and risk for type 2 diabetes mellitus in U.S. men. Ann Intern Med. 2002;136:201–209.
9. Snitker S, Mitchell BD, Shuldiner AR. Physical activity and prevention of type 2 diabetes. Lancet 2003;361(9351):87–88.
10. Hsueh WC, Mitchell BD, Aburomia R, et al. Diabetes in the Old Order Amish: characterization and heritability analysis of the Amish Family Diabetes Study. Diabetes Care. 2000;23:595–601.
11. The Diabetes Prevention Program (DPP): description of lifestyle intervention. Diabetes Care. 2002;25:2165–2171.
12. Anderson GH, Catherine NL, Woodend DM, Wolever TM. Inverse association between the effect of carbohydrates on blood glucose and subsequent short-term food intake in young men. Am J Clin Nutr. 2002;76(5): 1023–1030.

13. Willett W, Manson J, Liu S. Glycemic index, glycemic load, and risk of type 2 diabetes. Am J Clin Nutr. 2002;76(suppl):274S–280S.

14. Jenkins DJ, Kendall CW, Augustin LS, et al. Glycemic index: overview of implications in health and disease. Am J Clin Nutr. July 2002;76(1): 266S–273S.

15. Willett W, Manson J, Liu S. Glycemic index, glycemic load, and risk of type 2 diabetes. Am J Clin Nutr. 2002;76(suppl):274S–280S.

16. Wolever TM, Mehling C. High-carbohydrate-low-glycaemic index dietary advice improves glucose disposition index in subjects with impaired glucose tolerance. Br J Nutr. 2002;87:477–487.

17. Fung TT, Hu FB, Pereira MA, et al. Whole-grain intake and the risk of type 2 diabetes: a prospective study in men. Am J Clin Nutr. 2002;76:535–540.

18. Willett W, Manson J, Liu S. Glycemic index, glycemic load, and risk of type 2 diabetes. Am J Clin Nutr. 2002;76(suppl):274S–280S.

19. Liu S, Willett WC, Stampfer MJ, Hu FB, et al. A prospective study of dietary glycemic load, carbohydrate intake, and risk of coronary heart disease in US women. Am J Clin Nutr. 2000;71:1455–1461.

20. Wursch P, Pi-Sunyer FX. The role of viscous soluble fiber in the metabolic control of diabetes. A review with special emphasis on cereals rich in beta-glucan. Diabetes Care. 1997;20:1774–1780.

21. Slama G. Dietary therapy in type 2 diabetes oriented towards postprandial blood glucose improvement. Diabetes Metab Rev. 1998;14(suppl 1): S19–S24.

22. Montonen J, Knekt P, Jarvinen R, Aromaa A, Reunanen A. Whole-grain and fiber intake and the incidence of type 2 diabetes. Am J Clin Nutr. 2003;77:622–629.

23. Fung TT, Hu FB, Pereira MA, et al. Whole-grain intake and the risk of type 2 diabetes: a prospective study in men. Am J Clin Nutr. 2002;76: 535–540.

24. Hung T, Sievenpiper JL, Marchie A, Kendall CW, Jenkins DJ. Fat versus carbohydrate in insulin resistance, obesity, diabetes and cardiovascular disease. Curr Opin Clin Nutr Metab Care. 2003;6:165–176.

25. Salmeron J, Hu FB, Manson JE, et al. Dietary fat intake and risk of type 2 diabetes in women. Am J Clin Nutr. 2001;73:1019–1026.

26. Rivellese AA, De Natale C, Lilli S. Type of dietary fat and insulin resistance. Ann N Y Acad Sci. 2002;967:329–335.

27. Jiang R, Manson JE, Stampfer MJ, et al. Nut and peanut butter consumption and risk of type 2 diabetes in women. JAMA 2002;288(20):2554–2560.

28. Sargeant LA, Khaw KT, Bingham S, et al. Fruit and vegetable intake and population glycosylated haemoglobin levels: the EPIC-Norfolk Study. Eur J Clin Nutr. 2001;55:342–348.

29. Williams DE, Wareham NJ, Cox BD, et al. Frequent salad vegetable consumption is associated with a reduction in the risk of diabetes mellitus. J Clin Epidemiol. 1999;52:329–335.

30. Reunanen A, Knekt P, Aaran RK, Aromaa A. Serum antioxidants and risk of non-insulin dependent diabetes mellitus. Eur J Clin Nutr. 1998;52:89–93.

31. Feskens EJ, Virtanen SM, Rasanen L, et al. Dietary factors determining diabetes and impaired glucose tolerance. A 20-year follow-up of the Finnish and Dutch cohorts of the Seven Countries Study. Diabetes Care. 1995;18:1104–1112.

32. Ruhe RC, McDonald RB. Use of antioxidant nutrients in the prevention and treatment of type 2 diabetes. J Am Coll Nutr. 2001;5:363S–369S.

33. Facchini FS, Humphreys MH, DoNascimento CA, Abbasi F, Reaven GM. Relation between insulin resistance and plasma concentrations of lipid hydroperoxides, carotenoids, and tocopherols. Am J Clin Nutr. 2000;72:776–779.

34. Salonen JT, Jyyssonen K, Tuomainen TP. Increased risk of non-insulin diabetes mellitus at low plasma vitamin E concentrations. A four year follow-up study in men. Br Med J. 1995;311:1124–1127.

35. Maritim AC, Sanders RA, Watkins JB III. Diabetes, oxidative stress, and antioxidants: A review. J Biochem Mol Toxicol. 2003;17:24–38.

36. Evans JL, Goldfine ID, Maddux BA, Grodsky GM. Are oxidative stress-activated signaling pathways mediators of insulin resistance and beta-cell dysfunction? Diabetes. 2003;52:1–8.

37. Knowler WC, Barrett-Connor E, Fowler SE, et al. Reduction in the incidence of type 2 diabetes with lifestyle intervention or metformin. N Engl J Med. 2002;346:393–403.

Chapter 5. Preventing Type 2 Diabetes

1. Sato Y. Diabetes and life-styles: role of physical exercise for primary prevention. Br J Nutr. 2000;84(suppl 2):S187–S190.

2. Coon KA, Tucker KL. Television and children's consumption patterns. A review of the literature. Minerva Pediatr. 2002;54:423–436.

3. Boethel CD. Sleep and the endocrine system: new associations to old diseases. Curr Opin Pulm Med. 2002;8:502–505.

4. Al-Delaimy WK, Manson JE, Willett WC, Stampfer MJ, Hu FB. Snoring as a risk factor for type II diabetes mellitus: a prospective study. Am J Epidemiol. 2002;155:387–393.

5. Pevernagie D, Hamans E, Van Cauwenberge P, Pauwels R. External nasal dilation reduces snoring in chronic rhinitis patients: a randomized controlled trial. Eur Respir J. 2000;15:996–1000.

6. Kirkness JP, Wheatley JR, Amis TC. Nasal airflow dynamics: mechanisms and responses associated with an external nasal dilator strip. Eur Respir J. 2000;15:929–936.

7. Ulfberg J, Fenton G. Effect of Breathe Right nasal strip on snoring. Rhinology 1997;35:50–52.

8. Loth S, Petruson B. Improved nasal breathing reduces snoring and morning tiredness. A 6-month follow-up study. Arch Otolaryngol Head Neck Surg. 1996;122:1337–1340.

9. Suzuki K, Ito Y, Nakamura S, Ochiai J, Aoki K. Relationship between serum carotenoids and hyperglycemia: a population-based cross-sectional study. J Epidemiol. 2002;12:357–366.

10. Knekt P, Kumpulainen J, Jarvinen R, et al. Flavonoid intake and risk of chronic diseases. Am J Clin Nutr. 2002;76:560–568.

11. Belury MA. Dietary conjugated linoleic acid in health: physiological effects and mechanisms of action. Annu Rev Nutr. 2002;22:505–531.

12. van Dam RM, Willett WC, Rimm EB, Stampfer MJ, Hu FB. Dietary fat and meat intake in relation to risk of type 2 diabetes in men. Diabetes Care. 2002;25:417–424.

13. Alarcon de la Lastra C, Barranco MD, Motilva V, Herrerias JM. Mediterranean diet and health: biological importance of olive oil. Curr Pharm Des. 2001;7:933–950.

14. Perez-Jimenez F, Lopez-Miranda J, et al. A Mediterranean and a high-carbohydrate diet improve glucose metabolism in healthy young persons. Diabetologia. 2001;44:2038–2043.

15. Vessby B, Unsitupa M, Hermansen K, et al. Substituting dietary saturated for monounsaturated fat impairs insulin sensitivity in healthy men and women: The KANWU Study. Diabetologia. 2001;44:312–319.

16. Velazquez OC, Seto RW, Rombeau JL. The scientific rationale and clinical application of short-chain fatty acids and medium-chain triacylglycerols. Proc Nutr Soc. 1996;55:49–78.

17. Bucher HC, Hengstler P, Schindler C, Meier G. N-3 polyunsaturated fatty acids in coronary heart disease: a meta-analysis of randomized controlled trials. Am J Med. 2002;112:298–304.

18. Rose DP, Connolly JM. Omega-3 fatty acids as cancer chemopreventive agents. Pharmacol Therapeutics. 1999;83:217–244.

19. Ford ES. Vitamin supplement use and diabetes mellitus incidence among adults in the United States. J Epidemiol. 2001;153:892–897.

20. Hu FB, Bronner L, Willett WC, et al. Fish and omega-3 fatty acid intake and risk of coronary heart disease in women. JAMA. 2002;287:1815–1821.

Chapter 6. Monitoring Diabetes

1. Goldstein D, Little R. Monitoring glycemia in diabetes. Short-term assessment. Endocrinol Metab Clin North Am. 1997;26(3):475–486.
2. American Diabetes Association. Tests of glycemia in diabetes (position statement). Diabetes Care. 1997;20(suppl 1):518.
3. DCCT Research Group. The effect of intensive treatment of diabetes on the development and progression of long-term complications in insulin-dependent diabetes mellitus. N Engl J Med. 1993;329(14):977–986.
4. UK Prospective Diabetes Study (UKPDS) Group. Intensive blood-glucose control with sulphonylureas or insulin compared with conventional treatment and risk of complications in patients with type 2 diabetes (UKPDS 33). Lancet. 1998;352:837–853.
5. Bertrand S, Aris-Jilwan N, Reddy S, Yale J. Recommendations for the use of self-monitoring of blood glucose (SMBG) in diabetes mellitus. Canadian Diabetes 1996; 9:3–5.
6. DAFNE Study Group. Training in flexible, intensive insulin management to enable dietary freedom in people with type 1 diabetes: dose adjustment for normal eating (DAFNE) randomised controlled trial. BMJ. 2002;325(7367):746.
7. Ohkubo Y, Kishikawa H, Araki E, et al. Intensive insulin therapy prevents the progression of diabetic microvascular complications in Japanese patients with non-insulin-dependent diabetes mellitus: a randomized prospective 6-year study. Diabetes Res Clin Pract. 1995;28(2):103–117.
8. Formanek R. FDA approves watch-like device to monitor blood sugar levels. FDA Consumer Magazine. May–June 2001.
9. Tierney M, Tamada J, Potts R, Jovanovic L, Garg S; Cygnus Research Team. Clinical evaluation of the Glucowatch biographer: a continual, non-invasive glucose monitor for patients with diabetes. Biosen Bioelectron. 2002;16:621–629.
10. Holman R. Analysis of the United Kingdom Prospective Diabetes Study. Endocr Pract. 2002;8:33–34.
11. Austin GE. Usefulness of fructosamine for monitoring outpatients with diabetes. Am J Med Sci. 1999;318(5):316–323.
12. Bode B, Sabbah H, Davidson P. What's ahead in glucose monitoring? New techniques hold promise for improved ease and accuracy. Postgrad Med. 2001;109(4):41–49.
13. Bode BW, Gross TM, Thornton KR, et al. Continuous glucose monitoring used to adjust diabetes therapy improves glycosylated hemoglobin: a pilot study. Diabetes Res Clin Pract. 1999;46(3):183–190.
14. Sabbah H, McCulloch K, Davidson PC, et al. Reduction in severe hypoglycemia following use of continuous glucose monitoring to guide therapy adjustments: a pilot study. Diabetes. 2001;50(suppl 1):S14–20.

15. Katayama S, Inaba M. Importance of blood pressure control in patients with diabetes mellitus. J Diabetes Complications. 2002;16:87–91.

16. Hänninen JA. Blood pressure control in subjects with type 2 diabetes. J Hum Hypertens. 2000;14(2):111–115.

17. Grover SA, Coupal L, Zowall H, Dorais M. Cost effectiveness of testing hyperlipidemia in the presence of diabetes: who should be treated? Circulation. 2000;102:722–727.

18. Bakris GL. Preserving renal function in adults with hypertension and diabetes: a consensus approach. National Kidney Foundation Hypertension and Diabetes Executive Committees Working Group. Am J Kidney Dis. 2000;36(3):646–661.

19. Huerta MG, Nadler JL. Role of inflammatory pathways in the development and cardiovascular complications of type 2 diabetes. Curr Diab Rep. 2002;2:396–402.

20. Seshadri N, Robinson K. Homocysteine, B vitamins, and coronary artery disease. Med Clin North Am. 2000;84(1):215–237.

21. Cantin B, Despres JP, Lamarche B, et al. Association of fibrinogen and lipoprotein(a) as a coronary heart disease risk factor in men (The Quebec Cardiovascular Study). Am J Cardiol 2002;89(6):662–666.

Chapter 7. Diet Therapy in Managing Diabetes

1. Lafrance L, Rabasa-Lhoret R, Poisson D, Ducros F, Chiasson JL. Effects of different glycaemic index foods and dietary fibre intake on glycaemic control in type 1 diabetic patients on intensive insulin therapy. Diabet Med. 1998;15:972–978.

2. Gilbertson HR, Brand-Miller JC, Thorburn AW, Evans S, Chondros P, Werther GA. The effect of flexible low glycemic index dietary advice versus measured carbohydrate exchange diets on glycemic control in children with type 1 diabetes. Diabetes Care. 2001;24:1137–1143.

3. Giacco R, Parillo M, Rivellese AA, et al. Long-term dietary treatment with increased amounts of fiber-rich low-glycemic index natural foods improves blood glucose control and reduces the number of hypoglycemic events in type 1 diabetic patients. Diabetes Care. 2000;23:1461–1466.

4. Buyken AE, Toeller M, Heitkamp G, et al. Glycemic index in the diet of European outpatients with type 1 diabetes: relations to glycated hemoglobin and serum lipids. Am J Clin Nutr. 2001;73:574–581.

5. Toeller M, Buyken AE, Heitkamp G, Berg G, Scherbaum WA. Prevalence of chronic complications, metabolic control and nutritional intake in type 1 diabetes: comparison between different European regions. EURODIAB Complications Study group. Horm Metab Res. 1999;31:680–685.

6. Kalkwarf HJ, Bell RC, Khoury JC, Gouge AL, Miodovnik M. Dietary

fiber intakes and insulin requirements in pregnant women with type 1 diabetes. J Am Diet Assoc. 2001;101:305–310.

7. Hung T, Sievenpiper JL, Marchie A, Kendall CW, Jenkins DJ. Fat versus carbohydrate in insulin resistance, obesity, diabetes and cardiovascular disease. Curr Opin Clin Nutr Metab Care. 2003;6:165–176.

8. Chandalia M, Garg A, Lutjohann D, et al. Beneficial effects of high dietary fiber intake in patients with type 2 diabetes mellitus. N Engl J Med. 2000;342:1392–1398.

9. Jarvi AE, Karlstrom BE, Granfeldt YE, et al. Improved glycemic control and lipid profile and normalized fibrinolytic activity on a low-glycemic index diet in type 2 diabetic patients. Diabetes Care. 1999;22:10–18.

10. Brynes AE, Lee JL, Brighton RE, et al. A low glycemic diet significantly improves the 24-h blood glucose profile in people with type 2 diabetes, as assessed using the continuous glucose MiniMed monitor. Diabetes Care. 2003;26:548–549.

11. Barringer T, Kirk J, Santaniello A, et al. Effects of a multivitamin and mineral supplement on infection and quality of life. Ann Intern Med. 2003;138:365–371.

12. Althuis MD, Jordan NE, Ludington EA, Wittes JT. Glucose and insulin responses to dietary chromium supplements: a meta-analysis. Am J Clin Nutr. 2002;76:148–155.

13. Cunningham JJ. The glucose/insulin system and vitamin C: Implications in insulin-dependent diabetes mellitus. J Am Coll Nutr. 1998;17:105–108.

14. Eriksson J, Kohvakka A. Magnesium and ascorbic acid supplementation in diabetes mellitus. Ann Nutr Metab. 1995;39:217–223.

15. Mullan BA, Young IS, Fee H, McCance DR. Ascorbic acid reduces blood pressure and arterial stiffness in type 2 diabetes. Hypertension. 2002;40:804–809.

16. Anderson JW, Gowri MS, Turner J, et al. Antioxidant supplementation effects on low-density lipoprotein oxidation for individuals with type 2 diabetes mellitus. J Am Coll Nutr. 1999;18:451–461.

17. Astley S, Langrish-Smith A, Southon S, Sampson M. Vitamin E supplementation and oxidative damage to DNA and plasma LDL in type 1 diabetes. Diabetes Care. 1999;22:1626–1631.

18. Pinkney JH, Downs L, Hopton M, Mackness MI, Bolton CH. Endothelial dysfunction in Type 1 diabetes mellitus: relationship with LDL oxidation and the effects of vitamin E. Diabet Med. 1999;16:993–999.

19. Skyrme-Jones RA, O'Brien RC, Berry KL, Meredith IT. Vitamin E supplementation improves endothelial function in type I diabetes mellitus: a randomized, placebo-controlled study. J Am Coll Cardiol. 2000;36:94–102.

20. Gazis A, White DJ, Page SR, Cockcroft JR. Effect of oral vitamin E (alpha-tocopherol) supplementation on vascular endothelial function in Type 2 diabetes mellitus. Diabet Med. 1999;16:304–311.

21. Paolisso G, Tagliamonte MR, Barbieri M, et al. Chronic vitamin E administration improves brachial reactivity and increases intracellular magnesium concentration in type II diabetic patients. J Clin Endocrinol Metab. 2000;85:109–115.

22. Barbagallo M, Dominguez LJ, Tagliamonte MR, Resnick LM, Paolisso G. Effects of vitamin E and glutathione on glucose metabolism: role of magnesium. Hypertension. 1999;34:1002–1006.

23. Upritchard JE, Sutherland WH, Mann JI. Effect of supplementation with tomato juice, vitamin E, and vitamin C on LDL oxidation and products of inflammatory activity in type 2 diabetes. Diabetes Care. 2000;23: 733–738.

24. Devaraj S, Jialal I. Alpha tocopherol supplementation decreases serum C-reactive protein and monocyte interleukin-6 levels in normal volunteers and type 2 diabetic patients. Free Radic Biol Med. 2000;29:790–792.

25. Gokkusu C, Palanduz S, Ademoglu E, Tamer S. Oxidant and antioxidant systems in niddm patients: influence of vitamin E supplementation. Endocr Res 2001;27:377–386.

26. Tutuncu NB, Bayraktar M, Varli K. Reversal of defective nerve conduction with vitamin E supplementation in type 2 diabetes: a preliminary study. Diabetes Care. 1998;21:1915–1918.

27. Bursell SE, Clermont AC, Aiello LP, et al. High-dose vitamin E supplementation normalizes retinal blood flow and creatinine clearance in patients with type 1 diabetes. Diabetes Care. 1999;22:1245–1251.

28. Engelen W, Keenoy BM, Vertommen J, De Leeuw I. Effects of long-term supplementation with moderate pharmacologic doses of vitamin E are saturable and reversible in patients with type 1 diabetes. Am J Clin Nutr. 2000;72:1142–1149.

29. Upritchard JE, Sutherland WH, Mann JI. Effect of supplementation with tomato juice, vitamin E, and vitamin C on LDL oxidation and products of inflammatory activity in type 2 diabetes. Diabetes Care. 2000;23: 733–738.

30. Jones CL, Gonzalez V. Pyridoxine deficiency: a new factor in diabetic neuropathy. J Am Pod Assoc. 1978;68:646–653.

31. Solomon LR, Cohen K. Erythrocyte O_2 transport and metabolism and effects of vitamin B6 therapy in type II diabetes mellitus. Diabetes. 1989;38:881–886.

32. Coelingh-Bennick HJT, Schreurs WHP. Improvement of oral glucose tolerance in gestational diabetes. Br Med J. 1975;3:13–15.

33. Barbagallo M, Dominguez LJ, Galioto A, et al. Role of magnesium in insulin action, diabetes and cardio-metabolic syndrome X. Mol Aspects Med. 2003;24:39–52.

34. Lima Mde L, Cruz T, Pousada JC, et al. The effect of magnesium supplementation in increasing doses on the control of type 2 diabetes. Diabetes Care. 1998;21:682–686.

35. White JR, Campbell RK. Magnesium and diabetes: A review. Ann Pharmacother. 1993;27:775–780.

36. Salgueiro MJ, Krebs N, Zubillaga MB, et al. Zinc and diabetes mellitus: is there a need of zinc supplementation in diabetes mellitus patients? Biol Trace Elem Res. 2001;81:215–228.

37. Parikh P, Mani U, Iyer U. Role of spirulina in the control of glycemia and lipidemia in type 2 diabetes mellitus. J Med Food. 2001;4:193–199.

38. Yu YM, Chang WC, Chang CT, Hsieh CL, Tsai CE. Effects of young barley leaf extract and antioxidative vitamins on LDL oxidation and free radical scavenging activities in type 2 diabetes. Diabetes Metab. 2002;28:107–114.

39. Farmer A, Montori V, Dinneen S, Clar C. Fish oil in people with type 2 diabetes mellitus. Cochrane Database Syst Rev. 2001;(3):CD003205.

40. Montori VM, Farmer A, Wollan PC, Dinneen SF. Fish oil supplementation in type 2 diabetes: a quantitative systematic review. Diabetes Care. 2000;23:1407–1415.

41. Woodman RJ, Mori TA, Burke V, et al. Effects of purified eicosapentaenoic and docosahexaenoic acids on glycemic control, blood pressure, and serum lipids in type 2 diabetic patients with treated hypertension. Am J Clin Nutr. 2002;76:1007–1015.

Chapter 8. Natural Products for Type 1 Diabetes

1. Cox DJ, Gonder-Frederick L, Polonsky W, Schlundt D, Kovatchev B, Clarke W. Blood glucose awareness training (BGAT-2): long-term benefits. Diabetes Care. 2001;24(4):637–642.

2. Kretowski A, Mysliwiec J, Szelachowska M, Kinalski M, Kinalska I. Nicotinamide inhibits enhanced in vitro production of interleukin-12 and tumour necrosis factor-alpha in peripheral whole blood of people at high risk of developing type 1 diabetes and people with newly diagnosed type 1 diabetes. Diabetes Res Clin Pract. 2000;47:81–86.

3. Kolb H, Burkart V. Nicotinamide in type 1 diabetes. Mechanism of action revisited. Diabetes Care. 1999;22(suppl 2):B16–B20.

4. Cleary JP. Vitamin B3 in the treatment of diabetes mellitus: case reports and review of the literature. J Nutr Med. 1990;1:217–225.

5. Pocoit F, Reimers JI, Andersen HU. Nicotinamide—biological actions

and therapeutic potential in diabetes prevention. Diabetologia. 1993;36: 574–576.

6. Pozzilli P, Andreani D. The potential role of nicotinamide in the secondary prevention of IDDM. Diabetes Metabol Rev. 1993;9:219–230.

7. Schatz DA, Bingley PJ. Update on major trials for the prevention of type 1 diabetes mellitus: the American Diabetes Prevention Trial (DPT-1) and the European Nicotinamide Diabetes Intervention Trial (ENDIT). J Pediatr Endocrinol Metab. 2001;14(suppl 1):619–622.

8. Visalli N, Cavallo MG, Signore A, et al. A multi-centre randomized trial of two different doses of nicotinamide in patients with recent-onset type 1 diabetes (the IMDIAB VI). Diabetes Metab Res Rev. 1999;15:181–185.

9. Chakravarthy BK, Gupa S, Gambhir SS, Gode KD. Pancreatic beta-cell regeneration in rats by (–)-epicatechin. Lancet. 1981;2:759–760.

10. Chakravarthy BK, Gupa S, Gode KD. Functional beta cell regeneration in the islets of pancreas in alloxan induced diabetic rats by (–)-epicatechin. Life Sci. 1982;31:2693–2697.

11. Maebashi M, Makino Y, Furukawa Y, et al. Therapeutic evaluation of the effect of biotin on hyperglycemia in patients with non-insulin dependent diabetes mellitus. J Clin Biochem Nutr. 1993;14:211–218.

12. Koutsikos D, Agroyannis B, Tzanatos-Exarchou H. Biotin for diabetic peripheral neuropathy. Biomed Pharmacother. 1990;44:511–514.

13. Porchezhian E, Dobriyal RM. An overview on the advances of Gymnema sylvestre: chemistry, pharmacology and patents. Pharmazie. 2003;58: 5–12.

14. Shanmugasundaram ER, Rajeswari G, Baskaran K, et al. Use of Gymnema sylvestre leaf extract in the control of blood glucose in insulin-dependent diabetes mellitus. J Ethnopharmacol 1990;30:281–294.

15. Srivastava Y, Venkatakrishna-Bhatt H, Verma Y, et al. Antidiabetic and adaptogenic properties of Momordica charantia extract. An experimental and clinical evaluation. Phytotherapy Res. 1993;7:285–289.

16. Welihinda J, Karunanaya EH, Sheriff MHR, Jayasinghe KSA. Effect of Momardica charantia on the glucose tolerance in maturity onset diabetes. J Ethnopharmacol. 1986;17:277–282.

Chapter 9. Natural Products for Type 2 Diabetes

1. Bell DS. Importance of postprandial glucose control. Southern Med J. 2001;94:804–809.

2. Vuksan V, Jenkins DJ, Spadafora P, et al. Konjac-mannan (glucomannan) improves glycemia and other associated risk factors for coronary heart disease in type 2 diabetes. A randomized controlled metabolic trial. Diabetes Care. 1999;22:913–919.

3. Jenkins DJ, Kendall CW, Axelsen M, Augustin LS, Vuksan V. Viscous and nonviscous fibres, nonabsorbable and low glycaemic index carbohydrates, blood lipids and coronary heart disease. Curr Opin Lipidol. 2000;11:49–56.

4. Marlett JA, McBurney MI, Slavin JL. Position of the American Dietetic Association: health implications of dietary fiber. J Am Diet Assoc. 2002;102:993–1000.

5. Vuksan V, Sievenpiper JL, Owen R, et al. Beneficial effects of viscous dietary fiber from Konjac-mannan in subjects with the insulin resistance syndrome: results of a controlled metabolic trial. Diabetes Care. 2000; 23:9–14.

6. Vuksan V, Sievenpiper JL, Xu Z, et al. Konjac-Mannan and American ginseng: emerging alternative therapies for type 2 diabetes mellitus. J Am Coll Nutr. 2001;20(5 Suppl):370S–383S.

7. Fujita H, Yamagami T, Ohshima K. Fermented soybean-derived water-soluble Touchi extract inhibits alpha-glucosidase and is antiglycemic in rats and humans after single oral treatments. J Nutr. 2001;131:1211–1213.

8. Hiroyuki F, Tomohide Y, Kazunori O. Efficacy and safety of Touchi extract, an alpha-glucosidase inhibitor derived from fermented soybeans, in non-insulin-dependent diabetic mellitus. J Nutr Biochem. 2001;12:351–356.

9. Fujita H, Yamagami T, Ohshima K. Long-term ingestion of a fermented soybean-derived Touchi-extract with alpha-glucosidase inhibitory activity is safe and effective in humans with borderline and mild type-2 diabetes. J Nutr. 2001;131:2105–2108.

10. Asano N, Oseki K, Tomioka E, Kizu H, Matsui K. N-containing sugars from Morus alba and their glycosidase inhibitory activities. Carbohydr Res. 1994;259:243–255.

11. Chen F, Nakashima N, Kimura I, Kimura M. Hypoglycemic activity and mechanisms of extracts from mulberry leaves (folium mori) and cortex mori radicis in streptozotocin-induced diabetic mice. Yakugaku Zasshi. 1995;115:476–482.

12. Andallu B, Suryakantham V, Lakshmi Srikanthi B, Reddy GK. Effect of mulberry (Morus indica L.) therapy on plasma and erythrocyte membrane lipids in patients with type 2 diabetes. Clin Chim Acta. 2001; 314:47–53.

13. Baskaran K, Ahamath BK, Shanmugasundaram KR, Shanmugasundaram ERB. Antidiabetic effect of a leaf extract from *Gymnema sylvestre* in non-insulin dependent diabetes mellitus patients. J Ethnopharmacol. 1990;30: 295–305.

14. Vuksan V, Sievenpiper J, Koo V, et al. American ginseng (Panax quinquefolius) reduces postprandial glycemia in nondiabetic subjects with type 2 diabetes mellitus. Arch Intern Med. 2000;160:1009–1013.

15. Vuksan V, Stavro MP, Sievenpiper JL, et al. Similar postprandial glycemic reductions with escalation of dose and administration time of American ginseng in type 2 diabetes. Diabetes Care. 2000;23:1221–1226.

16. Vuksan V, Sievenpiper JL, Wong J, et al. American ginseng (Panax quinquefolius) attenuates postprandial glycemia in a time-dependent but not dose-dependent manner in healthy individuals. Am J Clin Nutr. 2001;73: 753–758.

17. Vuksan V, Stavro MP, Sievenpiper JL, et al. American ginseng improves glycemia in individuals with normal glucose tolerance: effect of dose and time escalation. J Am Coll Nutr. 2000;19(6):738–744.

18. Sievenpiper JL, Amason JT, Leiter LA, Vuksan V. Variable effects of American ginseng: a batch of American ginseng (Panax quinquefolius) with a depressed ginsenoside profile does not affect postprandial hypoglycemia. Eur J Clin Nutr. 2003;57:243–248.

19. Franz MJ, Bantle JP, Beebe CA, et al. Evidence-based nutrition principles and recommendations for the treatment and prevention of diabetes and related complications. Diabetes Care. 2002;25(1):148–198.

20. Sharma RD, Raghuram TC, Rao NS. Effect of fenugreek seeds on blood glucose and serum lipids in type I diabetes. Eur J Clin Nutr. 1990;44: 301–306.

21. Mada Z, Abel R, Samish S, Arad J. Glucose-lowering effect of fenugreek in non-insulin dependent diabetics. Eur J Clin Nutr. 1988;42:51–54.

22. Gupta A, Gupta R, Lal B. Effect of Trigonella foenum-graecum (fenugreek) seeds on glycaemic control and insulin resistance in type 2 diabetes mellitus: a double blind placebo controlled study. J Assoc Physicians India. 2001;49:1057–1061.

23. Sharma KK, Gupta RK, Gupta S, Samuel KC. Antihyperglycemic effect of onion: effect on fasting blood sugar and induced hyperglycemia in man. Ind J Med Res. 1977;65:422–429.

24. UKPDS 34. UK Prospective diabetes study group. Effect of intensive blood glucose control with metformin on complications in overweight patients with type 2 diabetes. Lancet. 1998;352:854–865.

25. Aventis Pharma Inc. Glucophage product monograph. Laval, Quebec: 2001.

26. Steppan CM, Bailey ST, Bhat S, et al. The hormone resistin links obesity to diabetes. Nature. 2001;409:307–312.

27. Polo V, Saibene A, Pontiroli AE. Nicotinamide improves insulin secretion and metabolic control in lean type 2 diabetic patients with secondary failure to sulphonylureas. Acta Diabetol. 1998;35:61–64.

Chapter 10. Lifestyle and Attitude in Managing Diabetes

1. Fournier M, de Ridder D, Bensing J. How optimism contributes to the adaptation of chronic illness. A prospective study into the enduring effects of optimism on adaptation moderated by the controllability of chronic illness. Pers Individ Dif. 2002. In press.

2. Anderson RJ, Freedland KE, Clouse RE, Lustman PJ. The prevalence of comorbid depression in adults with diabetes: a meta-analysis. Diabetes Care. 2001;24(6):1069–1078.

3. McGuire MT, Jeffery RW, French SA. The psychologic correlates of obesity. Clinics in Family Practice. 2002;4(2):319–331.

4. Maruta T, Colligan RC, Malichoc M, Offord KP. Optimists vs pessimists: Survival rate among medical patients over a 30-year period. Mayo Clin Proc. 2000;75:140–143.

5. Grey M, Boland EA, Davidson M, Yu C, Tamborlane WV. Coping skills training for youths with diabetes on intensive therapy. Appl Nurs Res. 1999;12:3–12.

6. Barglow P, Hatcher R, Edidin DV, Sloan–Rossiter M. Stress and metabolic control in diabetes: Psychosomatic evidence and evaluation of methods. Psychosom Med. 1984;46:127–144.

7. McGrady A, Bailey BK, Good MP. Controlled study of biofeedback-assisted relaxation in Type 1 diabetes. Diabetes Care. 1991;14:360–365.

8. Lane JD, McCaskill CC, Ross SL, Feinglos MN, Surwit RS. Relaxation training for NIDDM: Predicting who may benefit. Diabetes Care. 1993;16:1087–1094.

9. Gumbiner B. The treatment of obesity in Type II diabetes mellitus. Prim Care. 1999;26(4):869–883.

10. DeFronzo RA. The triumvirate: beta-cell, muscle, liver—a collusion responsible for NIDDM. Diabetes. 1988;37:667–687.

11. Henry RR, Wallace P, Olefsky JM. Effects of weight loss on mechanisms of hyperglycemia in obese non-insulin-dependent diabetes mellitus. Diabetes. 1986;35:990–998.

12. NHLBI Obesity Education Expert Panel. Clinical guidelines on the identification, evaluation, and treatment of overweight and obesity in adults. The evidence report. www.nhlbi.nih.gov, 1998;1–228.

13. Pronk NO, Wing RR. Physical activity and long term maintenance of weight loss. Obesity Res. 1994;2:587–589.

14. Boule NG, Haddad E, Kenny GP, Wells GA, Sigal RJ. Effects of exercise on glycemic control and body mass in type 2 diabetes mellitus: a meta-analysis of controlled clinical trials. JAMA. 2001;286(10):1218–1227.

Chapter 11. Diabetic Complications: An Overview

1. Lingenfelser T, Overcamp D, Renn W, et al. Insulin-associated modulation of neuroendocrine counterregulation, hypoglycemia perception, and cerebral function in insulin-dependent diabetes mellitus: evidence for an intrinsic effect of insulin on the central nervous system. J Clin Endocrinol Metab. 1996;81(3):1197–1205.
2. Vincent TE, Mendiratta S, May JM. Inhibition of aldose reductase in human erythrocytes by vitamin C. Diabetes Res Clin Pract. 1999;43:1–8.
3. Maxwell SRJ, Thomason H, Sandler D, et al. Antioxidant status in patients with uncomplicated insulin-dependent and non-insulin-dependent diabetes mellitus. Eur J Clin Invest. 1997;27:484–490.
4. Skra J, Hodinar A, Kvasnicka J, Hilgertova J. Relationship of oxidative stress and fibrinolysis in diabetes mellitus. Diabetic Med. 1996;13:800–805.
5. Reljanovic M, Reichel G, Rett K, et al. Treatment of diabetic polyneuropathy with the antioxidant thioctic acid (alpha-lipoic acid): a two year multicenter randomized double-blind placebo-controlled trial (ALADIN II). Alpha Lipoic Acid in Diabetic Neuropathy. Free Radic Res. 1999;31:171–179.
6. Jacob S, Ruus P, Hermann R, et al. Oral administration of RAC-alpha-lipoic acid modulates insulin sensitivity in patients with type-2 diabetes mellitus: a placebo-controlled pilot trial. Free Radic Biol Med. 1999;27:309–314.
7. Hoogeveeen EK, Kostense PJ, Eysink PED, et al. Hyperhomocysteinemia is associated with the presence of retinopathy in type 2 diabetes mellitus. Arch Intern Med. 2000;160:2984–2990.
8. Appel LJ, Moore TJ, Obarzanek E, et al. A clinical trial of the effects of dietary patterns on blood pressure. DASH Collaborative Research Group. N Engl J Med. 1997;336:1117–1124.
9. Sacks FM, Svetkey LP, Vollmer WM, et al. Effects on blood pressure of reduced dietary sodium and the Dietary Approaches to Stop Hypertension (DASH) diet. DASH-Sodium Collaborative Research Group. N Engl J Med. 2001;344:3–10.
10. Tsi D, Tan BKH. Cardiovascular pharmacology of 3-n-butylphthalide in spontaneously hypertensive rats. Phytother Res. 1997;11:576–582.
11. Le QT, Elliott WJ. Dose-response relationship of blood pressure and serum cholesterol to 3-n-butylphthalide, a component of celery oil. Clin Res. 1991;39:750A.
12. Silagy CA, Neil AW. A meta-analysis of the effect of garlic on blood pressure. J Hypertens. 1994;12:463–468.

13. Whelton PK, He J. Potassium in preventing and treating high blood pressure. Semin Nephrol. 1999;19:494–499.

14. Jee SH, Miller ER 3rd, Guallar E, et al. The effect of magnesium supplementation on blood pressure: a meta-analysis of randomized clinical trials. Am J Hypertens. 2002;15:691–696.

15. Fujita H, Yasumoto R, Hasegawa M, Ohshima K. Antihypertensive activity of "Katsuobushi Oligopeptide" in hypertensive and borderline hypertensive subjects. Jpn Pharmacol Ther. 1997;25:147–151.

16. Fujita H, Yamagami T, Ohshima K. Effect of an ACE-inhibitory agent, kastuobushi oligopeptide, in the spontaneously hypertensive rat and in borderline and mildly hypertensive subjects. Nutr Res. 2001;21:1149–1158.

17. Freis ED. Rationale against the drug treatment of marginal diastolic systemic hypertension. Am J Cardiol. 1990;66:368–371.

18. Neal B, MacMahon S, Chapman N. Effects of ACE inhibitors, calcium antagonists, and other blood-pressure-lowering drugs: results of prospectively designed overviews of randomised trials. Blood Pressure Lowering Treatment Trialists' Collaboration. Lancet. 2000;356:1955–1964.

19. Manuel y Keenoy B, Vertommen J, De Leeuw I. The effect of flavonoid treatment on the glycation and antioxidant status in Type 1 diabetic patients. Diabetes Nutr Metab. 1999;12:256–263.

Chapter 12. Recommendations for Specific Chronic Complications

1. Beckman JA, Creager MA, Libby P. Diabetes and atherosclerosis. JAMA. 2002;287:2570–2581.

2. De Mattia G, Laurenti O, Fava D. Diabetic endothelial dysfunction: effect of free radical scavenging in Type 2 diabetic patients. J Diabetes Complications. 2003;17(suppl 2):30–35.

3. Price KD, Price CS, Reynolds RD. Hyperglycemia-induced ascorbic acid deficiency promotes endothelial dysfunction and the development of atherosclerosis. Atherosclerosis. 2001;158:1–12.

4. Heitzer T, Finckh B, Albers S, et al. Beneficial effects of alpha–lipoic acid and ascorbic acid on endothelium-dependent, nitric oxide-mediated vasodilation in diabetic patients: relation to parameters of oxidative stress. Free Radic Biol Med. 2001;31:53–61.

5. Carr A, Frei B. The role of natural antioxidants in preserving the biological activity of endothelium-derived nitric oxide. Free Radic Biol Med. 2000;28:1806–1814.

6. Vuksan V, Jenkins DJ, Spadafora P, et al. Konjac-mannan (glucomannan) improves glycemia and other associated risk factors for coronary heart disease in type 2 diabetes. A randomized controlled metabolic trial. Diabetes Care. 1999;22:913–919.

7. Illingworth DR, Stein EA, Mitchel YB, et al. Comparative effects of lovastatin and niacin in primary hypercholesterolemia. Arch Intern Med. 1994;154:1586–1595.

8. Carlson LA, Hamsten A, Asplund A. Pronounced lowering of serum levels of lipoprotein Lp(a) in hyperlipidaemic subjects treated with nicotinic acid. J Intern Med. 1989;226:271–276.

9. Pan J, Lin M, Kesala RL, Van J, Charles MA. Niacin treatment of the atherogenic lipid profile and Lp(a) in diabetes. Diabetes Obes Metab. 2002;4:255–261.

10. Van JT, Pan J, Wasty T, et al. Comparison of extended-release niacin and atorvastatin monotherapies and combination treatment of the atherogenic lipid profile in diabetes mellitus. Am J Cardiol. 2002;89:1306–1308.

11. Rindone JP, Achacoso S. Effect of low-dose niacin on glucose control in patients with non-insulin-dependent diabetes mellitus and hyperlipidemia. Am J Ther. 1996;3:637–639.

12. Grundy SM, Vega GL, McGovern ME, et al. Efficacy, safety, and tolerability of once-daily niacin for the treatment of dyslipidemia associated with type 2 diabetes: results of the assessment of diabetes control and evaluation of the efficacy of Niaspan trial. Arch Intern Med. 2002;162:1568–1576.

13. Kane MP, Hamilton RA, Addesse E, Busch RS, Bakst G. Cholesterol and glycemic effects of Niaspan in patients with type 2 diabetes. Pharmacotherapy. 2001;21:1473–1478.

14. El-Enein AMA. The role of nicotinic acid and inositol hexaniacinate as anticholesterolemic and antilipemic agents. Nutr Rep Intl. 1983;28:899–911.

15. ETDRS Investigators. Aspirin effects on mortality and morbidity in patients with diabetes mellitus. Early Treatment Diabetic Retinopathy Study report 14. JAMA. 1992;268:1292–1300.

16. Lawson LD, Wang ZJ. Tablet quality: A major problem in clinical trials with garlic supplements. Forsch Kmplmentaermed 2000;7:45.

17. Lawson LD, Wang ZJ, Papdimitrou D. Allicin release under simulated gastrointestinal conditions from garlic powder tablets employed in clinical trials on serum cholesterol. Planta Medica. 2001;67:13–18.

18. Koch H, Lawson L, eds. *Garlic: The Science and Therapeutic Application of Allium Sativum L and Related Species.* 2nd ed. Baltimore, Md.: Williams & Wilkins; 1996.

19. Silagy CA, Neil HA. A meta-analysis of the effect of garlic on blood pressure. J Hypertens. 1994;12:463–468.

20. Stevinson C, Pittler MH, Erst E. Garlic for treating hypercholesterolemia: a meta-analysis of randomized clinical trials. Ann Intern Med. 2000;133:420–429.

21. Albert MA, Danielson E, Rifai N, Ridker PM. Effect of statin therapy on C-reactive protein levels: the pravastatin inflammation/CRP evaluation (PRINCE): a randomized trial and cohort study. JAMA. 2001;286:64–70.

22. Upritchard JE, Sutherland WH, Mann JI. Effect of supplementation with tomato juice, vitamin E, and vitamin C on LDL oxidation and products of inflammatory activity in type 2 diabetes. Diabetes Care. 2000;23:733–738.

23. Grundy SM, Vega GL, McGovern ME, et al. Efficacy, safety, and tolerability of once-daily niacin for the treatment of dyslipidemia associated with type 2 diabetes: results of the assessment of diabetes control and evaluation of the efficacy of Niaspan trial. Arch Intern Med. 2002;162:1568–1576.

24. Sarter B. Coenzyme Q10 and cardiovascular disease: a review. J Cardiovasc Nurs. 2002;16(4):9–20.

25. Bargossi AM, Grossi G, Fiorella PL, et al. Exogenous CoQ10 supplementation prevents plasma ubiquinone reduction induced by HMG–CoA reductase inhibitors. Mol Aspects Med. 1994;15(suppl):S187–S193.

26. Schonlau F, Rohdewald P. Pycnogenol for diabetic retinopathy. A review. Int Ophthalmol. 2001;24:161–171.

27. Passariello N, Bisesti V, Sgambato S. Influence of anthocyanosides on the microcirculation and lipid picture in diabetic and dyslipidic subjects. Gazz Med Ital. 1979;138:563–566.

28. Forst T, Pohlmann T, Kunt T, et al. The influence of local capsaicin treatment on small nerve fibre function and neurovascular control in symptomatic diabetic neuropathy. Acta Diabetol. 2002;39:1–6.

29. Rains C, Bryson HM. Topical capsaicin. A review of its pharmacological properties and therapeutic potential in post-herpetic neuralgia, diabetic neuropathy and osteoarthritis. Drugs Aging. 1995;7:317–328.

30. Reljanovic M, Reichel G, Rett K, et al. Treatment of diabetic polyneuropathy with the antioxidant thioctic acid (alpha-lipoic acid): a two year multicenter randomized double-blind placebo-controlled trial (ALADIN II). Alpha Lipoic Acid in Diabetic Neuropathy. Free Radic Res. 1999;31:171–179.

31. Jacob S, Ruus P, Hermann R, et al. Oral administration of RAC-alpha-lipoic acid modulates insulin sensitivity in patients with type-2 diabetes mellitus: a placebo-controlled pilot trial. Free Radic Biol Med. 1999;27:309–314.

32. Hui H. A review of treatment of diabetes by acupuncture during the past forty years. J Tradit Chin Med. 1995;15:145–154.

33. Abuaisha BB, Costanzi JB, Boulton AJ. Acupuncture for the treatment of

chronic painful peripheral diabetic neuropathy: a long-term study. Diabetes Res Clin Pract. 1998;39:115–121.

34. Campbell R, Ruggenti P, Remuzzi G. Halting the progression of chronic nephropathy. J Am Soc Nephrol. 2002;13(11):S190.

35. Younes H, Alphonse JC, Behr S, Demigne C, Remesy C. Role of fermentable carbohydrate supplements with a low-protein diet in the course of chronic renal failure: experimental bases. Am J Kidney Dis. 1999; 33(4):633–646.

36. Gaede P, Poulsen HE, Parving HH, Pedersen O. Double-blind, randomised study of the effect of combined treatment with vitamin C and E on albuminuria in Type 2 diabetic patients. Diabet Med. 2001;18:756–760.

Appendix H: What to Look for in a Multiple Vitamin and Mineral Supplement

1. National Research Council. Diet and Health: Implications for Reducing Chronic Disease Risk. Washington, D.C.: National Academy Press; 1989.

2. Ervin RB, Wright JD, Kennedy-Stephenson J. Use of dietary supplements in the United States, 1988–94. Vital Health Stat. 1999;(244):1–14.

3. Balluz LS, Kieszak SM, Philen RM, Mulinare J. Vitamin and mineral supplement use in the United States. Results from the third National Health and Nutrition Examination Survey. Arch Fam Med. 2000;9: 258–262.

4. Schlebusch L, Bosch BA, Polglase G, Kleinschmidt L, Pillay BJ, Cassimjee MH. Double-blind, placebo-controlled, double-centre study of the effects of an oral multivitamin-mineral combination on stress. S Afr Med J. 2000;90:1216–1223.

5. Carroll D, Ring C, Suter M, Willemsen G. The effects of an oral multivitamin combination with calcium, magnesium, and zinc on psychological well-being in healthy young male volunteers: a double-blind placebo-controlled trial. Psychopharmacology. 2000;150:220–225.

6. Benton D, Haller J, Fordy J. Vitamin supplementation for 1 year improves mood. Neuropsychobiology. 1995;32:98–105.

7. Benton D, Fordy J, Haller J. The impact of long-term vitamin supplementation on cognitive functioning. Psychopharmacology. 1995;117:298–305.

8. Johnson MA, Porter KH. Micronutrient supplementation and infection in institutionalized elders. Nutr Rev. 1997;55:400–404.

9. Meyer F, Bairati I, Dagenais GR. Lower ischemic heart disease incidence and mortality among vitamin supplement users. Can J Cardiol. 1996; 12:930–934.

10. Blot WJ. Vitamin/mineral supplementation and cancer risk: international chemoprevention trials. Proc Soc Exp Biol Med. 1997;216:291–296.

11. Jacques PF, Chylack LT Jr, Hankinson SE, et al. Long-term nutrient intake and early age-related nuclear lens opacities. Arch Ophthalmol. 2001;119:1009–1019.

12. Giovannucci E, Stampfer MJ, Colditz GA, et al. Multivitamin use, folate, and colon cancer in women in the Nurses' Health Study. Ann Intern Med. 1998;129:517–524.

Index